Sepsis-Associated Encephalopathy

Irina A. Savvina, Natalia V. Beloborodova and Tatyana N. Trofimova

Sepsis-Associated Encephalopathy

Clinical, Metabolomic, Neurophysiological and Neuroimaging Parallels

nova
science publishers
New York

Library of Congress Cataloging-in-Publication Data

Print ISBN: 979-8-89113-178-1
PDF ISBN: 979-8-89113-398-3
ePUB ISBN: 979-8-89113-399-0

Published by Nova Science Publishers, Inc. † New York

Contents

Foreword

I have the privilege of accepting an invitation from the editor and publisher of the manuscript *Sepsis-Associated Encephalopathy: Clinical, Metabolomic, Neurophysiological and Neuroimaging Parallels* to write this foreword.

As an anesthesiologist and intensive care specialist, I think it is of great importance to discuss the problem of acute brain damage due to sepsis in a combination of diagnostic and therapeutic approaches based on the latest knowledge in the field of fundamental medicine.

The manuscript *Sepsis-Associated Encephalopathy: Clinical, Metabolomic, Neurophysiological, and Neuroimaging Parallels* reviews the modern conception of pathogenesis, pathophysiology, morphology of sepsis-associated encephalopathy, clinical presentation, neurophysiological, radiological, and laboratory diagnosis, management, and therapeutic tactics of patients with brain injury due to sepsis.

In our high-tech twenty-first century, despite the powerful progress of medicine, there is probably not a single hospital in the world that has not been affected by the problem of sepsis as one of the most common causes of mortality in intensive care units or disability, leading to the permanent or prolonged social maladjustment.

The annual growth in the number of scientific publications devoted to the problem of sepsis indicates its high relevance and confirms the interest of researchers and clinicians in this topic.

In less than half a century of studying sepsis and septic conditions in intensive care units, more and more new approaches to accelerated diagnosis and treatment of septic conditions appear, and considerable attention is paid to methods for predicting and preventing the development of sepsis in patients in the ICU.

In recent years, not only clinicians, microbiologists, and pharmacologists, but also specialists in molecular genetics and genetic engineering have been actively involved in the study of the problem of sepsis. Proteomics, genomics, and metabolomics expand our understanding of the pathophysiology and pathogenesis of sepsis and, in particular, sepsis-associated encephalopathy as a variant of acute cerebral dysfunction, the early diagnosis of which makes it possible to start proactive intensive therapy and make cerebral damage reversible.

Clinical assessment of brain dysfunction of patients with sepsis using various neurological and resuscitation scales allows one to determine the level of cerebral damage and a patient's perspective according to the severity of the cerebral injury. This is detailed in the relevant chapter.

Biomarkers are a significant part of laboratory diagnostics of sepsis-associated encephalopathy in the different stages of the disease. It is essential to understand the role of microbiota and microbial metabolites in sepsis-associated encephalopathy. The authors did an excellent job of expressing their views on this matter.

Neurophysiological monitoring such as EEG and multimodal evoked potentials are the sensitive and predictive options to control the functional condition of the brain, and some of them can be used under sedation in critical patients with sepsis.

The chapter *Neuroradiology of Sepsis-Associated Encephalopathy* contains fundamental knowledge about neuroimaging findings in septic patients.

Positron emission tomography allows you to study brain metabolism, cerebral perfusion, neuronal damage, and neurotransmitter dysfunction which improves diagnostics and therapeutical tactics in sepsis-associated encephalopathy.

The important chapter for clinicians is *Sepsis-Associated Encephalopathy as a Component of Multiple Organ Failure in ICU Patients.*

Diagnosis and treatment of sepsis-associated encephalopathy in pediatric practice have some features that are discussed in the relevant chapter.

The need for improved treatment modalities is apparent. This is stated in the chapter on *Therapeutic Tactics in Sepsis-Associated Encephalopathy: Present and Prospects.*

Molecular genetic aspects of diagnosis and clinical approaches to sepsis-associated encephalopathy are reflected in the last chapter of the book.

"The sciences feed young men, they give joy to the old...", the great Russian scientist Mikhail Lomonosov wrote in the eighteenth century.

Russian team's manuscript highlights new insights into sepsis-associated encephalopathy and provides updates in both diagnostics and treatment approaches for improving outcomes in this state.

Prof. Mikhail Y. Kirov, MD, Ph.D,
Correspondent Member of the Russian Academy of Sciences,
Head of the Department of Anesthesiology and
Intensive Care,
North State Medical University, Arkhangelsk, Russia

Preface

Sepsis-associated encephalopathy belongs to the clinical spectrum of acute diffuse brain dysfunction with often irreversible cerebral damage but without clinical and/or laboratory signs of direct brain infection. Unfortunately, sepsis-induced encephalopathy is associated with an unfavorable outcome among septic patients. However, early diagnosis and timely correction of neurological disorders in sepsis can minimize the severity of cognitive deficits and affect the further social adaptation of survivors.

The title *Sepsis-Associated Encephalopathy: Clinical, Metabolomic, Neurophysiological, and Neuroimaging Parallels* represents a knowledge-based book that includes questions of modern conception about the pathogenesis of sepsis-associated encephalopathy, pathophysiological and pathomorphological aspects of sepsis-associated encephalopathy, clinical and neurophysiological assessment of acute cerebral damage in sepsis, neuroradiological patterns of cerebral injury in sepsis, features of laboratory diagnostics based on biomarker verification and the assessment of the role of microbiota and microbial metabolites in sepsis-associated encephalopathy. Peculiarities of neurological and radiological diagnosis, the role of neurophysiological monitoring in the early detection of sepsis-associated brain dysfunction, and present and prospects in therapeutic tactics in sepsis-associated encephalopathy are the important topics of the discussion. A special chapter is devoted to the features of sepsis-associated encephalopathy in children. Finally, it's a very interesting chapter regarding molecular genetic aspects of diagnosis and clinical approaches to sepsis-associated encephalopathy.

This book was written by anesthesiologists and intensive care, functional diagnostics specialists, neurologists, neuroradiologists, neurosurgeons, pathologists, laboratory diagnosticians, and microbiologists – 23 authors from the most reputable medical research centers and university clinics of Russia, whose daily work is to manage and treat patients of various profiles with infection and sepsis.

"When the brain is healthy and in a calm state, a person thinks sensibly", – wrote the great ancient Greek physician Hippocrates in the third-century BC. We sincerely hope that this manuscript will be useful to readers in solving the clinical problems of daily practical work on the diagnosis and treatment of acute brain damage in the structure of multiple organ dysfunction in sepsis.

Irina A. Savvina
Moscow, Saint Petersburg, Russia -Toronto, Canada *Natalia V. Beloborodova*
Tatyana N. Trofimova

Acknowledgments

I thank the departments of intensive care, neurophysiology and functional diagnosis, neuroradiology, laboratory diagnostics, and pathomorphology, each of which has provided opportunities for colleagues to contribute to the writing of the book using their knowledge and clinical experience.

Special thanks are also due to Correspondent Member of the Russian Academy of Sciences, Prof. Mikhail Y. Kirov for the Foreword.

I would like to acknowledge the publisher, editors, and support staff at Nova Science Publishers, they were very helpful in the various stages of developing and producing the volume.

And especially thanks to the contributing authors whose expertise has been particularly important in making this manuscript edition possible.

My heartfelt gratitude to the co-editors Prof. Natalia V. Beloborodova and Correspondent Member of the Russian Academy of Sciences, Prof. Tatyana N. Trofimova for their cooperation in writing the book. Their competence in the relevant fields of medical science and practice has allowed them to present the current state of the problem of sepsis-associated encephalopathy.

Irina A. Savvina, Professor, MD, Ph.D.

Chapter 1

Modern conception about the pathogenesis of sepsis-associated encephalopathy

Irina A. Savvina[1,2]*, MD., Ph.D., Kristina M. Bykova[1], MD., Anna O. Petrova[1], MD., Ph.D.

[1] Department of Anesthesiology and Intensive Care, Almazov National Medical Research Centre of Ministry of Health Care of Russian Federation, Saint Petersburg, Russian Federation

[2] Department of Anesthesiology and Intensive Care named after V.L. Vanevskiy of the North-Western State Medical University named after Ilya I. Mechnikov of the Ministry of Health of Russian Federation, Saint Petersburg, Russian Federation

Abstract

Sepsis-associated encephalopathy (SAE) is a transient and reversible dysfunction of the brain that develops in a patient if there is a focus on infection as a source of sepsis outside the central nervous system (CNS). The pathophysiological basis of SAE is diffuse neuroinflammation, ischemia, and neurotoxic processes.

Damage to the blood-brain barrier (BBB), activation of microglia, which performs the function of immunocompetent cells in the brain, neurotransmission imbalance, hypoperfusion, ischemic damage to neurons, and violation of their trophy, astrogliosis, neuronal pyroptosis and apoptosis, secondary neuroanatomic changes in the brain are known pathogenetic links in the development of acute cerebral damage in sepsis. An endothelial dysfunction is a central event in the pathogenesis of sepsis, contributing to increased vascular permeability and impaired autoregulation of cerebral blood flow. The infiltration of immune cells into brain tissue and an increase in the release of pro-inflammatory cytokines activate the endothelium, which triggers a cascade of coagulation. Intravascular micro thrombosis leads to the development of cerebral ischemia. In patients with sepsis, there is a discrepancy between neuronal activation, increased metabolic needs of the brain, and cerebral vascular reactivity. Complex and diverse pathophysiological ways of realization of acute cerebral damage in sepsis are the subject of discussion in this chapter.

---

* Corresponding author: Irina A. Savvina, Professor, MD., Ph.D.
e-mail address: irinasavvina@mail.ru

Editor: Irina A. Savvina, Natalia V. Beloborodova and Tatyana N. Trofimova
In: Sepsis-Associated Encephalopathy
ISBN: 979-8-89113-178-1

Keywords: sepsis-associated encephalopathy, damaged blood-brain barrier, hypoperfusion, cerebral ischemia, neuroinflammation, activated microglia, astrogliosis, neurotransmission, neuronal pyroptosis, apoptosis, neuroanatomic changes

Abbreviation

BBB – blood-brain barrier
BDNF – brain neurotrophic factor
CCL2 – C-chemokine ligand 2
CD-68 – cluster differentiation 68
CNS – central nervous system
COX-2 – cyclooxygenase-2
CypD – cyclophilin D
DIC – disseminated intravascular coagulation
EA – electroacupuncture
EEG – electroencephalography
GFAP – glial fibrillar acidic protein
GSDMD-NT – N-terminal GSDMD
HMGB1 – highly mobile protein group box 1
IF – immunofluorescence
IFN-γ – interferon-γ
IL-1β – interleukin-1β
IL-3 – interleukin-3
IL-6 – interleukin-6
IL-10 – interleukin-10
IL-13 – interleukin-13
IL-17A – interleukin-17A
IL-18 – interleukin-18
IRGM1 – immunity-related GTPase M1
LPS – lipopolysaccharide
MAPK – mitogen-activated protein kinase
MCP-1 – chemoattractant protein monocytes-1
NLRP3 – pyrin domain-containing-3
PBMC – peripheral blood mononuclear cells
SAE – sepsis-associated encephalopathy
TLR-2 – toll-like receptor-2
TNF-α – tumor necrosis factor-α
TrkB-FL – TrkB-full length
WB – western blotting
ZO-1 – zonula occludens-1

Introduction

Over the past two decades, sepsis-associated encephalopathy (SAE) has been identified as a clinically significant problem with high prevalence in patients with sepsis. The cellular pathophysiology of SAE remains insufficiently studied.

The mechanisms underlying the development of SAE in systemic inflammation have yet to be clarified. In the absence of infection foci in the patient's central nervous system, peripheral inflammation leads to the activation of the central immune system through several communication pathways between the immune system and the brain. There are some of the main factors of cerebral dysfunctions secondary to sepsis (Liu et al. 2022).

It is believed that the pathophysiological mechanisms of the development of cerebral dysfunction include neuroinflammation, impaired functioning of the blood-brain barrier (BBB), deterioration of brain perfusion, neuroanatomic changes, and death of neurons (Westhoff et al. 2019; Ehler et al. 2017) (Figure 1.1). Neuroinflammation is mainly realized through the infiltration of neutrophils into the brain, and activation of microglia and astrocytes, which enhances the mechanisms of excitotoxicity in the brain and BBB dysfunction. Hypoperfusion is often observed in patients with SAE and can be caused by abnormal vasodilation, impaired autoregulation of cerebral blood flow, and inflammatory processes. Pyroptosis and apoptosis are common pathways of neuronal death associated with brain dysfunction in sepsis. Neuroanatomic changes, including vasogenic edema of the white matter, expansion of perivascular spaces, increased axial diffusion of water in the corpus callosum, and fractional anisotropy in the ventral striatum, were found in patients with SAE (Liu et al. 2022). Against the background of sepsis, BBB damage is caused by severe systemic inflammation, which can lead to ischemic

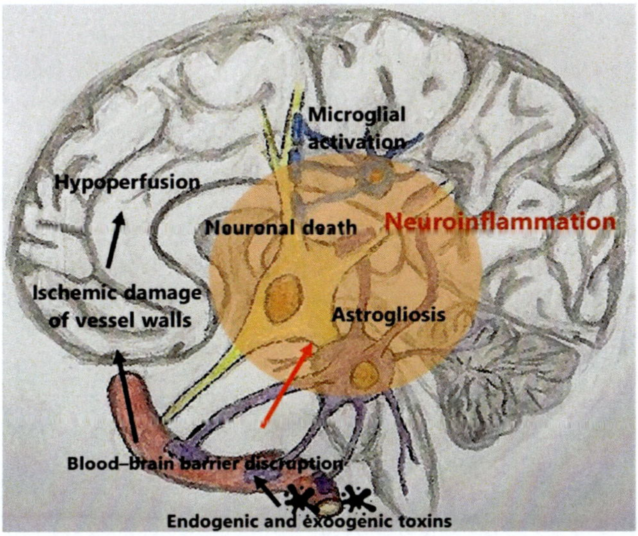

Figure 1.1. The main pathophysiological changes in sepsis-associated encephalopathy are neuroinflammation, ischemic damage to the vascular wall and BBB, hypoperfusion, activation of microglia, astrogliosis, and death of neurons. (Author's drawing Kristina M. Bykova, 2023)

damage to the endothelial wall of blood vessels, the formation of microabscesses, infiltration with immune cells, and toxins in the parenchyma of the brain. These changes can cause abnormal reactivation of astrocytes, which exacerbates brain damage, including aberrant neurotransmission. Micro- and macrovascular lesions in various brain regions and local and global hypoperfusion can lead to various cognitive and behavioral disorders secondary to septic problems. Below we will take a closer look at the main pathogenetic mechanisms of sepsis-associated encephalopathy.

Experimental models of septic encephalopathy

Various experimental models are used to study sepsis, ranging from large animals such as sheep and pigs to smaller mammals such as rats (Im Kafa and Ma 2007) and mice (Baumgart et al. 2009). To study the pathogenesis of septic encephalopathy, the model of ligation and perforation of the cecum is most often used. This model is well known in the international literature for reproducing polymicrobial sepsis and allows inducing various degrees of severity, similar to what occurs in humans. This model is also effective for studying neurological dysfunction in the acute period of sepsis and after sepsis (Savi Felipe Figueredo et al. 2021).

Animal models, although not ideal, are of some value for understanding the main pathogenetic mechanisms and testing potential treatments. Similar to the development of acute cerebral dysfunction in the form of neurological deficits in patients, animal models of sepsis also demonstrate a deficit in long-term memory and suggest the loss of neurons, as well as a decrease in cortical cholinergic innervation as physical manifestations (El Streck et al. 2008).

Neuroinflammation

Previously, hypotheses were put forward about numerous pathophysiological mechanisms of sepsis-associated encephalopathy, but at the moment it is quite established that systemic inflammation is the starting point for the violation of cerebral homeostasis.

Uncontrolled neuroinflammation is an important marker of septic encephalopathy. With the development of sepsis, peripheral and local inflammation can cause neutrophil migration to the brain and activate astrocytes and microglia (Michels, Vieira 2015; Greenhalgh, David, and Bennett 2020; Shulyatnikova and Verkhratsky 2020). Then activated immune cells in the central nervous system can release an increased amount of pro-inflammatory mediators, alter oxidative stress, and increase the number of neurotransmitters that aggravate central and peripheral inflammatory reactions.

Glial cells are numerous in the central nervous system and are necessary for brain development and maintenance of homeostasis. These cells also regulate tissue repair after injury, and their dysfunction is a factor possibly contributing to neurodegenerative and mental diseases.

Microglia are the main immune cells of the brain. In addition, peripheral immune cells entering the central nervous system after injury and disease can directly affect the function of microglia, astrocytes, and oligodendrocytes, which indicates a connection between immune cells and glial cells (Greenhalgh, David, and Bennett 2020). Microglia make up 6–18% of human brain cells (Pelvig et al. 2008). Microglia is the first cell that reacts to neuroinflammation. These cells regulate neuronal functions and the process of brain inflammation by secreting cytokines and interacting with other nerve cells.

There are two types of activated microglia phenotypes: pro-inflammatory phenotype M1 and anti-inflammatory M2 (Tang and Le 2016). Microglia with different phenotypes have either an adverse or positive effect on neurological function (Yan et al. 2020). M1 is activated by interferon-γ (IFN-γ) and lipopolysaccharide (LPS) with the formation of IL-6 and CC-chemokine ligand 2 (CCL2).

Microglia M2 is activated by anti-inflammatory cellular mediators, including IL-13 and IL-3. It produces IL-10 and neurotrophic factors to repair brain tissue and neurons (Colonna and Butovsky 2017) (Figure 1.2).

It is well known that M2 microglia can protect nerve cells from inflammatory damage, while activated M1 microglia can exacerbate neuroinflammation and oxidative stress by increasing the synthesis of inflammatory mediators and reducing ATP production in sepsis. Thus, the increase of microglia M2 or inhibition of microglia M1 can alleviate inflammation and dysfunction of the brain after the development of sepsis.

Under normal conditions, microglia with branched morphology are at rest, responsible for monitoring the microenvironment (Figure 1.1). Peripheral inflammation activates microglia with the help of inflammatory mediators, and interactions between microglia and neighboring cells (Li et al. 2020).

Activation of microglial cells and their migration into the vessels of the brain at the beginning of systemic inflammation is one of the earliest pathophysiological changes observed in SAE. After activation of the microglia, their morphology and functions change (they acquire an amoeboid form).

In one study it was shown that in patients who died from septic shock, an increase in amoeboid-form microglia was observed in the hippocampus and cerebral cortex (Polito et al. 2011).

Also, researchers (Ye et al. 2009) reported that during sepsis IL-17A, secreted by peripheral immune cells, can activate microglia, and then inflammatory mediators produced by activated

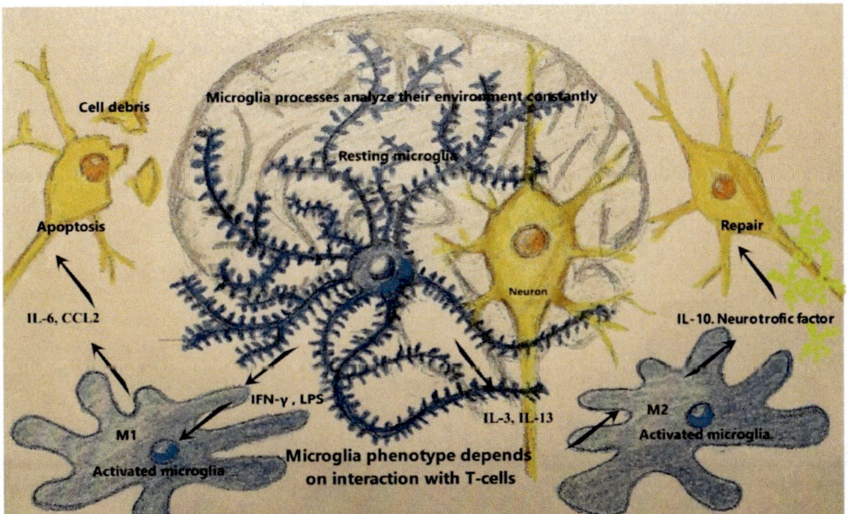

Figure 1.2. Phenotypic types of microglia depend on the microenvironment. (Author's drawing by Kristina M. Bykova, 2023)

microglia enhance the release of IL-17A from immune cells, which creates a vicious circle to increase brain inflammation (Ye et al. 2019).

Some studies have demonstrated that activation of microglia in sepsis leads to brain dysfunction, including delirium, memory impairment, long-term cognitive impairment due to the secretion of a large number of pro-inflammatory cytokines, increased expression of many neurotransmitters and changes in the energy metabolism of the brain in sepsis (Ye et al. 2019; Tauber et al. 2021). Besides, microglia can significantly contribute to glucose uptake and glycolysis due to the expression of glucose transporters 1 (GLUT), increased production of IL-1ß, and enhanced oxidative/nitrosative enzymes in inflammation (Lauro and Limatola 2020).

Yan et al. (2020) found that the induction of microglia from the M1 phenotype to the M2 phenotype by stimulating IL-4/IL-13 inhibits the release of inflammatory cytokines and facilitates brain dysfunction in SAE by increasing the content of mitochondria. Thus, regulating the polarization of microglia and inhibiting the secretion of proinflammatory mediators may be a promising targeted therapeutic method for improving long-term cognitive impairment caused by sepsis.

Highly mobile protein group box 1 (HMGB1), as a late pro-inflammatory factor, is significantly increased in sepsis in various parts of the brain, including the hippocampus (Wu et al. 2023). HMGB1 causes neuroinflammation and cognitive impairment due to direct binding to the end products of enhanced glycation (RAGE – receptor of the end products of increased glycosylation) and Toll-like receptor 4 (TLR4). In an experimental study by Xin et al. (2022), electroacupuncture (EA) was used as a treatment for SAE in male rats with a model of sepsis caused by lipopolysaccharide. Immunofluorescence (IF) and Western blotting (WB) were used to determine neuroinflammation and the HMGB1 signaling pathway. The results showed that EA can improve the decline in working memory in rats with SAE.

EA facilitated neuroinflammation by suppressing the transmission of HMGB1/TLR4 signals and HMGB1/RAGE in the hippocampus, reducing the levels of pro-inflammatory factors and reducing the activation of microglia and astrocytes. However, EA did not affect the expression of dense contacts of the blood-brain barrier in the hippocampus (Xin et al. 2022).

Westhoff et al. (2019) showed that in patients who died from septic shock, systemic inflammation was accompanied by powerful activation of microglia (revealed by using antibodies against cluster differentiation 68 (CD-68)). Local differences in the brain with increased activation of microglia in the shell, hippocampus, and cerebellum have also been identified. This discovery indicates the activation of the immune system in the brain, which may explain the long-term cognitive deficit in patients who have experienced severe systemic inflammation (Westhoff et al. 2019).

Damage to the BBB

BBB is a highly selective and dynamic interaction between the parenchyma of the brain and cerebral circulation.

The role of BBB dysfunction in sepsis has been widely studied, and it is known that the violation of BBB permeability plays an important role in the development of acute neuroinflammation and long-term brain damage after sepsis (Lucineia Gainski Danielski et al. 2018) in the form of neurocognitive deficit.

BBB is formed by endothelial brain cells, pericytes, astrocytes, and surrounding microglial cells. Among the components of the BBB, an important role is played by proteins creating tight contacts that provide a strong binding between cells and the transmission of information. The main proteins of dense contacts include transmembrane proteins such as occludin, claudin, and JAM-1, as well as cytoplasmic attachment proteins such as zonula occludens-1 (ZO-1) (Sun et al. 2021). Under normal conditions, the BBB serves as a physical barrier. Tight junctions between adjacent endothelial cells restrict molecules from diffusing through the endothelium (Kadry, Noorani, and Cucullo 2020). BBB also plays an important role in immunological protection preventing the infiltration of leukocytes from the periphery into the central nervous system (Gao and Hernandes 2021). In brain tissue samples obtained from deceased patients with sepsis, significant suppression of dense compound proteins – occludin, claudin-5, and ZO-1 – in endothelial cells of microvessels was revealed, which indicates a violation of the BBB function (Erikson et al. 2020).

Astrocytes, being a structural element of the blood-brain barrier and the main homeostatic cells of the central nervous system, contribute to the protection of the brain from infections. Forming multifunctional anatomical barriers, astroglial cells support the interaction of the central and peripheral links of the nervous system, limiting damage to nervous tissue (Lucinéia Gainski Danielski et al. 2022).

Until recently, it was believed that astrocytes represent a homogeneous population, but this hypothesis now is refuted (Chaboub and Deneen 2013). Like microglia, astrocytes can have different morphologies (Chaboub and Deneen 2013), and based on their morphology and spatial organization, astrocytes are divided into two main subtypes: protoplasmic and fibrous astrocytes (Villarreal and Vogel 2021). Fibrous astrocytes express high levels of glial fibrillar acidic protein (GFAP) compared to protoplasmic astrocytes (Escartin et al. 2021).

Despite the high metabolic activity, astrocytes use less than 15% of the total brain energy in the form of glucose. The rate of glucose uptake and glycolysis is high; however, since the rate of oxidative phosphorylation is low compared to the metabolic rate of astrocytes, they serve as a source of lactate production (Bordone et al. 2019).

Astrocytes detect, produce, and integrate inflammatory signals between immune cells and brain parenchyma cells, thereby regulating the brain's immune response. Astrocytes exhibit various activities to maintain the normal functioning of the central nervous system, for example, they provide almost complete coverage of the cerebral vessels (Mathiisen et al. 2010).

In SAE, astrocytes are present in both the reactive and astrogliopathic states; the balance between these states determines the evolution of pathology and neurological outcomes. In humans, pathophysiological models of SAE are complicated by the frequent presence of concomitant diseases, as well as age-related remodeling of brain tissue associated with astroglia aging; these mixed factors additionally affect the progression of SAE and the formation of neurological deficits (Shulyatnikova and Verkhratsky 2020).

With sepsis, pathogens, mediators of inflammation, and oxidation are released into the blood. These mediators interact with BBB cells, increasing their selective permeability (van der Poll et al. 2017). The entry of LPS and other molecules into the parenchyma of the brain (Rudd et al. 2020) leads to the activation of glial cells, such as astrocytes and microglia (Figure 1.3). Activated astrocytes can activate microglial cells (Lucineia Gainski Danielski et al. 2018) in addition to the release of reactive oxygen species (Barichello et al. 2021) and cytokines (Mazeraud et al. 2020). These events result in damage to neurons. On the other hand, activated microglia can increase neuronal damage. There is also data on astrogliosis during sepsis (Michels et al. 2015).

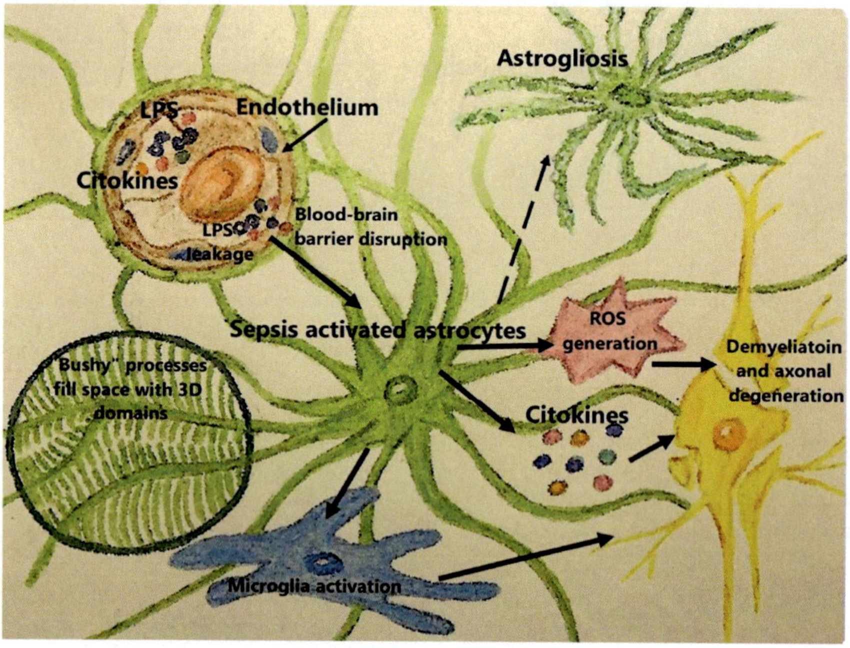

Figure 1.3. The role of astrocytes in the development of sepsis. LPS – lipopolysaccharides, ROS – reactive oxygen species. (Author's drawing by Kristina M. Bykova, 2023)

In experiments on animals with sepsis, it was shown that astrocytes demonstrate increased expression of proinflammatory cytokine genes, such as TNF-α, interleukins IL-1ß, IL-6, IL-18, chemoattractant protein monocytes-1 (MCP-1), and cyclooxygenase-2 (COX-2) with a decrease of IL-10, accompanied by an increased level of mRNA expression of a TLR-2 (Bellaver et al. 2018). These results are similar to the results obtained in the homogenate of brain tissue of a rat with sepsis (Lucineia Gainski Danielski et al. 2020). This cytokine profile was closely related to the action of microglial cells (Moraes et al. 2021), but interestingly, the study provided evidence that mediators released by peripheral blood mononuclear cells (PBMC) directly contribute to the reactivity of astrocytes during sepsis independently of microglia (Bellaver et al. 2019). Data on astrocyte activation in humans is limited. However, the available information indicates that, as in the case of microglia, astrocytes also move from a resting to an activated state during stimulation (Shulyatnikova and Verkhratsky 2020). Astrocytes of the human brain are more diverse, more complex, and more present in the central nervous system compared to the brains of rodents (Vasile, Dossi, and Rouach 2017).

Pathoanatomic analysis of the tissue of the right frontal lobe in three cases in patients with sepsis revealed an increase in the GFAP marker, which indicates a higher activity of astrocytes in this area compared to the control (Warford et al. 2017).

Other studies involving children, adults, and elderly patients with sepsis show a general increase in the s-100ß marker due not only to the activation of microglia but also the activation of astrocytes. This activation was associated with a longer duration of delirium, greater severity of delirium, and in-hospital mortality (Villarreal and Vogel 2021; Khan et al. 2020). Thus, there are convincing preclinical data on astrocyte activation after sepsis and several clinical studies, confirming this fact (Lucinéia Gainski Danielski et al. 2022). Some questions still need scientific evidence, for example, how the homeostatic functions of astrocytes are disrupted in sepsis, how astrocytes are activated after BBB activation, and how astrocytes interact with BBB after that. The answers to these and other questions will be able to explain how astroglia activation can contribute to the formation of long-term neurological consequences of sepsis.

Hypoperfusion: ischemic injury

Many studies have shown that ischemic brain damage often occurs against the background of sepsis (Villéga et al. 2017; Sekino, Selim, and Shehadah 2022). Hemodynamic changes precede cognitive impairment and structural changes in the brain (Catarina et al. 2021). Clinical data have shown that cerebral blood flow is significantly reduced in patients with SAE (Pierrakos et al. 2014).

Inadequate cerebral blood flow can lead to the realization of a cascade of cerebral ischemia, which is controlled by three main processes: a decrease in oxygen and energy delivery (Kinoshita et al. 2019), an increase in stress signals, and activation of microglia (Greenhalgh, David, and Bennett 2020).

Hypoxic or ischemic changes are the most common injuries detected during the autopsy of the brain of patients with sepsis (Janz et al. 2010).

Decreased cerebral blood flow and hypercoagulation are the main factors in the development of cerebral ischemia in patients with sepsis (Pfister et al. 2008). Violation of cerebral blood flow autoregulation is also common in patients with septic shock, especially in the presence of hypercapnia (Taccone et al. 2010).

Acute unregulated inflammatory reactions aimed at eradication of an infectious agent in patients with sepsis can cause hypercoagulation and vasculopathy of cerebral blood vessels, leading to cerebral ischemia.

Acute vascular endothelial dysfunction is a central event in the pathogenesis of sepsis and contributes to increased vascular permeability and impaired autoregulation of cerebral blood flow (Bermejo-Martin et al. 2018). The infiltration of immune cells into brain tissue and an increase in the release of pro-inflammatory cytokines activate endothelial cells, which leads to the activation of the coagulation cascade. Then microthrombi can form in the blood vessels, which can cause cerebral ischemia (Nwafor et al. 2019).

Septic shock leads to severe hypoperfusion, causing an imbalance of the brain's oxygen demand, cellular metabolism, and energy production.

Available studies show that hypoperfusion and ischemia can induce changes in white matter and may contribute to long-term cognitive impairment in patients with ischemic stroke. It has also been suggested that hypoperfusion may also cause long-term cognitive impairment in stroke due to the accumulation of tau protein pathology (Miners, Kehoe, and Love 2020). Further studies are needed to study the role of ischemia/hypoperfusion in the formation of cognitive disorders associated with sepsis.

Patients with sepsis may have focal lesions that cause direct brain damage. Sharshar et al. (2004) reported various focal lesions in 23 patients who died in the ICU from septic shock: ischemia (100%), hemorrhages (26%), hypercoagulation syndrome (9%), microabscesses (9%), and multi-focal necrotizing leukoencephalopathy (9%). Sepsis can cause life-threatening coagulopathy, including disseminated intravascular coagulation (DIC) and intracerebral hemorrhage (Valderrama et al. 2020).

Neuroanatomic changes

Two different pathways transmit signals of inflammation to the brain in the absence of a violation of the permeability of the BBB: the vagus nerve receives a signal of local inflammation and transmits information to the autonomous nuclei of the medulla oblongata (Reyes et al. 2012); brain structures devoid of BBB – the periventricular zone of the IY ventricle, III ventricles, neurohypophysis, pineal gland, lamina terminals – ensure the flow of inflammatory mediators to the brain (Sharshar et al. 2005).

Vagus nerve stimulation occurs shortly after lipopolysaccharide administration. Signals from the vagus nerve reach the autonomic and neuroendocrine systems (Reyes et al. 2012; Sharshar et al. 2005). Deprived of the BBB, the periventricular regions are located near the third ventricle and include the area postrema, which controls nausea and transmits information from the peripheral branches of the vagus nerve to the central block – the dorsal vagal nuclear complex located in the caudal parts of the brainstem. “Painful” behavior is induced by the action of pro-inflammatory cytokines in the brain.

In rodents, systemic or central administration of IL-1ß induces all behavioral, endocrine, and vegetative features of “painful” behavior (Anforth et al. 1998).

The brain stem is involved in three main functions: the formation of wakefulness, stem reflexes and control of vital functions, and modulation of the immune response. Dysfunction of the brain stem can lead to impaired wakefulness and disruption of the cardiovascular and immune systems, which will lead to an increase in mortality. We found that the early disappearance of the cough reflex and the oculocephalic reaction was independently associated with an increase in mortality in ICU in critically ill patients under sedation (Sharshar et al. 2011). A decrease in heart rate variability, reflecting a violation of sympathetic activity emanating from the autonomic nuclei of the brain stem, is also associated with a worse outcome in sepsis. The absence of EEG reactivity, indicating dysfunction of the ascending activating reticular formation, is a predictor of death in septic patients (Azabou et al. 2015).

Sepsis is associated with multiple neuroendocrine disorders (Aboab et al. 2008; Siami et al. 2013). While the initial stage of sepsis is characterized by increased secretion of pituitary hormones, especially in response to decreased sensitivity of peripheral hormone receptors, prolonged sepsis is characterized by decreased secretion of pituitary hormones (Siami et al. 2013). For example, septic shock is associated with relative adrenal insufficiency and increased mortality (Aboab et al. 2008). Septic shock may also be associated with a violation of the production of vasopressin due to the hyperpolarization of neurons in the terminal plate region (Stare et al. 2015).

The psychological consequences of sepsis include anxiety, depression, and post-traumatic stress disorder (Muscatell et al. 2015), all of which affect the amygdala and its network-neuronal connections to the prefrontal cortex, hypothalamus, and brainstem. The amygdala is particularly affected by the activation of microglia in sepsis (Muscatell et al. 2015). Memory impairment can be caused by damage to the hippocampus or frontal cortex. Hippocampal atrophy is associated with memory loss, for example, in Alzheimer’s disease. In rodents, sepsis also causes hippocampal dysfunction and subsequent changes in spatial memory, confirmed by the Morris water maze test (Liu et al. 2014), which correlate with long-term cognitive dysfunction, neuronal death, gliosis, and increased production of reactive oxygen species.

The prefrontal cortex and other sensorimotor areas make up the frontal cortex. Cognitive defects that occur after injuries to the frontal cortex include, mainly, impaired memorization, attention, and executive functions. Ultrastructural abnormalities of neurons were shown in the sensorimotor cortex on a model of endotoxic shock in dogs. Cognitive functions associated with the prefrontal cortex, including memorization and fluency of speech, are often impaired after sepsis (Iwashyna et al. 2010).

Neuroinflammation in the frontal cortex leads to cognitive impairment. Due to the reversibility of SAE, no obvious changes in the brain and spinal cord were observed in most histological studies (Molnár et al. 2018). Nevertheless, new data suggest that a violation of cerebral autoregulation may contribute to the development of edema and changes in white matter in sepsis (Griton et al. 2020). Neuroanatomic changes were noted in patients with SAE, including vasogenic edema of the white matter, separation of myelin, expansion of perivascular spaces, increased axial diffusion of water in the corpus callosum, and fractional anisotropy in the ventral striatum (Zrzavy et al. 2019). Dysfunction in different areas of the brain can cause various behavioral disorders. Violation of the organization of white matter causes delirium (Azabou et al. 2018). Impaired brain stem function can lead to dysphagia, impaired regulation of the neuroendocrine system, and somnipathy, which is associated with multiple organ dysfunction and higher mortality in patients (Azabou et al. 2018). Disorder of the hypothalamus or amygdala is associated with behavioral changes, including depression, fear, and anxiety (Tovote, Fadok, and Lüthi 2015). As is known, the hippocampus and frontal cortex play a vital role in memory formation; thus, disruption of the hippocampus and frontal cortex causes deterioration of memory and executive functions (Zhu et al. 2014). To date, changes in the microstructure of the brain caused by sepsis are largely unknown, but it can be assumed that these changes may contribute to the development of brain dysfunction and the formation of long-term cognitive impairment.

Thus, further study of neuroanatomic changes in the septic process is important for the study of clinical features and psychocognitive disorders in SAE.

Death of nerve cells

An increasing number of studies show that cell death is an important factor in brain dysfunction in SAE. Apoptosis and pyroptosis of brain cells caused by inflammation play a crucial role in the occurrence and progression of SAE (Chen et al. 2020; Tsuchiya 2020; Wang et al. 2022).

Apoptosis is a kind of regulated cell death, accompanied by cell contraction and the formation of foamy cells in the cellular membrane. It is well known that mitochondria are the main organelles associated with apoptosis. With the development of sepsis, mitochondrial dysfunction is found in various areas of the brain, especially in the hippocampus, which can cause an imbalance of reactive oxygen/nitrogen species, apoptosis of hippocampal cells, and severe neurocognitive disorders.

Excessive apoptosis of neurons is characterized by an increased content of enhanced proapoptotic proteins that are released from mitochondrial levels of split caspase. More recently, mitochondrial cyclophilin D isomerase (CypD) is associated with mitochondrial dysfunction and cellular apoptosis in SAE. Suppression of CypD synthesis can protect brain cells from apoptosis since the possibility of fluctuations in mitochondrial permeability is reduced and the release of free radicals from mitochondria is suppressed, which can reduce the degree of brain damage and improve survival (Kobayashi et al. 2022). Similarly, the inhibition of ceramide significantly weakened the process of apoptosis neurons and reduced cognitive impairment in septic animals (Zhang et al. 2021).

In a study by Wang et al. (2022), potential mechanisms underlying the development of cognitive dysfunction in SAE have been identified (Wang et al. 2022).

A significant role is given to the Foxcl gene, which belongs to the family of transcription factors regulating cell migration.

Transcription nuclear factor NF-kB regulates genes involved in immune and inflammatory reactions, in the coding of cytokines (IL-1, IL-2, IL-6, IL-12, TNF), chemokines, acute phase proteins, and adhesion molecules. NF-kB is the central link of immune responses with the possibility of activating genes encoding apoptosis and cell proliferation. With a decrease in the expression of the Foxcl and IqBa gene (inhibits apoptosis of transcription factor NF-kB) and an increase in the expression of IL-1ß and TNFa, increased apoptosis of hippocampal neurons was observed in mice with sepsis previously caused by ligation and perforation of the cecum. It was found that overexpression of Foxcl contributed to the expression of IqBa; at the same time neuronal apoptosis, microglial migration, and inflammation were suppressed both in vitro and in vivo in mice (Wang et al. 2022). Activation of the endothelium in sepsis causes the expression of nuclear factor kappa bi (NF-kB), a pro-inflammatory signaling pathway in the endothelial cells of the brain microvessels. This signaling process promotes transcription of the inflammatory mediator cyclooxygenase-2, which leads to an increase in BBB permeability through the synthesis of prostaglandin E2, which was shown in a study on mice (Yang et al. 2022).

There is an obvious link between apoptosis of neuronal cells and abnormalities of proinflammatory signaling pathways, including NF-kB, mitogen-activated protein kinase (MAPK), and brain neurotrophic factor (BDNF) in SAE.

Activation of NF-kB is considered a central event in sepsis, which can trigger inflammatory mediators (Figure 1.3).

In addition, p65, a subunit of the NF-kB heterodimer, can induce transcription of Nod-like receptor protein microglia 3 (NLRP3) by direct binding to the promoter region of NLRP3 in SAE. Being an important component of the inflammasome NLRP3, activation of NLRP3 induces cellular apoptosis. Data are accumulating demonstrating that suppressive activation of NF-kB/p65-induced NLRP3 inflammasome inhibits apoptosis of neurons induced by LPS in vivo and in vitro (Chen et al. 2020; Tsuchiya 2020).

Toll-like receptor 4 (TLR4) belongs to the family of receptors involved in innate immunity. These are highly selective receptors that recognize pathogen-associated molecular complexes, representing the first line of defense against infections (Figure 1.4). TLR4 has long been recognized as a sensitive receptor for gram-negative lipopolysaccharides (Zhang et al. 2021). In a study by Zhang et al. (2021), sodium butyrate blocked the activation of TLR4 and thereby inhibited nuclear transcription of NF-kB, which reduced microglial activation and secretion of inflammatory factors and, ultimately, led to the relief of inflammation in the hippocampus of septic mice and a decrease in anxiety behavior (Zhang et al. 2021).

Microglia has many receptors for various stimuli, such as receptors for ATP, and toll-like receptors (TLRs) that react to molecules of dying cells (damage-associated molecular patterns (DAMPs)) or pathogens (pathogen-associated molecular patterns (PAMPs)).

Mitogen-activated protein kinase (MAPK) plays a key role in apoptosis, developing due to inflammation. Apoptosis of cells in the cortex and hippocampus of animals with sepsis can be weakened by p38 MAPK inhibitors (Gu, Mei, and Zhao 2021). Zhou et al. (2020) found that neuronal apoptosis and autophagy were closely related to the p38 MAPK signaling pathway in a mouse sepsis model, while the immunity-related GTPase M1 (IRGM1) partially improved neuronal apoptosis through the p38 MAPK signaling pathway.

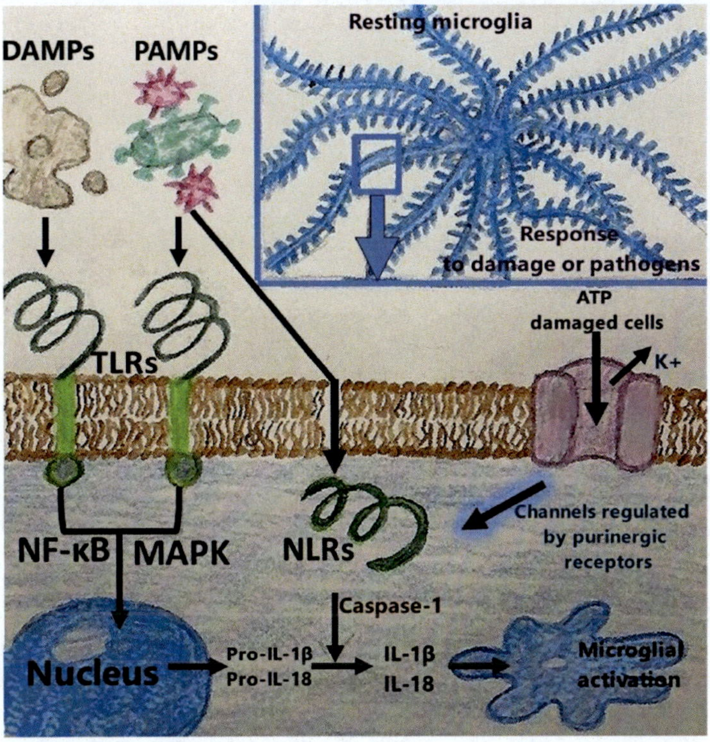

Figure 1.4. Response of microglia for damage or pathogen.

Nuclear factor kappa B (NF-κB), mitogen-activated protein kinase (MAPK), NOD-like receptors (NLRs), Toll-like receptors (TLRs), damage-associated molecular patterns (DAMPs), pathogen-associated molecular patterns (PAMPs). (Author's drawing by Kristina M. Bykova, 2023)

BDNF plays an important role in neuron plasticity, learning, and memory through the activation of TrkB-full length (TrkB-FL) receptors. It has been reported that abnormal TrkB shortening mediated by calpain results in a violation of the regulation of BDNF/TrkB signaling and is associated with cognitive impairment in some neurodegenerative disorders.

It has been documented that inactivation of BDNF/TrkB signaling after brain injury is involved in apoptosis and autophagy of neuronal cells. For example, activation of BDNF/TrkB facilitated brain damage caused by SAE, while impaired BDNF/TrkB signaling was associated with brain dysfunction in aging mice (Qiu et al. 2020). Probably, treatment with emodin, a chemical compound from rhubarb, reduced apoptosis of hippocampal neurons in mice with sepsis by activating the BDNF/TrkB pathway (Gao et al. 2022).

Pyroptosis is defined as regulated necrosis with rapid damage to the plasma membrane and release of intracellular contents (Tsuchiya 2020), and this is a common model of cell death in sepsis, which may worsen inflammation. In one study, scientists observed pyroptosis of splenic dendritic cells in mice with sepsis (Wang et al. 2021). Similarly, Xu et al. (2019) noticed pyroptosis of nerve cells in septic mice and found that inhibition of pyroptosis can reduce brain damage and cognitive impairment in SAE. They suggested that pyroptosis of nerve cells is induced by inflammatory mediators, which are secreted by peripheral blood in the central nervous system during SAE (Xu et al. 2019).

Pyroptosis can develop in canonical or non-canonical signaling pathways. In the non-canonical signaling pathway, lipopolysaccharides can activate caspases-11, -4, and -5 to form the N-terminal GSDMD (GSDMD-NT). Then GSDMD-NT acquires a ring-shaped structure and forms holes in the cell membrane, which causes the production of IL-1ß and IL-18 and leads to cell lysis. The canonical signaling pathway plays a potential role in the pathogenesis of SAE, and inhibition of pyroptosis may be a useful therapeutic target for SAE (Wang et al. 2020).

The canonical signaling pathway is based on the preliminary activation of inflammasomes.

As a key canonical inflammasome, the NLRP3 inflammasome is closely related to brain damage in SAE. Mice with induced sepsis had increased expression of NLRP3, GSDMD-NT was revealed, and activation of NLRP3 in the hippocampus led to cognitive impairment by induction of pyroptosis (Fu et al. 2019).

Recently, it was found that Sestrin 2 improves the outcome of sepsis by reducing NLRP3/caspase-1-dependent pyroptosis (Wang et al. 2020).

One study examined the role of the P2X7R receptor in the occurrence of cognitive dysfunction in SAE and its molecular mechanism (Wang et al. 2022).

As is known, the P2X7R receptor is a three-dimensional ion channel controlled by extracellular adenosine-5-triphosphate. The receptor is present in different types of cells, including stem, blood, glial, nerve, endothelial, muscle, and others. The P2X7 receptor induces the release of pro-inflammatory molecules, cell proliferation and death, metabolic changes, and phagocytosis. In an experiment on mice with SAE, it was shown that P2X7R inhibitors dramatically improved the survival of animal individuals, facilitated cognitive dysfunction, and decreased apoptosis of brain cells (Wang et al. 2022).

Lei et al. (2021) investigated the relationship between autophagy and pyroptosis in mice with SAE. The results showed that both autophagy and pyroptosis are involved in the development of SAE, and pannexin-1 reduces the occurrence of pyroptosis due to autophagy. Collectively, it has been suggested that both canonical and non-canonical pathways of cellular pyroptosis are associated with cellular apoptosis (Wang et al. 2020). However, the exact functions of the canonical and non-canonical pathways of pyroptosis and their relationship with apoptosis and autophagy in SAE require further investigation.

Conclusion

Sepsis-associated encephalopathy is a disease caused by the disconnection of the work, primarily of the immune and nervous systems. We hope that a deeper understanding of the pathogenesis of septic encephalopathy will lead to new cellular and molecular targets, which, in turn, will allow the development of specific drugs and prevent the negative impact of SAE on survival.

Sepsis affects the brain in many unique ways, so it is necessary to conduct further studies in vitro and in vivo to get a deeper and more comprehensive view of the pathophysiology of SAE. There is a need for specific treatment methods that will affect the main links of pathogenesis along with a personalized approach to intensive therapy of clinical manifestations of SAE.

Conflict of interest: The authors declare that there is no conflict of interest.
Acknowledgment: The authors express their deep gratitude to the university

Teachers, alma mater – Pavlov University, Voronezh State Medical University named after N. N. Burdenko, for instilled love for the study of fundamental medical sciences – pathophysiology, pathological anatomy, histology – the knowledge without which the clinical practice of a doctor is unthinkable.

References

Aboab, Jerome, Andrea Polito, David Orlikowski, Tarek Sharshar, Muriel Castel, and Djillali Annane. 2008. «Hydrocortisone Effects on Cardiovascular Variability in Septic Shock: A Spectral Analysis Approach». *Critical Care Medicine* 36 (5): 1481–86. https://doi.org/10.1097/CCM.0b013e31816f48f2.

Anforth, H. R., R. M. Bluthe, A. Bristow, S. Hopkins, M. J. Lenczowski, G. Luheshi, J. Lundkvist, et al. 1998. «Biological Activity and Brain Actions of Recombinant Rat Interleukin-1alpha and Interleukin-1beta». *European Cytokine Network* 9 (3): 279–88.

Azabou, Eric, Eric Magalhaes, Antoine Braconnier, Lyria Yahiaoui, Guy Moneger, Nicholas Heming, Djillali Annane, et al. 2015. «Early Standard Electroencephalogram Abnormalities Predict Mortality in Septic Intensive Care Unit Patients». *PloS One* 10 (10): e0139969. https://doi.org/10.1371/journal.pone.0139969.

Azabou, Eric, Vincent Navarro, Nathalie Kubis, Martine Gavaret, Nicholas Heming, Alain Cariou, Djillali Annane, Fréderic Lofaso, Lionel Naccache, and Tarek Sharshar. 2018. «Value and Mechanisms of EEG Reactivity in the Prognosis of Patients with Impaired Consciousness: A Systematic Review». *Critical Care (London, England)* 22 (1): 184. https://doi.org/10.1186/s13054-018-2104-z.

Barichello, Tatiana, Jaqueline S. Generoso, Allan Collodel, Fabricia Petronilho, and Felipe Dal-Pizzol. 2021. «The Blood-Brain Barrier Dysfunction in Sepsis». *Tissue Barriers* 9 (1): 1840912. https://doi.org/10.1080/21688370.2020.1840912.

Bellaver, Bruna, Andréia S. Rocha, Débora G. Souza, Douglas T. Leffa, Marco Antônio De Bastiani, Guilherme Schu, Pâmela C. Lukasewicz Ferreira, et al. 2019. «Activated Peripheral Blood Mononuclear Cell Mediators Trigger Astrocyte Reactivity». *Brain, Behavior, and Immunity* 80 (August): 879–88. https://doi.org/10.1016/j.bbi.2019.05.041.

Bellaver, Bruna, João Paulo dos Santos, Douglas Teixeira Leffa, Larissa Daniele Bobermin, Paola Haack Amaral Roppa, Iraci Lucena da Silva Torres, Carlos-Alberto Gonçalves, Diogo Onofre Souza, and André Quincozes-Santos. 2018. «Systemic Inflammation as a Driver of Brain Injury: The Astrocyte as an Emerging Player». *Molecular Neurobiology* 55 (3): 2685–95. https://doi.org/10.1007/s12035-017-0526-2.

Bermejo-Martin, Jesus F., Marta Martín-Fernandez, Cristina López-Mestanza, Patricia Duque, and Raquel Almansa. 2018. «Shared Features of Endothelial Dysfunction between Sepsis and Its Preceding Risk Factors (Aging and Chronic Disease)». *Journal of Clinical Medicine* 7 (11): 400. https://doi.org/10.3390/jcm7110400.

Bordone, Melina Paula, Mootaz M. Salman, Haley E. Titus, Elham Amini, Jens V. Andersen, Barnali Chakraborti, Artem V. Diuba, et al. 2019. «The Energetic Brain - A Review from Students to Students». *Journal of Neurochemistry* 151 (2): 139–65. https://doi.org/10.1111/jnc.14829.

Catarina, Anderson Velasque, Gisele Branchini, Lais Bettoni, Jarbas Rodrigues De Oliveira, and Fernanda Bordignon Nunes. 2021. «Sepsis-Associated Encephalopathy: From Pathophysiology to Progress in Experimental Studies». *Molecular Neurobiology* 58 (6): 2770–79. https://doi.org/10.1007/s12035-021-02303-2.

Chaboub, Lesley S., and Benjamin Deneen. 2013. «Astrocyte Form and Function in the Developing Central Nervous System». *Seminars in Pediatric Neurology* 20 (4): 230–35. https://doi.org/10.1016/j.spen.2013.10.003.

Chen, Shenglong, Chaogang Tang, Hongguang Ding, Zhonghua Wang, Xinqiang Liu, Yunfei Chai, Wenqiang Jiang, Yongli Han, and Hongke Zeng. 2020. «Maf1 Ameliorates Sepsis-Associated Encephalopathy by Suppressing the NF-KB/NLRP3 Inflammasome Signaling Pathway». *Frontiers in Immunology* 11: 594071. https://doi.org/10.3389/fimmu.2020.594071.

Colonna, Marco, and Oleg Butovsky. 2017. «Microglia Function in the Central Nervous System During Health and Neurodegeneration». *Annual Review of Immunology* 35 (April): 441–68. https://doi.org/10.1146/annurev-immunol-051116-052358.

Danielski, Lucineia Gainski, Amanda Della Giustina, Marwa Badawy, Tatiana Barichello, João Quevedo, Felipe Dal-Pizzol, and Fabrícia Petronilho. 2018. «Brain Barrier Breakdown as a Cause and Consequence of Neuroinflammation in Sepsis». *Molecular Neurobiology* 55 (2): 1045–53. https://doi.org/10.1007/s12035-016-0356-7.

Danielski, Lucineia Gainski, Amanda Della Giustina, Sandra Bonfante, Mariana Pereira de Souza Goldim, Larissa Joaquim, Kiuanne Lobo Metzker, Erica Bernardo Biehl, et al. 2020. «NLRP3 Activation Contributes to Acute Brain Damage Leading to Memory Impairment in Sepsis-Surviving Rats». *Molecular Neurobiology* 57 (12): 5247–62. https://doi.org/10.1007/s12035-020-02089-9.

Danielski, Lucinéia Gainski, Amanda Della Giustina, Fernanda Frederico Gava, Tatiana Barichello, and Fabricia Petronilho. 2022. «The Many Faces of Astrocytes in the Septic Brain». *Molecular Neurobiology* 59 (12): 7229–35. https://doi.org/10.1007/s12035-022-03027-7.

Ehler, Johannes, Lucinda K. Barrett, Valerie Taylor, Michael Groves, Francesco Scaravilli, Matthias Wittstock, Stephan Kolbaske, et al. 2017. «Translational Evidence for Two Distinct Patterns of Neuroaxonal Injury in Sepsis: A Longitudinal, Prospective Translational Study». *Critical Care (London, England)* 21 (1): 262. https://doi.org/10.1186/s13054-017-1850-7.

El, Streck, Comim Cm, Barichello T, and Quevedo J. 2008. «The Septic Brain». *Neurochemical Research* 33 (11). https://doi.org/10.1007/s11064-008-9671-3.

Erikson, Kristo, Hannu Tuominen, Merja Vakkala, Janne Henrik Liisanantti, Tuomo Karttunen, Hannu Syrjälä, and Tero Ilmari Ala-Kokko. 2020. «Brain Tight Junction Protein Expression in Sepsis in an Autopsy Series». *Critical Care (London, England)* 24 (1): 385. https://doi.org/10.1186/s13054-020-03101-3.

Escartin, Carole, Elena Galea, András Lakatos, James P. O'Callaghan, Gabor C. Petzold, Alberto Serrano-Pozo, Christian Steinhäuser, et al. 2021. «Reactive Astrocyte Nomenclature, Definitions, and Future Directions». *Nature Neuroscience* 24 (3): 312–25. https://doi.org/10.1038/s41593-020-00783-4.

Fu, Qun, Jing Wu, Xiao-Yan Zhou, Mu-Huo Ji, Qing-Hong Mao, Qing Li, Man-Man Zong, Zhi-Qiang Zhou, and Jian-Jun Yang. 2019. «NLRP3/Caspase-1 Pathway-Induced Pyroptosis Mediated Cognitive Deficits in a Mouse Model of Sepsis-Associated Encephalopathy». *Inflammation* 42 (1): 306–18. https://doi.org/10.1007/s10753-018-0894-4.

Gao, Li-Li, Zhi-Hao Wang, Yu-Hang Mu, Zuo-Long Liu, and Li Pang. 2022. «Emodin Promotes Autophagy and Prevents Apoptosis in Sepsis-Associated Encephalopathy through Activating BDNF/TrkB Signaling». *Pathobiology: Journal of Immunopathology, Molecular, and Cellular Biology* 89 (3): 135–45. https://doi.org/10.1159/000520281.

Gao, Qingzeng, and Marina Sorrentino Hernandes. 2021. «Sepsis-Associated Encephalopathy and Blood-Brain Barrier Dysfunction». *Inflammation* 44 (6): 2143–50. https://doi.org/10.1007/s10753-021-01501-3.

Greenhalgh, Andrew D., Sam David, and F. Chris Bennett. 2020. «Immune Cell Regulation of Glia during CNS Injury and Disease». *Nature Reviews: Neuroscience* 21 (3): 139–52. https://doi.org/10.1038/s41583-020-0263-9.

Griton, Marion, Ibtihel Dhaya, Renaud Nicolas, Gérard Raffard, Olivier Periot, Bassem Hiba, and Jan Pieter Konsman. 2020. «Experimental Sepsis-Associated Encephalopathy Is Accompanied by Altered Cerebral Blood Perfusion and Water Diffusion and Related to Changes in Cyclooxygenase-2 Expression and Glial Cell Morphology but Not to Blood-Brain Barrier Breakdown». *Brain, Behavior, and Immunity* 83 (январь): 200–213. https://doi.org/10.1016/j.bbi.2019.10.012.

Gu, Ming, Xiang-Lin Mei, and Ya-Nan Zhao. 2021. «Sepsis and Cerebral Dysfunction: BBB Damage, Neuroinflammation, Oxidative Stress, Apoptosis, and Autophagy as Key Mediators and the Potential Therapeutic Approaches». *Neurotoxicity Research* 39 (2): 489–503. https://doi.org/10.1007/s12640-020-00270-5.

Im Kafa, Ari I., and Kurt Ma. 2007. «The Peri-Microvascular Edema in Hippocampal CA1 Area in a Rat Model of Sepsis». *Neuropathology : Official Journal of the Japanese Society of Neuropathology* 27 (3). https://doi.org/10.1111/j.1440-1789.2007.00757.x.

Iwashyna, Theodore J., E. Wesley Ely, Dylan M. Smith, and Kenneth M. Langa. 2010. «Long-Term Cognitive Impairment and Functional Disability among Survivors of Severe Sepsis». *JAMA* 304 (16): 1787–94. https://doi.org/10.1001/jama.2010.1553.

Janz, David R., Ty W. Abel, James C. Jackson, Max L. Gunther, Stephan Heckers, and E. Wesley Ely. 2010. «Brain Autopsy Findings in Intensive Care Unit Patients Previously Suffering from Delirium: A Pilot Study». *Journal of Critical Care* 25 (3): 538.e7-12. https://doi.org/10.1016/j.jcrc.2010.05.004.

Baumgart, K., V. Simkova, F. Wagner, S. Weber, M. Georgieff, P. Radermacher, G. Albuszies, and E. Barth. 2009. «Effect of SOD-1 Over-Expression on Myocardial Function During Resuscitated Murine Septic Shock». *Intensive Care Medicine* 35 (2). https://doi.org/10.1007/s00134-008-1319-x.

Kadry, Hossam, Behnam Noorani, and Luca Cucullo. 2020. «A Blood-Brain Barrier Overview on Structure, Function, Impairment, and Biomarkers of Integrity». *Fluids and Barriers of the CNS* 17 (1): 69. https://doi.org/10.1186/s12987-020-00230-3.

Khan, Babar A., Anthony J. Perkins, Nagendra K. Prasad, Anantha Shekhar, Noll L. Campbell, Sujuan Gao, Sophia Wang, et al. 2020. «Biomarkers of Delirium Duration and Delirium Severity in the ICU». *Critical Care Medicine* 48 (3): 353–61. https://doi.org/10.1097/CCM.0000000000004139.

Kinoshita, Hisanori, Takakuni Maki, Ken Yasuda, Natsue Kishida, Norio Sasaoka, Yasushi Takagi, Akira Kakizuka, and Ryosuke Takahashi. 2019. «KUS121, a Valosin-Containing Protein Modulator, Attenuates Ischemic Stroke via Preventing ATP Depletion». *Scientific Reports* 9 (1): 11519. https://doi.org/10.1038/s41598-019-47993-w.

Kobayashi, Takayuki, Hiroyuki Uchino, Eskil Elmér, Yukihiko Ogihara, Hidetoshi Fujita, Shusuke Sekine, Yusuke Ishida, Iwao Saiki, Shoichiro Shibata, and Aya Kawachi. 2022. «Disease Outcome and Brain Metabolomics of Cyclophilin-D Knockout Mice in Sepsis». *International Journal of Molecular Sciences* 23 (2): 961. https://doi.org/10.3390/ijms23020961.

Lauro, Clotilde, and Cristina Limatola. 2020. «Metabolic Reprograming of Microglia in the Regulation of the Innate Inflammatory Response». *Frontiers in Immunology* 11: 493. https://doi.org/10.3389/fimmu.2020.00493.

Lei, Yupeng, Ruixi Zhou, Xuemei Sun, Fajuan Tang, Hu Gao, Lin Chen, and Xihong Li. 2021. «The Pannexin-1 Channel Regulates Pyroptosis Through Autophagy in a Mouse Model of Sepsis-Associated Encephalopathy». *Annals of Translational Medicine* 9 (24): 1802. https://doi.org/10.21037/atm-21-6579.

Li, Yi, Lu Yin, Zhongmin Fan, Binxiao Su, Yu Chen, Yan Ma, Ya Zhong, Wugang Hou, Zongping Fang, and Xijing Zhang. 2020. «Microglia: A Potential Therapeutic Target for Sepsis-Associated Encephalopathy and Sepsis-Associated Chronic Pain». *Frontiers in Pharmacology* 11: 600421. https://doi.org/10.3389/fphar.2020.600421.

Liu, Lingling, Keliang Xie, Hongguang Chen, Xiaoqing Dong, Yuan Li, Yang Yu, Guolin Wang, and Yonghao Yu. 2014. «Inhalation of Hydrogen Gas Attenuates Brain Injury in Mice with Cecal Ligation and Puncture via Inhibiting Neuroinflammation, Oxidative Stress, and Neuronal Apoptosis». *Brain Research* 1589 (November): 78–92. https://doi.org/10.1016/j.brainres.2014.09.030.

Liu, Yu-xiao, Yang Yu, Jing-peng Liu, Wen-jia Liu, Yang Cao, Run-min Yan, and Yong-ming Yao. 2022. «Neuroimmune Regulation in Sepsis-Associated Encephalopathy: The Interaction Between the Brain and Peripheral Immunity». *Frontiers in Neurology* 13. https://www.frontiersin.org/articles/10.3389/fneur.2022.892480.

Mathiisen, Thomas Misje, Knut Petter Lehre, Niels Christian Danbolt, and Ole Petter Ottersen. 2010. «The Perivascular Astroglial Sheath Provides a Complete Covering of the Brain Microvessels: An Electron Microscopic 3D Reconstruction». *Glia* 58 (9): 1094–1103. https://doi.org/10.1002/glia.20990.

Mazeraud, Aurélien, Cássia Righy, Eleonore Bouchereau, Sarah Benghanem, Fernando Augusto Bozza, and Tarek Sharshar. 2020. «Septic-Associated Encephalopathy: A Comprehensive Review». *Neurotherapeutics* 17 (2): 392–403. https://doi.org/10.1007/s13311-020-00862-1.

Michels, Monique, Amanda V. Steckert, João Quevedo, Tatiana Barichello, and Felipe Dal-Pizzol. 2015. «Mechanisms of Long-Term Cognitive Dysfunction of Sepsis: From Blood-Borne Leukocytes to Glial Cells». *Intensive Care Medicine Experimental* 3 (1): 30. https://doi.org/10.1186/s40635-015-0066-x.

Michels, Monique, Andriele S. Vieira, Francieli Vuolo, Hugo Galvane Zapelini, Bruna Mendonça, Francielle Mina, Diogo Dominguini, et al. 2015. «The Role of Microglia Activation in the Development of Sepsis-Induced Long-Term Cognitive Impairment». *Brain, Behavior, and Immunity* 43 (January): 54–59. https://doi.org/10.1016/j.bbi.2014.07.002.

Miners, Scott, Patrick G. Kehoe, and Seth Love. 2020. «Cognitive Impact of COVID-19: Looking Beyond the Short Term». *Alzheimer's Research & Therapy* 12 (1): 170. https://doi.org/10.1186/s13195-020-00744-w.

Molnár, Levente, Béla Fülesdi, Norbert Németh, and Csilla Molnár. 2018. «Sepsis-Associated Encephalopathy: A Review of Literature». *Neurology India* 66 (2): 352–61. https://doi.org/10.4103/0028-3886.227299.

Moraes, Carolina Araújo, Camila Zaverucha-do-Valle, Renaud Fleurance, Tarek Sharshar, Fernando Augusto Bozza, and Joana Costa d'Avila. 2021. «Neuroinflammation in Sepsis: Molecular Pathways of Microglia Activation». *Pharmaceuticals* 14 (5): 416. https://doi.org/10.3390/ph14050416.

Muscatell, Keely A., Katarina Dedovic, George M. Slavich, Michael R. Jarcho, Elizabeth C. Breen, Julienne E. Bower, Michael R. Irwin, and Naomi I. Eisenberger. 2015. «Greater Amygdala Activity and Dorsomedial Prefrontal-Amygdala Coupling Are Associated with Enhanced Inflammatory Responses to Stress». *Brain, Behavior, and Immunity* 43 (January): 46–53. https://doi.org/10.1016/j.bbi.2014.06.201.

Nwafor, Divine C., Allison L. Brichacek, Afroz S. Mohammad, Jessica Griffith, Brandon P. Lucke-Wold, Stanley A. Benkovic, Werner J. Geldenhuys, Paul R. Lockman, and Candice M. Brown. 2019. «Targeting the Blood-Brain Barrier to Prevent Sepsis-Associated Cognitive Impairment». *Journal of Central Nervous System Disease* 11: 1179573519840652. https://doi.org/10.1177/1179573519840652.

Pelvig, D. P., H. Pakkenberg, A. K. Stark, and B. Pakkenberg. 2008. «Neocortical Glial Cell Numbers in Human Brains». *Neurobiology of Aging* 29 (11): 1754–62. https://doi.org/10.1016/j.neurobiolaging.2007.04.013.

Pfister, David, Martin Siegemund, Salome Dell-Kuster, Peter Smielewski, Stephan Rüegg, Stephan P. Strebel, Stephan C. U. Marsch, Hans Pargger, and Luzius A. Steiner. 2008. «Cerebral Perfusion in Sepsis-Associated Delirium». *Critical Care (London, England)* 12 (3): R63. https://doi.org/10.1186/cc6891.

Pierrakos, Charalampos, Rachid Attou, Laurence Decorte, Athanasios Kolyviras, Stefano Malinverni, Philippe Gottignies, Jacques Devriendt, and David De Bels. 2014. «Transcranial Doppler to Assess Sepsis-Associated Encephalopathy in Critically Ill Patients». *BMC Anesthesiology* 14: 45. https://doi.org/10.1186/1471-2253-14-45.

Polito, Andrea, Jean-Philippe Brouland, Raphael Porcher, Romain Sonneville, Shidasp Siami, Robert D. Stevens, Céline Guidoux, et al. 2011. «Hyperglycaemia and Apoptosis of Microglial Cells in Human Septic Shock». *Critical Care (London, England)* 15 (3): R131. https://doi.org/10.1186/cc10244.

Poll, Tom van der, Frank L. van de Veerdonk, Brendon P. Scicluna, and Mihai G. Netea. 2017. «The Immunopathology of Sepsis and Potential Therapeutic Targets». *Nature Reviews Immunology* 17 (7): 407–20. https://doi.org/10.1038/nri.2017.36.

Qiu, Li-Li, Wei Pan, Dan Luo, Guang-Fen Zhang, Zhi-Qiang Zhou, Xiao-Yun Sun, Jian-Jun Yang, and Mu-Huo Ji. 2020. «Dysregulation of BDNF/TrkB Signaling Mediated by NMDAR/Ca2+/Calpain Might Contribute to Postoperative Cognitive Dysfunction in Aging Mice». *Journal of Neuroinflammation* 17 (1): 23. https://doi.org/10.1186/s12974-019-1695-x.

Reyes, Edison-Pablo, Sebastián Abarzúa, Aldo Martin, Jorge Rodríguez, Paula P. Cortés, and Ricardo Fernández. 2012. «LPS-Induced c-Fos Activation in NTS Neurons and Plasmatic Cortisol Increases in Septic Rats Are Suppressed by Bilateral Carotid Chemodenervation». *Advances in Experimental Medicine and Biology* 758: 185–90. https://doi.org/10.1007/978-94-007-4584-1_26.

Rudd, Kristina E., Sarah Charlotte Johnson, Kareha M. Agesa, Katya Anne Shackelford, Derrick Tsoi, Daniel Rhodes Kievlan, Danny V. Colombara, et al. 2020. «Global, Regional, and National Sepsis Incidence and Mortality, 1990–2017: Analysis for the Global Burden of Disease Study». *The Lancet* 395 (10219): 200–211. https://doi.org/10.1016/S0140-6736(19)32989-7.

Savi, Felipe Figueredo, Alexandre de Oliveira, Gabriela Ferreira de Medeiros, Fernando Augusto Bozza, Monique Michels, Tarek Sharshar, Felipe Dal-Pizzol, and Cristiane Ritter. 2021. «What Animal Models Can Tell Us about Long-Term Cognitive Dysfunction Following Sepsis: A Systematic Review». *Neuroscience & Biobehavioral Reviews* 124 (May): 386–404. https://doi.org/10.1016/j.neubiorev.2020.12.005.

Sekino, Nobufumi, Magdy Selim, and Amjad Shehadah. 2022. «Sepsis-Associated Brain Injury: Underlying Mechanisms and Potential Therapeutic Strategies for Acute and Long-Term Cognitive Impairments». *Journal of Neuroinflammation* 19 (1): 101. https://doi.org/10.1186/s12974-022-02464-4.

Sharshar, Tarek, Djillali Annane, Geoffroy Lorin de la Grandmaison, Jean Philippe Brouland, Nicholas S. Hopkinson, and Gray Françoise. 2004. «The Neuropathology of Septic Shock». *Brain Pathology (Zurich, Switzerland)* 14 (1): 21–33. https://doi.org/10.1111/j.1750-3639.2004.tb00494.x.

Sharshar, Tarek, Nicholas S. Hopkinson, David Orlikowski, and Djillali Annane. 2005. «Science Review: The Brain in Sepsis–Culprit and Victim». *Critical Care (London, England)* 9 (1): 37–44. https://doi.org/10.1186/cc2951.

Sharshar, Tarek, Raphaël Porcher, Shidasp Siami, Benjamim Rohaut, Juliette Bailly-Salin, Nicholas S. Hopkinson, Bernard Clair, et al. 2011. «Brainstem Responses Can Predict Death and Delirium in Sedated Patients in Intensive Care Unit». *Critical Care Medicine* 39 (8): 1960–67. https://doi.org/10.1097/CCM.0b013e31821b843b.

Shulyatnikova, Tatyana, and Alexei Verkhratsky. 2020. «Astroglia in Sepsis Associated Encephalopathy». *Neurochemical Research* 45 (1): 83–99. https://doi.org/10.1007/s11064-019-02743-2.

Siami, Shidasp, Andrea Polito, Raphael Porcher, Tarik Hissem, Anne Blanchard, Catherine Boucly, Robert Carlier, Djillali Annane, Jean-Philippe Haymann, and Tarek Sharshar. 2013. «Thirst Perception and Osmoregulation of Vasopressin Secretion Are Altered During Recovery from Septic Shock». *PloS One* 8 (11): e80190. https://doi.org/10.1371/journal.pone.0080190.

Stare, Jerneja, Shidasp Siami, Eric Trudel, Masha Prager-Khoutorsky, Tarek Sharshar, and Charles W. Bourque. 2015. «Effects of Peritoneal Sepsis on Rat Central Osmoregulatory Neurons Mediating Thirst and Vasopressin Release». *The Journal of Neuroscience: The Official Journal of the Society for Neuroscience* 35 (35): 12188–97. https://doi.org/10.1523/JNEUROSCI.5420-13.2015.

Sun, Qing, Xiang Xu, Tianyi Wang, Zhongmou Xu, Xiaocheng Lu, Xiang Li, and Gang Chen. 2021. «Neurovascular Units and Neural-Glia Networks in Intracerebral Hemorrhage: From Mechanisms to Translation». *Translational Stroke Research* 12 (3): 447–60. https://doi.org/10.1007/s12975-021-00897-2.

Taccone, Fabio Silvio, Diego Castanares-Zapatero, Daliana Peres-Bota, Jean-Louis Vincent, Jacques Berre', and Christian Melot. 2010. «Cerebral Autoregulation Is Influenced by Carbon Dioxide Levels in Patients with Septic Shock». *Neurocritical Care* 12 (1): 35–42. https://doi.org/10.1007/s12028-009-9289-6.

Tang, Yu, and Weidong Le. 2016. «Differential Roles of M1 and M2 Microglia in Neurodegenerative Diseases». *Molecular Neurobiology* 53 (2): 1181–94. https://doi.org/10.1007/s12035-014-9070-5.

Tauber, Simone C., Marija Djukic, Johannes Gossner, Helmut Eiffert, Wolfgang Brück, and Roland Nau. 2021. «Sepsis Associated Encephalopathy and Septic Encephalitis: An Update». *Expert Review of Anti-Infective Therapy* 19 (2): 215–31. https://doi.org/10.1080/14787210.2020.1812384.

Tovote, Philip, Jonathan Paul Fadok, and Andreas Lüthi. 2015. «Neuronal Circuits for Fear and Anxiety». *Nature Reviews: Neuroscience* 16 (6): 317–31. https://doi.org/10.1038/nrn3945.

Tsuchiya, Kohsuke. 2020. «Inflammasome-Associated Cell Death: Pyroptosis, Apoptosis, and Physiological Implications». *Microbiology and Immunology* 64 (4): 252–69. https://doi.org/10.1111/1348-0421.12771.

Valderrama, Eduard Valdes, Kelley Humbert, Aaron Lord, Jennifer Frontera, and Shadi Yaghi. 2020. «Severe Acute Respiratory Syndrome Coronavirus 2 Infection and Ischemic Stroke». *Stroke* 51 (7): e124–27. https://doi.org/10.1161/STROKEAHA.120.030153.

Vasile, Flora, Elena Dossi, and Nathalie Rouach. 2017. «Human Astrocytes: Structure and Functions in the Healthy Brain». *Brain Structure and Function* 222 (5): 2017–29. https://doi.org/10.1007/s00429-017-1383-5.

Villarreal, Alejandro, and Tanja Vogel. 2021. «Different Flavors of Astrocytes: Revising the Origins of Astrocyte Diversity and Epigenetic Signatures to Understand Heterogeneity after Injury». *International Journal of Molecular Sciences* 22 (13): 6867. https://doi.org/10.3390/ijms22136867.

Villéga, Frédéric, Jean-Christophe Delpech, Marion Griton, Caroline André, Jean-Michel Franconi, Sylvain Miraux, and Jan Pieter Konsman. 2017. «Circulating Bacterial Lipopolysaccharide-Induced Inflammation Reduces Flow in Brain-Irrigating Arteries Independently from Cerebrovascular Prostaglandin Production». *Neuroscience* 346 (March): 160–72. https://doi.org/10.1016/j.neuroscience.2017.01.018.

Wang, Hongyu, Hongwei Wang, Yinsen Song, Congyan Liu, Xinling Qian, Dalong Zhang, Xin Jiang, and Sisen Zhang. 2022. «Overexpression of Foxc1 Ameliorates Sepsis-Associated Encephalopathy by Inhibiting Microglial Migration and Neuroinflammation Through the IκBα/NF-κB Pathway». *Molecular Medicine Reports* 25 (3): 107. https://doi.org/10.3892/mmr.2022.12623.

Wang, Kaifang, Meiyan Sun, Zhaodong Juan, Jianxin Zhang, Yingui Sun, Guizhi Wang, Chunling Wang, et al. 2022. «The Improvement of Sepsis-Associated Encephalopathy by P2X7R Inhibitor Through Inhibiting the Omi/HtrA2 Apoptotic Signaling Pathway». *Behavioural Neurology* 2022 (January): 3777351. https://doi.org/10.1155/2022/3777351.

Wang, Li-Xue, Chao Ren, Ren-Qi Yao, Yi-Nan Luo, Yue Yin, Yao Wu, Ning Dong, Xiao-Mei Zhu, and Yong-Ming Yao. 2021. «Sestrin2 Protects Against Lethal Sepsis by Suppressing the Pyroptosis of Dendritic Cells». *Cellular and Molecular Life Sciences: CMLS* 78 (24): 8209–27. https://doi.org/10.1007/s00018-021-03970-z.

Wang, Yan, Xueyan Liu, Qiang Wang, and Xin Yang. 2020. «Roles of the Pyroptosis Signaling Pathway in a Sepsis-Associated Encephalopathy Cell Model». *The Journal of International Medical Research* 48 (8): 300060520949767. https://doi.org/10.1177/0300060520949767.

Warford, Jordan, Anna-Claire Lamport, Barry Kennedy, and Alexander S. Easton. 2017. «Human Brain Chemokine and Cytokine Expression in Sepsis: A Report of Three Cases». *Canadian Journal of Neurological Sciences* 44 (1): 96–104. https://doi.org/10.1017/cjn.2016.310.

Westhoff, D., J. Y. Engelen-Lee, I. C. M. Hoogland, E. M. A. Aronica, D. J. van Westerloo, D. van de Beek, and W. A. van Gool. 2019. «Systemic Infection and Microglia Activation: A Prospective Postmortem Study in Sepsis Patients». *Immunity & Ageing: I & A* 16: 18. https://doi.org/10.1186/s12979-019-0158-7.

Wu, Tiantian, Chao Ren, Xiaowei Dou, Yao Wu, Ning Dong, Hui Zhang, and Yongming Yao. 2023. «Interleukin-35 Downregulates the Immune Response of Effector CD4 + T Cells Via Restricting High Mobility Group Box-1 Protein-Dependent Autophagy in Sepsis». *Shock (Augusta, GA.)* 59 (2): 277–87. https://doi.org/10.1097/SHK.0000000000001990.

Xin, Yueyang, Jinxu Wang, Tiantian Chu, Yaqun Zhou, Cheng Liu, and Aijun Xu. 2022. «Electroacupuncture Alleviates Neuroinflammation by Inhibiting the HMGB1 Signaling Pathway in Rats with Sepsis-Associated Encephalopathy». *Brain Sciences* 12 (12): 1732. https://doi.org/10.3390/brainsci12121732.

Xu, Xi-E., Lu Liu, Yu-Chang Wang, Chun-Tao Wang, Qiang Zheng, Qin-Xin Liu, Zhan-Fei Li, Xiang-Jun Bai, and Xing-Hua Liu. 2019. «Caspase-1 Inhibitor Exerts Brain-Protective Effects against Sepsis-Associated Encephalopathy and Cognitive Impairments in a Mouse Model of Sepsis». *Brain, Behavior, and Immunity* 80 (August): 859–70. https://doi.org/10.1016/j.bbi.2019.05.038.

Yan, Chaoying, Zhi Ma, Hongli Ma, Qing Li, Qian Zhai, Tao Jiang, Zhanqin Zhang, and Qiang Wang. 2020. «Mitochondrial Transplantation Attenuates Brain Dysfunction in Sepsis by Driving Microglial M2 Polarization». *Molecular Neurobiology* 57 (9): 3875–90. https://doi.org/10.1007/s12035-020-01994-3.

Yang, Chien-Chung, Li-Der Hsiao, Ya-Fang Shih, Mei-Hsiu Su, and Chuen-Mao Yang. 2022. «Sphingosine 1-Phosphate-Upregulated COX-2/PGE2 System Contributes to Human Cardiac Fibroblast Apoptosis: Involvement of MMP-9-Dependent Transactivation of EGFR Cascade». *Oxidative Medicine and Cellular Longevity* 2022: 7664290. https://doi.org/10.1155/2022/7664290.

Ye, Bo, Tianzhu Tao, Andong Zhao, Liyuan Wen, Xiaofei He, Yi Liu, Qiang Fu, Weidong Mi, and Jingsheng Lou. 2019. «Blockade of IL-17A/IL-17R Pathway Protected Mice from Sepsis-Associated Encephalopathy by Inhibition of Microglia Activation». *Mediators of Inflammation* 2019: 8461725. https://doi.org/10.1155/2019/8461725.

Zhang, Huidan, Heng Fang, Yirong Wang, Jing Xu, and Chunbo Chen. 2021. «Mechanisms of Sodium Butyrate Inhibition of Microglia Inflammatory Activation in Hippocampus Via Toll-Like Receptor 4/Nuclear Factor-κB p65 Pathway». *Zhonghua Wei Zhong Bing Ji Jiu Yi Xue* 33 (12): 1471–78. https://doi.org/10.3760/cma.j.cn121430-20211105-01647.

Zhang, Lina, Yuan Jiang, Songyun Deng, Yunan Mo, Yan Huang, Wenchao Li, Chenglong Ge, et al. 2021. «S100B/RAGE/Ceramide Signaling Pathway Is Involved in Sepsis-Associated Encephalopathy». *Life Sciences* 277 (July): 119490. https://doi.org/10.1016/j.lfs.2021.119490.

Zhou, Rui-Xi, Yu-Yao Li, Yi Qu, Qun Huang, Xue-Mei Sun, De-Zhi Mu, and Xi-Hong Li. 2020. «Regulation of Hippocampal Neuronal Apoptosis and Autophagy in Mice with Sepsis-Associated Encephalopathy by Immunity-Related GTPase M1». *CNS Neuroscience & Therapeutics* 26 (2): 177–88. https://doi.org/10.1111/cns.13229.

Zhu, Furong, Yingjun Zheng, Yu Qiang Ding, Yong Liu, Xianghui Zhang, Renrong Wu, Xiaofeng Guo, and Jingping Zhao. 2014. «Minocycline and Risperidone Prevent Microglia Activation and Rescue Behavioral Deficits Induced by Neonatal Intrahippocampal Injection of Lipopolysaccharide in Rats». *PloS One* 9 (4): e93966. https://doi.org/10.1371/journal.pone.0093966.

Zrzavy, T., R. Höftberger, T. Berger, H. Rauschka, O. Butovsky, H. Weiner, and H. Lassmann. 2019. «Pro-Inflammatory Activation of Microglia in the Brain of Patients with Sepsis». *Neuropathology and Applied Neurobiology* 45 (3): 278–90. https://doi.org/10.1111/nan.12502.

Chapter 2

Biomarkers of sepsis-associated encephalopathy

Irina V. Ostrova, Ph.D., and
Natalia V. Beloborodova*, MD., Ph.D.
Federal Research and Clinical Center of Intensive Care Medicine and Rehabilitology,
Negovsky V.A. Research Institute of General Reanimatology, Moscow, Russia

Abstract

Early detection of brain dysfunction is of great importance, since encephalopathy, in many cases, is the first manifestation of organ dysfunction in septic patients. Early diagnosis of SAE can help identify those patients with more severe diseases who require enhanced follow-up and immediate intervention. However, to date, there are no clear laboratory criteria for SAE. Therefore, clinical criteria should be used for the diagnosis of SE, in combination with electrophysiological and biochemical tests. Biomarkers are an additional instrument in the diagnosis of SAE. Some SE biomarkers can be irreplaceable for objective monitoring of the degree of brain changes. Due to the complex etiopathogenesis of SAE, it turns out that each marker is influenced by numerous factors. Summarizing the results of recent studies, the authors believe that individual groups of biomarkers following their participation in the pathophysiological process may be more useful for assessing the degree and dynamics of SAE during treatment. The exact role of biomarkers in the management of patients with sepsis has not been definitively determined; however, their use for the diagnosis of brain dysfunction and prediction of mortality in sepsis seems very promising. In this chapter, SAE biomarkers are considered from the point of view of various stages of SAE pathophysiology.

Keywords: sepsis, encephalopathy, brain dysfunction, delirium, biomarker, diagnosis, inflammation

* Corresponding author: Natalia V. Beloborodova, Professor, MD., Ph.D.
e-mail address: nvbeloborodova@yandex.ru

Editor: Irina A. Savvina, Natalia V. Beloborodova and Tatyana N. Trofimova
In: Sepsis-Associated Encephalopathy
ISBN: 979-8-89113-178-1

Abbreviations

BBB	blood-brain barrier
CAM-ICU	Intensive Care Confusion Assessment Method
CNS	central nervous system
CT	computed tomography
CRP	C-reactive protein
CSF	cerebrospinal fluid
ICDSC	Intensive Care Delirium Screening Checklist
FOUR	Full Outline of UnResponsiveness
GCS	Glasgow Coma Scale
ICAM-1	intercellular adhesion molecule-1
ICU	intensive care unit
miRNA/miR	microRNA
MRI	magnetic resonance imaging
NT-proCNP	amino-terminal pro-C-type natriuretic peptide
NSE	neuron-specific enolase
Nf	neurofilament protein
PCT	Procalcitonin
ROS	reactive oxygen species
SAD	sepsis-associated delirium
SAE	sepsis-associated encephalopathy
SOFA	Sequential Organ Failure Assessment score
TNF-α	tumor necrosis factor-α
TRAF6	tumor necrosis factor receptor-associated factor 6
VCAM-1	vascular cell adhesion molecule-1

Introduction

In the twenty-first century, sepsis remains the leading cause of death in intensive care units (ICU) equipped with multicomponent monitoring, despite the use of potent antimicrobial drugs and high-tech organ-substituting technologies [1]. Sepsis-associated encephalopathy (SAE), also known as septic encephalopathy (SE), sepsis-induced encephalopathy, sepsis-associated delirium (SAD), sepsis-induced brain dysfunction (SIBD), and sepsis-induced brain damage, is one of the most frequent and severe complications of sepsis [1–3]. SAE is a multifactorial syndrome belonging to the category of diffuse cerebral dysfunction, late form with often irreversible brain damage associated with sepsis, but without clinical and/or laboratory signs of direct brain infection [4–6]. SAE is associated with an unfavorable outcome among sepsis patients [1, 7–9].

Literature review

The rationale for the search for SAE biomarkers

The brain has a crucial role in sepsis because it mediates the immune response and acts as a susceptible target of the process. Early detection of delirium is of great importance, since delirium, in many cases, is the first manifestation of organ dysfunction in septic patients. Moreover, it can be the first symptom of sepsis and can even precede the fulfillment of sepsis criteria [1, 6]. However, there are still no clear diagnostic methods or biomarkers to identify such patients [5]. Clinically, SAE manifests itself in two different forms: an early predictable form and a late form, which is usually accompanied by complex metabolic encephalopathy, which can lead to irreversible brain damage [10].

SAE is associated with an increased duration of mechanical ventilation and a long stay in the intensive care unit, and in general, in the hospital [11]. Survivors of the acute stage have an increased risk of developing persistent neurocognitive dysfunction up to dementia [1, 12, 13].

Early diagnosis of SAE can help identify those patients with more severe diseases who require enhanced follow-up and immediate intervention. In critically ill patients, impaired consciousness is the earliest symptom of SAE, which should serve as a basis for finding the source of infection and an impetus for starting appropriate therapy [10, 14]. Unfortunately, SAE remains a “diagnosis of exclusion” and can only be diagnosed if other causes (infectious, metabolic, and toxic) are excluded [1, 15]. The main problem remains the inability to correctly determine the signs of SAE. This is because most resuscitation patients are under medical sedation. Nevertheless, the following scales are used to diagnose SAE in the clinic: CAM-ICU (Intensive Care Confusion Assessment Method), ICDSC (Intensive Care Delirium Screening Checklist), coma scales such as FOUR (Full Outline of UnResponsiveness) or GCS (Glasgow coma scale). However, the above scoring scales are non-specific methods and can therefore only be used for screening rather than diagnosis [3, 16, 17].

Electroencephalography (EEG) and evoked potentials (EPs) measures are used to obtain additional information about the mental status of the patient. A slowing of the normal alpha rhythm with the appearance of theta activity occurs in patients with no evidence of encephalopathy or with mild to moderate encephalopathy (confusion, delirium) and reflects cortical dysfunction. More pronounced changes in the electroencephalogram indicate the impaired function of deeper brain structures, such as the basal ganglia and the diencephalon [18]. In addition, the results of the EEG studies do not allow to answer the question whether the detected brain damages are irreversible or they indicate temporary brain dysfunction in patients with sepsis [18].

Neuroimaging techniques such as computed tomography (CT) and magnetic resonance imaging (MRI) are useful for detecting some abnormalities in brain structure. CT scans are most commonly used to detect structural damage to the brain due to the simplicity and convenience of the procedure. MRI of the brain allows you to get much more information, including the primary mechanisms of sepsis-associated brain damage (e.g., cytotoxic or vasogenic edema) or the development of delayed encephalopathy. MRI helps to identify cerebral infarction, leukoencephalopathy, and vascular edema. However, at an early stage, it is not common to screen for SAE by using neurophysiological or imaging methods [19].

Thus, the above examinations have drawbacks. Biomarkers are an additional instrument in the diagnosis of SAE. Biomarkers are commonly used for diagnosis because they are objective, convenient, and cheap. Therefore, biomarkers can be useful in prognostication, diagnosis of SAE, and, in the future, for the development of methods for its prevention and treatment [20].

The pathophysiology of SAE is not fully understood. Its etiology is likely multi-factorial, and several pathological mechanisms are involved in parallel, influence each other, and contribute to a varying degree to the development of SAE [1, 10]. The main disorders in sepsis include disrupted autoregulation of cerebral blood flow and ischemia caused by circulatory disorders;

dysfunction of the neuroendocrine network; inflammation-induced damage to neurons and glial cells; neurotransmitter imbalance [11, 21, 22]. Ehler J et al. (2020) proposed to single out three stages of development of the SAE [20]. First, systemic inflammation leads to endothelial dysfunction of the cerebrovascular system and blood-brain barrier (BBB) damage. It causes the entrance of proinflammatory cytokines in the brain parenchyma. The next stage is the activation of microglial cells, which most likely augments the inflammatory response in the brain and damages its cells – neurons, astroglia, and vascular endothelium. The consequence of this process is injury of brain structures, manifested in neurocognitive deficit (Figure 2.1).

This figure shows the stages of SAE pathophysiology. First, systemic inflammation leads to endothelial dysfunction in the cerebrovascular system and blood-brain barrier (*BBB*) damage; validated biomarkers – *CRP* (C-reactive protein); *PCT* (procalcitonin), *NT-proCNP* (amino-terminal pro-C-type natriuretic peptide), *ILs* (interleukins), *TNF-α* (tumor necrosis factor-α), *TRAF6* (tumor necrosis factor receptor-associated factor 6), *ICAM-1* (intercellular adhesion molecule-1), and *VCAM-1* (vascular cell adhesion molecule-1). Second, activated microglia augment inflammatory response in the brain; validated biomarker – *MiR* (microRNA). The third stage is astroglial and neuronal injury, manifesting as a neurocognitive deficit; validated biomarkers – *S100β*, *NSE* (neuron-specific enolase), *UCH-L1* (ubiquitin carboxyl-terminal hydrolase L1), *Nf* (neurofilament protein), and *Aβ* (beta-amyloid).

Biomarkers can be considered from the point of view of various stages of SAE pathophysiology [1, 20]. It should be borne in mind that each of the markers discussed below undergoes changes in the course of the disease and depends on numerous factors in such complex pathological conditions as sepsis and SAE. Summarizing the results of recent studies, the authors believe that individual groups of biomarkers following their participation in the pathophysiological process may be more useful for assessing the degree and dynamics of SAE during treatment (Table 2.1).

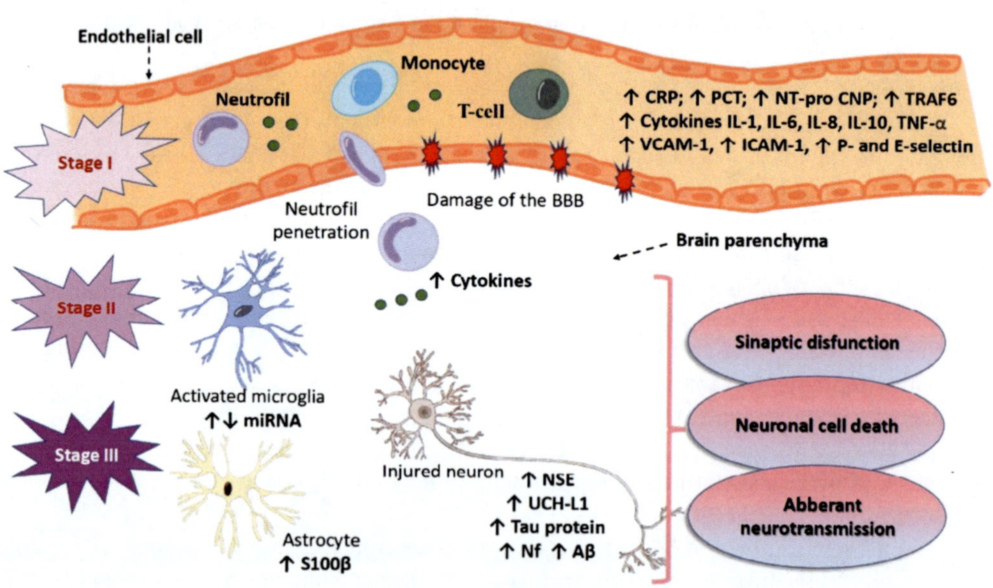

Figure 2.1 Biomarkers of SAE at the different stages of the pathophysiological process.

Table 2.1 Summary of biomarkers in different stages of SAE.

Biomarker/ source	Features of study	Findings	Reference
Inflammation			
CRP / liver	Data from 16 patients with sepsis, severe sepsis, or septic shock, of whom 12 had SAE.	Elevated CRP was associated with SAE and correlated with disturbed cerebrovascular autoregulation.	*Pfister D et al. 2008* [23]
PCT / the thyroid	50 delirious and 50 nondelirious ICU patients were included.	Procalcitonin was significantly associated with delirium in inflamed patients.	*van den Boogaard M et al. 2011* [24]
NT-proCNP / endothelium	CSF and plasma samples from 12 septic patients with SAE and 9 non-septic controls without encephalopathy were analyzed.	Plasma NT-proCNP levels were significantly higher in the sepsis cohort compared to controls with peak concentrations at study day 1 and a decrease over time.	*Ehler J et al. 2019* [25]
TRAF6 / PBMC	Data from 57 septic patients, of whom 29 were diagnosed with SAE.	Higher peripheral blood levels of TRAF6 in SAE patients than that in no-encephalopathy patients.	*Zhang Li-Na et al. 2016* [26]
Interleukins / leukocytes, TNF- α / monocytes	16 septic patients with encephalopathy, 10 septic patients without encephalopathy, and 20 healthy controls.	Increased plasma IL-6 levels in septic patients with encephalopathy in comparison to those in septic patients without encephalopathy and those in healthy controls within 12 h of the onset of SE.	*Nakamura T et al. 2003* [27]
	Data 41 burn sepsis patients, of whom 21 had SAE.	Higher serum levels of IL-10, IL-6, and TNF-α in SAE patients than those in the non-SAE group at 12, 24, 48, 72, and 120 h after diagnosis.	*Li XL et al. 2022* [28]
CD4+ / CD8+ T lymphocytes	Clinical data of 86 patients with severe sepsis. The incidence of SE in the patients was 39.5%.	The lower proportion of CD4+ T lymphocytes is a powerful predictor of SE in patients with severe sepsis.	*Lu ChX et al. 2016* [29]
	The study of 1,010 enrolled ICU patients (age ≥65 years), of whom 297 were diagnosed with delirium.	Natural killer cell count may be valuable for the prediction of SAD within elderly patient cohorts.	*Li D et al. 2021* [30]
Endothelial dysfunction, BBB injury			
VCAM-1, ICAM-1, P- & E-selectin / endothelium	A total of 30 patients presenting with CAP-induced sepsis were included. 10 (33%) developed SAE. 8 patients were included in the delirium, non-sepsis group.	SAE patients presented higher levels of VCAM-1, and ICAM-1 when compared to delirium patients.	*Tomasi CD et al. 2017* [31]
	Meta-analysis of SAE biomarkers in four case-control studies with 160 patients.	Plasma glycocalyx-associated molecules are elevated at SAE and may be useful for early identification of cognitive decline in sepsis patients.	*Baby Sh et al. 2023* [15]
Microglial activation			
MiR-370 / macrophages, monocytes, and microglia	Transcriptomic analyses of mouse brains at 24h and 120h after CLP. Candidate miRs were validated in mouse and patient samples (17 patients with SAE and 12 patients with sepsis without encephalopathy).	MiR-370-3p increased at 24h after CLP in SAE mouse brains (compared with the recovery phase). High plasma miR-370-3p in patients with SAE (but not sepsis alone).	*Visitchanakun P et al. 2020* [32]

(*Continued*)

Table 2.1 (Continued)

Biomarker/ source	Features of study	Findings	Reference
Neuronal and astroglial injury			
S100 proteins (S100β, S100A8, S100A9)	50 delirious and 50 nondelirious ICU patients.	S100β is associated with delirium in inflamed patients.	*van den Boogaard M at al. 2011* [24]
	16 patients with sepsis, of whom 12 had SAE.	Elevated S100β is associated with SAE.	*Pfister D et al. 2008* [23]
	A retrospective case series study included 41 burn sepsis, of whom 21 have SAE.	Higher serum levels of 100β and NSE of patients in the SAE group than that in the non-SAE group at 12, 24, and 48 h after diagnosis.	*Li XL et al. 2022* [28]
	Data from 57 septic patients, 29 were diagnosed with SAE.	Peripheral blood levels of S100A8 in SAE patients might be related to the severity of SAE and predict the outcome of SAE.	*Zhang Li-Na et al. 2016* [26]
NSE / neurons	A retrospective analysis of 124 patients with sepsis.	Higher plasma NSE concentrations are associated with mortality and delirium in critically ill septic patients.	*Anderson BJ et al. 2016* [33]
	Clinical data of 59 patients admitted to ICU with sepsis. SAE group (36 cases) non-SAE group (23 cases).	NSE combined with IL-6 on the third day in ICU demonstrates high diagnostic significance for SAE.	*Feng Q et al. 2017* [34]
Tau protein/neurons	109 patients with severe sepsis, 27 of whom developed SAE.	The close association between the serum Tau protein levels with the appearance of SAE in patients with severe sepsis.	*Zhao T et al. 2019* [35]
	41 burn sepsis patients. SAE group (21 cases) and non-SAE group (20 cases).	Higher serum levels of Tau protein of patients in the SAE group than that in the non-SAE group 5 days after diagnosis.	*Li XL et al. 2022* [28]
UCH-L1 / neurons	A prospective single-center study entailed 105 patients who suffered from sepsis.	Serum concentrations of UCH-L1 early elevated and associated with SAE and poor prognosis.	*Wu L et al. 2019* [36]
Nf, NfL / neurons	A prospective, pilot observational study included 20 patients with septic shock and 5 patients without sepsis serving as controls. The assessment of SAE.	Nf levels provide complementary prognostic information in SAE patients indicating a higher chance of death and poorer functional/cognitive outcomes in survivors.	*Ehler J et al. 2019* [37]
	A prospective observational study included 11 SAE patients and controls.	SAE patients showed higher CSF NfL levels than controls.	*Orhun G et al. 2021* [38]

SAE sepsis-associated encephalopathy; *CRP* C-reactive protein; *ICU* intensive care unit; *PCT* procalcitonin; *PBMC* peripheral blood mononuclear cells; *CSF* cerebrospinal fluid; *NT-proCNP* amino-terminal pro-C-type natriuretic peptide; *TRAF6* tumor necrosis factor receptor associated factor 6; *IL* interleukins; *TNF-α* tumor necrosis factor-α; *CLP* cecal ligation and puncture; *ICAM-1* intercellular adhesion molecule-1; *VCAM-1* vascular cell adhesion molecule-1; *MiR* microRNA; *NSE* neuron-specific enolase; *UCH-L1* ubiquitin carboxyl-terminal hydrolase L1; *Nf* neurofilament protein; *NfL* neurofilament light chains

In this chapter, SAE biomarkers will be considered sequentially depending on their participation in various stages of the pathogenesis of SAE.

Neuroinflammation

Inflammation is believed to be the starting point of some functional disorders of the brain [21, 39]. Systemic inflammation caused by infection and sepsis leads to profound changes in brain homeostasis. Inflammation in the brain is unlikely to be caused by bacterial products circulating in the blood, as only a small fraction of them enter the brain [40]. Although inflammatory processes in the nervous tissue are aimed at protecting the brain from foreign organisms, they are often detrimental to neurons. This is associated with microgliocytes – the main resident immune cells of the central nervous system (CNS). In sepsis, microglial activation occurs, caused by the interaction between the resident immune cells of the brain, the vascular endothelium, and blood leukocytes [41]. Numerous animal and human studies confirm the activation of microglia in the brain during sepsis [42–45].

Activated microglia secretes various cytotoxic substances, such as cyto- and chemokines, and reactive oxygen species (ROS), aimed at combating pathogens. However, excessive activation of microglia creates a vicious cycle of increased BBB permeability and neuronal death, which is one of the pathological mechanisms of neurodegenerative diseases, including SAE [46–48].

Potential biomarkers of neuroinflammation and delirium are ***markers of systemic inflammation*** that are often used in clinical practice, such as proinflammatory plasma cytokines, including ***tumor necrosis factor-α (TNF-α)***, ***interleukins (IL-1β, IL-2, IL-6, IL-8, IL-12, IL-10)***, ***C-reactive protein (CRP)***, and ***procalcitonin (PCT)***. Cytokine levels are measured in serum, but their levels in the brain cannot be easily quantified, and their low availability in the central nervous system limits research [47]. However, in many cases, there was a direct correlation between these biomarkers' levels with the duration of delirium, its severity, and nosocomial mortality [49, 50].

In their clinical study, McGrane et al. (2011) showed that high plasma concentrations of PCT and CRP predict prolonged periods of acute brain dysfunction, implicating inflammation as an important mechanism in the pathophysiology of delirium and coma during critical illness, irrespective of whether patients had sepsis or not [49]. Levels of PCT and IL-6 were higher in delirious patients in comparison to patients without delirium at 24 h after extubation following mechanical ventilation but not at 0 h [51]. Pfister et al. (2008) didn't find any difference in IL-6 levels between patients with and without SAD but showed a significant association between elevated CRP ($p = 0.008$) and SAD [23]. In the observational study by van den Boogaard M et al. (2011) 100 patients in the intensive care unit (ICU) with or without sepsis/SIRS and delirium were included. IL-8 levels in the blood were associated with delirium in patients with infection, while IL-10 blood concentrations were associated with delirium in noninfected individuals [24]. In the clinical trial of Tomasi et al. (2017), IL-10 levels were elevated in patients with SAE compared to a group of patients without it. It was shown that higher IL-8 levels were associated with increased mortality among delirious patients [31]. In the experimental study (a mouse model of SAE) the abnormal behavioral changes co-occurred with significant increases in hippocampal Iba1-positive cells (microglia) and IL-1β and IL-6 serum levels [43]. A clinical study by Nakamura et al. (2003) (16 septic patients with encephalopathy, 10 septic patients without encephalopathy, and 20 healthy controls) revealed within 12 h of the onset of SE increased plasma levels of IL-6 in septic patients with encephalopathy in comparison to those without encephalopathy ($p < 0.01$) and those in healthy controls ($p < 0.001$) [27]. In a prospective cohort study ($n = 138$) of Girard et al. (2012) higher concentrations of soluble tumor necrosis factor receptor-1 (sTNFR1) were associated with an increased probability of delirium ($p < 0.01$) during critical illness [52]. Tumor necrosis factor receptor-associated factor 6 (TRAF6) could be useful in diagnosing SAE and predicting its prognosis. TRAF6 levels in peripheral blood mononuclear cells (PBMC) in SAE patients were significantly higher than that in no-encephalopathy patients. TRAF6-relative levels of 1.44 were diagnostic of SAE with 85.70% specificity and 86.20% sensitivity. Besides TRAF6 relative levels of 2.94 predicted 28-day mortality of SAE with 80.00% specificity and 68.40% sensitivity [26].

Thus, high baseline inflammatory biomarkers predicted prolonged periods of acute brain dysfunction, implicating inflammation as an important mechanism in the pathophysiology of delirium and SAE [53].

Amino-terminal pro-C-type natriuretic peptide (***NT-proCNP***) is considered one of the good markers of SAE. NT-proCNP is the N-terminal fragment of the CNP precursor. NT-proCNP occurs in an equimolar concentration with CNP in human plasma and is considered to be a marker of the extent of CNP biosynthesis [54]. C-type NP is expressed primarily in the CNS and vascular tissues. It is suggested that this peptide acts primarily as a neurotransmitter in a paracrine way. CNP plays an important role in cardiovascular physiology as a potent vasorelaxant, as well as an inhibitor of vascular smooth muscle proliferation and endothelial cell migration [55]. Koch et al. (2011) found elevated NT-proCNP to be a predictor of mortality in patients with sepsis [56]. It revealed a positive correlation between delirium and preoperative plasma levels of NT-proCNP in cardiac surgery patients [57]. Changes in serum or cerebrospinal fluid (CSF) levels of NT-proCNP must reflect only inflammatory states related to general inflammation. Local inflammation does not trigger an increase in the NT-proCNP level [54]. The release of NT-proCNP may be caused by pro-inflammatory mediators such as IL-1β and TNF-α [58] and largely reflects vascular integrity [59]. These facts indicate the involvement of NT-proCNP in systemic inflammation and sepsis. Bíró et al. (1996) described in rats that the release of NT-proCNP causes an anxiolytic effect [60]. This indicates the importance of this peptide for the assessment of behavior changes. Therefore, NT-proCNP can be used as a specific biomarker of SAE.

The high peak concentration of plasma NT-proCNP in the early phase of sepsis might help to predict the emergence of SAE during the further course of the disease. In the clinical study (12 septic patients with SAE and 9 non-septic controls without encephalopathy) NSE, S100β, and NT-proCNP were measured in plasma at days 1, 3, and 7 in sepsis patients, once in controls and once in the CSF of both groups. Plasma NT-proCNP levels were significantly higher in SAE patients compared to controls with peak concentrations at study day 1 (10.1 ± 6.6 pmol/l vs. 3.3 ± 0.9 pmol/l; $p < 0.01$) and a decrease over time. It should be noted that no differences were detected between both groups for NSE and S100β levels in CSF [25].

Circulating blood inflammatory cells may also be involved in the pathogenesis of SAE. In particular, the proportion of CD4+ T lymphocytes is a powerful predictor of SE in patients with severe sepsis. Lu et al. (2016) showed that septic patients with SAE have fewer CD4+ T lymphocyte counts, a lower CD4+/CD8+ ratio, and a higher percentage of natural killer cells (NK cells) in the systemic circulation. An inverse relationship was found between CD4+ T lymphocyte percentage and the development of SAE [29]. NK cell count in the peripheral blood may be valuable for the prediction of SAD within elderly patient cohorts. The study of 1,010 enrolled ICU patients (age ≥65 years), of whom 297 were diagnosed with delirium NK cell count cut-off value of 87 cells/ml in septic patients at ICU admission, was predictive of delirium with a sensitivity of 80.2% and specificity of 80.8% [30].

An important role in the pathogenesis of sepsis is played by ***the complement system***. The complement system is a component of innate immunity and provides induction and control of inflammation. The infection causes activation of complement with subsequent release and accumulation of anaphylatoxins C3a and C5a. The latter are mediators of inflammation with a wide spectrum of action on various types of cells. In many clinical studies, elevated levels of C3a and C5a in the blood are associated with severe course and adverse outcomes in critical conditions [61, 62]. C5a has been associated with increased blood-brain barrier disruption, hyperactivation of inflammatory mediators, enhanced gliosis, and consumptive coagulopathy [62, 63]. The significance of C5a is well-known in sepsis and may be related to sepsis-associated brain damage [64, 65].

MicroRNA (miRNAs) are proposed as potential biomarkers of SAE. MiRNAs are small non-coding RNA molecules. They induce mRNA degradation or repress protein translation by binding to target messenger RNAs (mRNAs). MiRNAs such as ***miR-155, miR-27a, and miR-210*** are some of the most important regulators mediating microglial activation, polarization, and autophagy and, as a result, affecting neuroinflammation and CNS outcome (47). As mentioned above, microglia play a key role in neuroinflammation. It can cause neuronal damage by releasing inflammatory mediators, ROS, neurotransmitters, and other substances. Therefore, some microRNAs that are involved in the regulation of microglial activity are also expected to influence the development of SAE. In this regard, some miRNAs have been postulated as biomarkers of SAE [5, 17]. In particular, circulating ***miR-370***, alone or in combination with other miRNAs, has been proposed as a suitable candidate for the diagnosis of SAE. MiR-370-3p was shown to aggravate BBB disruption and neuron apoptosis in an in vitro model of SAE [66]. Transcriptomic analyses of mouse brains at 24 h and 120 h after cecal ligation and puncture (CLP) were performed. It was revealed that increased miR-370-3p levels in brains as well as in plasma of 24h-post-CLP mice compared with the recovery phase (120 h). In parallel, high plasma miR-370-3p was demonstrated in patients with SAE (n=17) (but not sepsis alone, n=12) suggesting the specificity toward SAE [32]. MiR-370 is very specific to SAE because its levels are not found in patients with sepsis and other inflammatory diseases. ***miR-130a-3p*** was also upregulated in SAE [67]. miR-25-3p on the contrary was downregulated in the cerebral cortex in the SAE mouse model at 12 h, 24 h, or 48 h after CLP operation [68]. MiR-155 is considered a pro-inflammatory mediator of the CNS and is upregulated in the brain of patients affected by many neurodegenerative diseases [17]. This miRNA was shown to be upregulated in macrophages, monocytes, and microglia in response to several proinflammatory stimuli, such as lipopolysaccharides (LPS), interferon-γ (IFN-γ), and TNF-α. Proinflammatory miRNAs also include miR-206 and miR36 [69].

Thus, microRNAs in the future can be excellent biomarkers of SAE, as they have important advantages, such as high bioavailability: they are present in various body fluids, including blood, urine, and saliva, which allows for relatively non-invasive sample collection; stability – they can be detected with a high probability by PCR analysis or RNA sequencing [17]. In addition, the small size of miRNAs allows them to easily penetrate the BBB, which makes them potential markers of CNS diseases [5]. The identification of new miRNAs and their combinations as biomarkers may help to improve SAE diagnosis and prognosis and to design new therapies.

Damage to the blood-brain barrier (BBB)

BBB is a highly selective semipermeable membrane that consists of a physical barrier (endothelial tight junctions) and a transport barrier (receptor-mediated transcytosis) that protects the brain from toxins and pathogens in blood circulation during sepsis. Sepsis-induced BBB defects are considered a major cause of SAE that allows the influx-transmigration of circulating molecules into the brain and, conversely, the translocation of several brain-specific molecules into the blood circulation [32].

Endothelial cells are an important component of the BBB. They maintain vascular integrity, tone, and patency and have important roles in hemostasis and inflammatory responses. Endothelial dysfunction plays a central role in the pathogenesis of sepsis-related organ dysfunction and failure as it results in dysregulated inflammation, vascular leakage, and abnormal coagulation [70]. Under inflammatory conditions, the endothelial cells become activated in response to proinflammatory stimuli and increase the surface expression of endothelial adhesion molecules such as E- and P-selectins, intercellular adhesion molecule-1 (ICAM-1), and vascular cell adhesion molecule-1 (VCAM-1).

ICAM-1 and ***VCAM-1*** are considered biomarkers that induce SAE. It has been confirmed a role for these molecules in sepsis and septic shock [71, 72]. Current studies suggest that the expression of these adhesion molecules may be a useful marker for active inflammation and endothelial dysfunction following sepsis. Their excessive expression in cerebrovascular endothelial cells increases the permeability of the BBB and allows the transfer of toxic factors from the peripheral circulation to the brain, leading to neuroinflammation [15]. The clinical study of Su Ch-M et al. (2014) involved 70 patients with severe sepsis, of whom 23 had SE. By stepwise logistic regression model, VCAM-1 level was independently associated with septic encephalopathy. It was revealed that VCAM-1 is a more powerful predictor of SE than lactate concentration and other adhesion molecules on admission [8]. Similar results were obtained in a study by Tomasi et al. (2017), which included 30 sepsis patients, 33% of whom developed SAE. Eight patients were included in the delirium, non-sepsis group. SAE patients presented higher levels of VCAM-1 and ICAM-1 when compared to delirium patients [31]. In another large cohort of critically ill patients, E-selectin, a cell adhesion molecule and a marker of endothelial injury, was associated with cognitive impairment and disability [73]. Meta-analysis of the four case-control studies with 160 patients revealed the higher pooled mean concentration of ICAM-1 ($p = 0.03$) and VCAM-1 ($p = 0.01$) in patients with SAE compared to the patients with sepsis alone. Single studies reported elevated levels of P-selectin, and E-selectin in patients with SAE compared to the patients with sepsis alone [15].

Thus, plasma glycocalyx-associated molecules are elevated in SAE and may be useful for early identification of cognitive decline in sepsis patients.

Astroglial and neuronal damage

S100β and **NSE** are brain injury biomarkers, mainly used in brain trauma, cerebral stroke, and hypoxic ischemia encephalopathy [1]. These proteins are most commonly investigated as biomarkers of SE. NSE and especially S100β are potential serum biomarkers for diagnosing and monitoring SE [74]. At the same time, many studies conduct a comparative analysis of the diagnostic abilities of these proteins.

NSE is an intracellular glycolytic enzyme of the CNS, which has a molecular weight of 78 kDa; it is found in neurons, neuroendocrine cells of the nervous system, as well as in erythrocytes and platelets. NSE γγ-isomer is known as a marker for all differentiated neurons, it is one of the intracellular enzymes of the CNS. Studies have confirmed the possibility of using the NSE enzyme activity parameter as a clinical diagnostic criterion for assessing the degree of damage to brain neurons due to ischemic and hemorrhagic strokes, epilepsy, traumatic brain injuries, and other destructive diseases of the central nervous system [75]. A few studies demonstrated increased levels of NSE at SAE [33, 34, 66, 76–79].

S100β is a calcium-binding protein that belongs to the S100 family, which is composed of low-molecular-weight, multigene proteins [74]. Most of the S100 proteins (up to 85–90% of the total content in the nervous tissue) are concentrated in astrocytes, 10–15% of proteins are located in neurons, and the minimum number of proteins is found in oligodendrocytes. S100 proteins are considered to be one of the key molecular components of complex intracellular systems providing functional homeostasis of the brain cells. They are synthesized by glial cells and then transported to neurons thus affecting metabolic processes and specific reception of neurotransmitters, changing the level of the specific binding of dopamine, serotonin, GABA, and norepinephrine with receptors. Experiments have confirmed the involvement of S100 group proteins in the regulation of neuron process-oriented growth.

S100β is predominately detected in astrocytes and Schwann cells. It can regulate intracellular enzyme activity, interact with cytoskeletal elements, and is involved in calcium homeostasis [79]. However, extracellular S100β in micromolar quantity may have deleterious effects such as inducing apoptosis in neurons [80]. Elevated levels of protein S100 in serum may be due to both its upregulated secretion following cell stress or activation and its release from injured cells [81].

Many studies have identified an association between the level of S100β and SAE [23, 73, 76, 79, 82, 83]. For example, we can cite the results of a relatively small clinical study involving 40 children with sepsis, of which 40% had moderate to severe septic encephalopathy, and a group of 25 healthy children as a control. It was found that children with septic encephalopathy had elevated serum and CSF levels of S100β compared to ones who had sepsis only [84]. In an observational study including 22 septic shock patients delirium was associated with elevated levels of serum protein S100β when using a laboratory cut-off value of 0.15 μg/L [83]. Similar results about the association of S100β with delirium were previously obtained also in a small cohort of septic shock patients [76]. In another large cohort of critically ill patients S100β was associated with cognitive impairment and disability [73]. Pfister D et al. (2008) analyzed data from 16 patients with sepsis, severe sepsis, or septic shock of whom 12 had SAD. They reported a significant association between elevated levels of S100β and delirium associated with sepsis ($p = 0{,}029$) [23]. Interesting data were obtained in a pilot single-center prospective cohort study in which 187 adult intensive care unit patients with diagnosed sepsis were observed: S100β protein levels were closely correlated with the duration of delirium ($R=0.8$; $p < 0.05$) in patients with sepsis [39].

It is possible to cite a fairly large list of studies that have confirmed the feasibility of measuring the level of S100β as a method of monitoring brain damage in sepsis [82, 85] or shown that higher S100β levels were associated with increased mortality among delirious patients [50, 79, 82, 86, 87]. Interestingly, some studies revealed the association of changes in EEG data with an increase in the concentration of S100β in blood serum [50, 88]. Some works indicate a relationship between an increased level of S100β and low scores on the scale GCS [82, 85, 86, 88]. A good example of using this biomarker to monitor patients is the clinical trial of Spapen et al. (2010): high concentrations of S100β were found in patients with GCS scores <13, which is consistent with the results reported in other studies that evaluated S100β as is a diagnostic criterion for SE [89]. However, some studies found no correlation between the increased S100β serum concentrations and SE [34, 90, 91].

In a large prospective study by Yao Bo et al. (2014), the clinical significance of serum S100β and NSE in the diagnosis of SAE and the prognosis of its course was evaluated in a cohort of 112 patients with severe sepsis and septic shock. Levels of S100β but not NSE were associated with increased mortality. Among patients who developed encephalopathy after withdrawal from sedation, elevated S100β levels were associated with encephalopathy, while no relationship was recorded with NSE levels [79]. In the study of Nguyen et al. (2006) in 170 patients with severe sepsis and septic shock, serum S100β and NSE were measured daily for four consecutive days after ICU admission. High biomarker levels were associated with the maximum SOFA scores ($p = 0.001$), and the highest values were found in patients who died early, within 4 days of inclusion ($p = 0.005$). Low consciousness encephalopathy type B (acute encephalopathy which is characterized by somnolence, stupor, and coma) was more frequently observed in patients with elevated S100β ($p = 0.004$) [76]. In a retrospective analysis of 124 patients with sepsis was revealed that an NSE concentration >12.5 μg/L is independently associated with a 23.3% (95% CI 6.7-39.9, $p = 0.006$) increased risk of 30-day mortality and a 29.3% (95% CI 8.8-49.8, $p = 0.005$) increased risk of delirium. The results show that NSE may have utility as a marker of neuronal injury in sepsis [33]. The study of Feng et al. (2017) (clinical data of 59 patients admitted to ICU with sepsis, SAE group, n=36 and non-SAE group, n=23) showed the increased levels of NSE, S100β, and IL-6 in the two groups on the first day of ICU admitting and decreased ones on the third day. Herewith the level of NSE and IL-6 on the first day and the third day of the SAE group was significantly higher than those of the non-SAE group. NSE combined with IL-6 on the third day in ICU demonstrated high diagnostic significance for SAE [34].

Other proteins of the S100 family (S100A8 and S100A9) are also proposed as biomarkers of SAE [26, 92].

Thus, despite the huge number of studies on these biomarkers, their results are not always unambiguous, but sometimes contradictory. Nevertheless, the established relationship between elevated levels of these biomarkers and increased mortality indicates the need for monitoring these patients, starting from the moment their admission to the ICU. It would be useful to establish a prognosis and stratify patients according to their disease severity.

Tau protein is also one of the potential biomarkers of brain injury. Tau protein (tubulin binding protein) is one of the microtubule-associated proteins (MAPs), which is located mainly in the axons of mature neurons. MAPs play an important role in cell differentiation and polarization promoting assembly and stability of microtubules. However, excessive accumulation of Tau protein in neurons has a toxic effect on the brain and is associated with the development of some neurodegenerative diseases [93]. For example, Tau protein makes up the neurofibrillary tangles, which are one of the two pathological signs of Alzheimer's disease [94]. Hyperphosphorylation of Tau depresses its biological activity and induces its accumulation in brain tissue [95, 96]. Tau levels were correlated with the occurrence of brain atrophy on MRI. Activated microglia and TNF-α have been shown to cause Tau protein accumulation in neurons [94]. There was identified a close association between the serum Tau protein levels with the appearance of SAE in patients with severe sepsis [28, 35]. The serum Tau protein levels and the SOFA score were independent factors that were associated with SAE. At the same time, the combined use of the serum Tau protein levels with the SOFA score improved the accuracy in distinguishing SAE from non-SAE patients. A cutoff value serum tau protein level of 75.92 pg/mL had 81.1% sensitivity and 86.1% specificity in predicting the 28-day mortality in patients with severe sepsis [35]. In a retrospective case series study that included 41 burn sepsis patients (SAE group – 21 cases and non-SAE group – 20 cases) the serum levels of Tau protein were higher in SAE patients than in the non-SAE group ($p < 0.01$). Multi-factor logistic regression analysis showed a sensitivity of 97% and a specificity of 99% for Tau protein [28]. Thus, serum Tau protein levels have higher clinical diagnostic value for sepsis patients complicated with SAE.

The impaired metabolism of ***beta-amyloid (Aß)*** can serve as a marker of neurodegeneration – this assumption can also be found in several publications. Aß is the main component of amyloid plaques found in the brains of people with Alzheimer's disease. In clinical and experimental studies, a link between beta-amyloid and delirium in sepsis has been identified [24]. In the brains of rats undergoing severe sepsis, an increased Aß content was found in brain tissue, namely in the hippocampus and in the prefrontal cortex, which was associated with long-term cognitive impairment [53].

The neurofilament protein (Nf protein), a specific biomarker for neuroaxonal injury, is consistently correlated with brain injury, disease severity, and survival in a range of neurological diseases [37]. Nf proteins are an important part of the axonal cytoskeleton and represent an architectonic stable tube system [97]. As a consequence of axonal injury Nf proteins are released into the extracellular fluid and can be measured by ELISA technique. Ehler et al. (2017) demonstrated that two different types of lesions are important in SAE – scattered ischemic lesions and diffuse neuroaxonal damage, and they showed in an experiment that the time from the onset of sepsis correlated with the levels of Nf protein in tissue ($R = 0.53$, $p = 0.045$) [98].

Neurofilament light chain (***NfL***) levels also are elevated in several neurological disorders [99]. A prospective pilot observational study including 20 patients with septic shock and five patients without sepsis serving as controls showed that plasma NfL (neurofilament light chains) levels increased in sepsis patients over time ($p = 0.0063$) and remained stable in patients without sepsis. Wherein plasma NfL values were significantly higher in patients with SAE ($p = 0.011$), correlated with the severity of SAE represented by ICDSC values ($R = 0.534$, $p = 0.022$), and associated with a poorer functional outcome after 100 days ($R = -0.535$, $p = 0.0003$). In another prospective observational study, which included 11 SAE patients and controls higher CSF NfL levels were revealed in SAE patients ($p = 0.0006$, in comparison with controls) [38]. Thus, Nf protein and NfL can be used as diagnostic and prognostic biomarkers of SAE, and their elevated levels indicate a higher probability of death and a worse functional/cognitive outcome in survivors.

There are some other proteins required for the maintenance of axonal integrity, for example, ***ubiquitin carboxyl-terminal hydrolase L1 (UCH-L1)***, which may be helpful for diagnosis of SAE, prediction of the outcome and evaluating the long-term quality of life of patients with sepsis [36]. In addition, it has been demonstrated in a prospective single-center study involving 105 patients suffering from sepsis that UCH-L1 is a reliable marker of brain injury: the serum concentrations of UCH-L1 were higher in the SAE group than in the no-SAE group ($p < 0.001$). UCH-L1 produced an AUC 0.812 for diagnosis of SAE with optimal cut-off values of 7.72 ng/ml [36].

Dysfunction of the neuroendocrine network

Stress hormones, such as cortisol, catecholamines, prolactin, and growth hormone, are known to down-regulate inflammation, but, according to many authors, their excessive release can have a detrimental effect on cognitive functions [100, 101].

One of the main components of the neuroendocrine network is the hypothalamic-pituitary-adrenal axis [11]. Sepsis is known to induce an abnormal pituitary response, resulting in profound hormonal changes in adrenocorticotropic hormone (ACTH), growth hormone, vasopressin, cortisol, mineralocorticoids, and thyroid hormones [47, 102, 103]. This system regulates the release of corticotropin-releasing hormone in the hypothalamus, ACTH in the adenohypophysis, and eventually the release of glucocorticoids into the systemic circulation by the adrenal glands. The level of cortisol in the blood is a key indicator of the activity of the hypothalamic-pituitary-adrenal system [11].

The combination of high levels of glucocorticoids in the conditions of manifestation of inflammation can be particularly harmful. It was shown that inflammation directly affects the integrity of the hippocampus and prefrontal cortex, and high levels of glucocorticoids may exacerbate these effects and can also aggravate the damage, at least partially, increasing neuroinflammation. Glucocorticoids have been found to inhibit anti-inflammatory signaling molecules in the hippocampus, thereby enhancing the inflammatory response to excitotoxic damage and exacerbating the death of hippocampal neurons [100]. Thus, sustained high levels of glucocorticoids during and after illness could contribute to structural hippocampal and prefrontal core damage, leading to cognitive impairment [101].

According to clinical studies, ***ACTH*** and ***cortisol*** are considered potential biomarkers of SAE. For example, in a retrospective case series study of 41 burn patients with sepsis, the serum levels of ACTH and cortisol in the SAE group were significantly higher than those in the non-SAE group. In this study, ACTH and cortisol were measured in dynamics 12, 24, and 48 hours after diagnosis, and turned out to be independent risk factors for the development of SAE as a complication of sepsis in patients with burns [28].

Nguyen et al. (2016) investigated whether high ***prolactin*** levels were associated with delirium in septic patients. It is known that similar to cortisol, prolactin is a stress hormone that can affect behavioral or cognitive function and is involved in the regulation of the immune system, beyond its sexual reproductive and lactogenesis properties. Hyperprolactinemia has often been reported in neuropsychiatric disorders, including schizophrenia, bipolar disorder, and altered mood. High prolactin levels also may be a risk factor for delirium in septic patients. So, in a clinical study, prolactin levels were measured daily for 4 days in 101 patients with sepsis, and it was found that prolactin levels were higher in patients with delirium than in patients without it ($p = 0.032$). There was a significant correlation between prolactin levels and the duration of delirium ($r = 0.49$, $p = 0.004$), serum creatinine levels ($r = 0.4$, $p = 0.001$), and the renal SOFA score ($r = 0.4$, $p = 0.001$) but not with age, APACHE III, or total SOFA scores. A prolactin cut-off value of 450 pmol/L predicted the development of delirium with a sensitivity of 65% and a specificity of 63% [9]. Thus, elevated prolactin release may be involved in the development of delirium in septic patients.

Conclusion

Early diagnosis of SAE can help identify those patients with more severe diseases who require enhanced follow-up and immediate intervention. However, to date, there are no clear laboratory criteria for SAE, therefore, clinical criteria should be used for the diagnosis of SE, in combination with electrophysiological and biochemical tests. At the same time, some SE biomarkers can be useful and irreplaceable for objective monitoring of the degree of brain changes. It should be noted that a single biomarker may not be sufficient to diagnose SAE, and a combination of biomarkers can improve the effectiveness of diagnostic methods. Due to the complex etiopathogenesis of SAE, it turns out that each marker is influenced by numerous factors; at the same time, the assessment of several biomarkers corresponding to a particular stage of the pathophysiological process can be useful both for diagnosis and for assessing the severity of SAE.

The exact role of biomarkers in the management of patients with sepsis has not been definitively determined; however, their use for the diagnosis of brain dysfunction and prediction of mortality in sepsis seems very promising.

References

1. Chung HY, Wickel J, Brunkhorst FM, Geis C. Sepsis-Associated Encephalopathy: From Delirium to Dementia? *J Clin Med.* 2020 Mar 5;9(3):703. DOI: 10.3390/jcm9030703
2. Jacob A, Brorson JR, Alexander JJ. Septic Encephalopathy: Inflammation in Man and Mouse. *Neurochem Int.* 2011 Mar;58(4):472–6. DOI: 10.1016/j.neuint.2011.01.004
3. Piva S, McCreadie V, Latronico N. Neuroinflammation in Sepsis: Sepsis Associated Delirium. *Cardiovasc Hematol Disord Drug Targets.* 2015 Jan 24;15(1):10–8. DOI: 10.2174/1871529X15666150108112452
4. Wilson JX, Young GB. Progress in Clinical Neurosciences: Sepsis-Associated Encephalopathy: Evolving Concepts. *Can J Neurol Sci.* 2003 May 16;30(2):98–105. DOI: 10.1017/S031716710005335X
5. Osca-Verdegal R, Beltrán-García J, Pallardó FV, García-Giménez JL. Role of microRNAs As Biomarkers in Sepsis-Associated Encephalopathy. *Mol Neurobiol.* 2021 Sep 23;58(9):4682–93. DOI: 10.1007/s12035-021-02445-3
6. Tang C, Zhou W, Chen X, Wang F, Men W, Liu J, et al. Research Progress of Biomarkers of Sepsis-Associated Encephalopathy. *Intensive Care Res.* 2023 Jan 11;3(1):69–76. DOI: 10.1007/s44231-022-00023-2
7. Hotchkiss RS, Karl IE. The Pathophysiology and Treatment of Sepsis. *N Engl J Med.* 2003 Jan 9;348(2):138–50. DOI: 10.1056/NEJMra021333
8. Su CM, Cheng HH, Tsai TC, Hsiao SY, Tsai NW, Chang WN, et al. Elevated Serum Vascular Cell Adhesion Molecule-1 Is Associated with Septic Encephalopathy in Adult Community-Onset Severe Sepsis Patients. *Biomed Res Int.* 2014;2014:1–10. DOI: 10.1155/2014/598762
9. Nguyen DN, Huyghens L, Schiettecatte J, Smitz J, Vincent JL. High Prolactin Levels are Associated with More Delirium in Septic Patients. *J Crit Care.* 2016 Jun;33:56–61. DOI: 10.1016/j.jcrc.2015.12.021
10. Molnar L, Fülesdi B, Németh N, Molnár C. Sepsis Associated Encephalopathy: A Review of the Literature. *Neurol India.* 2018;66(2):352. DOI: 10.4103/0028-3886.227299
11. Tauber SC, Djukic M, Gossner J, Eiffert H, Brück W, Nau R. Sepsis-Associated Encephalopathy and Septic Encephalitis: An Update. *Expert Rev Anti Infect Ther.* 2021 Feb 1;19(2):215–31. DOI: 10.1080/14787210.2020.1812384
12. Pinheiro da Silva F, Machado MCC, Velasco IT. Neuropeptides in Sepsis: From Brain Pathology to Systemic Inflammation. *Peptides (NY).* 2013 Jun;44:135–8. DOI: 10.1016/j.peptides.2013.03.029
13. Kaur J, Singhi P, Singhi S, Malhi P, Saini AG. Neurodevelopmental and Behavioral Outcomes in Children with Sepsis-Associated Encephalopathy Admitted to Pediatric Intensive Care Unit. *J Child Neurol.* 2016 May 23;31(6):683–90. DOI: 10.1177/0883073815610431
14. Gofton TE, Young GB. Sepsis-Associated Encephalopathy. *Nat Rev Neurol.* 2012 Oct 18;8(10):557–66. DOI: 10.1038/nrneurol.2012.183
15. Baby S, Reljic T, Villalba N, Kumar A, Yuan SY. Endothelial Glycocalyx-Associated Molecules as Potential Serological Markers for Sepsis-Associated Encephalopathy: A Systematic Review and Meta-Analysis. *PLoS One.* 2023 Feb 21;18(2):e0281941. DOI: 10.1371/journal.pone.0281941
16. Chaudhry N, Duggal AK. Sepsis Associated Encephalopathy. *Adv Med.* 2014;2014:1–16. DOI: 10.1155/2014/762320

17. Yuechen Z, Shaosong X, Zhouxing Z, Fuli G, Wei H. A Summary of the Current Diagnostic Methods for, and Exploration of the Value of microRNAs as Biomarkers in, Sepsis-Associated Encephalopathy. *Front Neurosci.* 2023 Mar 16;17. DOI: 10.3389/fnins.2023.1125888
18. Hosokawa K, Gaspard N, Su F, Oddo M, Vincent JL, Taccone FS. Clinical Neurophysiological Assessment of Sepsis-Associated Brain Dysfunction: A Systematic Review. *Crit Care.* 2014 Dec 8;18(6):674. DOI: 10.1186/s13054-014-0674-y
19. Zhu J, Zhang M, Han T, Wu H, Xiao Z, Lin S, et al. Exploring the Biomarkers of Sepsis-Associated Encephalopathy (SAE): Metabolomics Evidence from Gas Chromatography-Mass Spectrometry. *Biomed Res Int.* 2019 Nov 12;2019:1–10. DOI: 10.1155/2019/2612849
20. Ehler J, Petzold A, Sharshar T, Ely EW, Saller T. Biomarker Panel to Differentiate Brain Injury from Brain Dysfunction in Patients with Sepsis-Associated Encephalopathy. *Crit Care Med.* 2020 May;48(5):e436–7. DOI: 10.1097/CCM.0000000000004266
21. Heming N, Mazeraud A, Verdonk F, Bozza FA, Chrétien F, Sharshar T. Neuroanatomy of Sepsis-Associated Encephalopathy. *Crit Care.* 2017 Dec 21;21(1):65. DOI: 10.1186/s13054-017-1643-z
22. Atterton B, Paulino MC, Povoa P, Martin-Loeches I. Sepsis Associated Delirium. *Medicina (B Aires).* 2020 May 18;56(5):240. DOI: 10.3390/medicina56050240
23. Pfister D, Siegemund M, Dell-Kuster S, Smielewski P, Rüegg S, Strebel SP, et al. Cerebral Perfusion in Sepsis-Associated Delirium. *Crit Care.* 2008;12(3):R63. DOI: 10.1186/cc6891
24. van den Boogaard M, Kox M, Quinn KL, van Achterberg T, van der Hoeven JG, Schoonhoven L, et al. Biomarkers Associated with Delirium in Critically Ill Patients and their Relation with Long-Term Subjective Cognitive Dysfunction; Indications for Different Pathways Governing Delirium in Inflamed and Noninflamed Patients. *Crit Care.* 2011;15(6):R297. DOI: 10.1186/cc10598
25. Ehler J, Saller T, Wittstock M, Rommer PS, Chappell D, Zwissler B, et al. Diagnostic Value of NT-proCNP Compared to NSE and S100B in Cerebrospinal Fluid and Plasma of Patients with Sepsis-Associated Encephalopathy. *Neurosci Lett.* 2019 Jan;692:167–73. DOI: 10.1016/j.neulet.2018.11.014
26. Zhang LN, Wang XH, Wu L, Huang L, Zhao CG, Peng QY, et al. Diagnostic and Predictive Levels of Calcium-Binding Protein A8 and Tumor Necrosis Factor Receptor-Associated Factor 6 in Sepsis-Associated Encephalopathy. *Chin Med J (Engl).* 2016 Jul 20;129(14):1674–81. DOI: 10.4103/0366-6999.185860
27. Nakamura T, Kawagoe Y, Matsuda T, Ebihara I, Koide H. Effects of Polymyxin B-Immobilized Fiber Hemoperfusion on Amino Acid Imbalance in Septic Encephalopathy. *Blood Purif.* 2003;21(4–5):282–6. DOI: 10.1159/000072546
28. Li XL et al. Value of Cerebral Hypoxic-Ischemic Injury Markers in the Early Diagnosis of Sepsis-Associated Encephalopathy in Burn Patients with Sepsis. *Zhonghua Shao Shang Za Zhi.* 2022;38(1):21–8.
29. Lu CX, Qiu T, Tong HS, Liu ZF, Su L, Cheng B. Peripheral T-Lymphocyte, and Natural Killer Cell Population Imbalance is Associated with Septic Encephalopathy in Patients with Severe Sepsis. *Exp Ther Med.* 2016 Mar;11(3):1077–84. DOI: 10.3892/etm.2016.3000
30. Li D, Zhang J, Bai G, Chen J, Cheng W, Cui N. Lymphocyte and NK Cell Counts Can Predict Sepsis-Associated Delirium in Elderly Patients. *Front Aging Neurosci.* 2021 Jan 11;12. DOI: 10.3389/fnagi.2020.621298
31. Tomasi CD, Vuolo F, Generoso J, Soares M, Barichello T, Quevedo J, et al. Biomarkers of Delirium in a Low-Risk Community-Acquired Pneumonia-Induced Sepsis. *Mol Neurobiol.* 2017 Jan 14;54(1):722–6. DOI: 10.1007/s12035-016-9708-6
32. Visitchanakun P, Tangtanatakul P, Trithiphen O, Soonthornchai W, Wongphoom J, Tachaboon S, et al. Plasma miR-370-3P as a Biomarker of Sepsis-Associated Encephalopathy, the Transcriptomic Profiling Analysis of Microrna-Arrays From Mouse Brains. *Shock.* 2020 Sep;54(3):347–57. DOI: 10.1097/SHK.0000000000001473
33. Anderson BJ, Reilly JP, Shashaty MGS, Palakshappa JA, Wysoczanski A, Dunn TG, et al. Admission Plasma Levels of the Neuronal Injury Marker Neuron-Specific Enolase are Associated with Mortality and Delirium in Sepsis. *J Crit Care.* 2016 Dec;36:18–23. DOI: 10.1016/j.jcrc.2016.06.012
34. Feng Q et al. The Diagnostic Value of Neuron-Specific Enolase, Central Nervous System-Specific Protein, and Interleukin-6 in Sepsis-Associated Encephalopathy. *Zhonghua nei ke za zhi.* 2017;56(10):747–51. DOI: 10.3760/cma.j.issn.0578-1426.2017.10.008

35. Zhao T, Xia Y, Wang D, Pang L. Association between Elevated Serum Tau Protein Level and Sepsis-Associated Encephalopathy in Patients with Severe Sepsis. *Can. J. Infect. Dis. Med. Microbiol.* 2019 Jul 17;2019:1–6. DOI: 10.1155/2019/1876174
36. Wu L, Ai ML, Feng Q, Deng S, Liu ZY, Zhang LN, et al. Serum Glial Fibrillary Acidic Protein and Ubiquitin C-Terminal Hydrolase-L1 for Diagnosis of Sepsis-Associated Encephalopathy and Outcome Prognostication. *J Crit Care.* 2019 Aug;52:172–9. DOI: 10.1016/j.jcrc.2019.04.018
37. Ehler J, Petzold A, Wittstock M, Kolbaske S, Gloger M, Henschel J, et al. The Prognostic Value of Neurofilament Levels in Patients with Sepsis-Associated Encephalopathy – A Prospective, Pilot Observational Study. *PLoS One.* 2019 Jan 24;14(1):e0211184.
38. Orhun G, Esen F, Yilmaz V, Ulusoy C, Şanlı E, Yıldırım E, et al. Elevated sTREM2 and NFL Levels in Patients with Sepsis-Associated Encephalopathy. *Int. J. Neurosci.* 2023 Mar 4;133(3):327–33. DOI: 10.1080/00207454.2021.1916489
39. Rezepov NA, Skripkin Yu V., Ulitkina ON, Grebenchikov OA, Likhvantsev VV. Predictors of the Severity and Duration of Treatment of Sepsis-Associated Delirium. *Gen. Reanimatol.* 2017 Jan 1;13(6):28–37. DOI: 10.15360/1813-9779-2017-6-28-37
40. Banks WA, Robinson SM. Minimal Penetration of Lipopolysaccharide Across the Murine Blood-Brain Barrier. *Brain Behav Immun.* 2010 Jan;24(1):102–9. DOI: 10.1016/j.bbi.2009.09.001
41. Perry VH, Newman TA, Cunningham C. The Impact of Systemic Infection on the Progression of Neurodegenerative Disease. *Nat Rev Neurosci.* 2003 Feb;4(2):103–12. DOI: 10.1038/nrn1032
42. Hoogland ICM, Houbolt C, van Westerloo DJ, van Gool WA, van de Beek D. Systemic Inflammation and Microglial Activation: A Systematic Review of Animal Experiments. *J Neuroinflammation.* 2015 Dec 6;12(1):114. DOI: 10.1186/s12974-015-0332-6
43. Gao R, Huo JM, Peng GD, Hua YR, Gang ZS, Jun YJ, et al. Neuroinflammation-Induced Downregulation of Hippocampacal Neuregulin 1-ErbB4 Signaling in the Parvalbumin Interneurons Might Contribute to Cognitive Impairment in a Mouse Model of Sepsis-Associated Encephalopathy. *Inflammation.* 2017 Apr 2;40(2):387–400. DOI: 10.1007/s10753-016-0484-2
44. Zrzavy T, Höftberger R, Berger T, Rauschka H, Butovsky O, Weiner H, et al. Pro-Inflammatory Activation of Microglia in the Brain of Patients with Sepsis. *Neuropathol Appl Neurobiol.* 2019 Apr 19;45(3):278–90. DOI: 10.1111/nan.12502
45. Mazeraud A, Righy C, Bouchereau E, Benghanem S, Bozza FA, Sharshar T. Septic-Associated Encephalopathy: A Comprehensive Review. *Neurotherapeutics.* 2020 Apr 6;17(2):392–403. DOI: 10.1007/s13311-020-00862-1
46. Michels M, Danielski L, Dal-Pizzol F, Petronilho F. Neuroinflammation: Microglial Activation During Sepsis. *Curr Neurovasc Res.* 2014 Aug 25;11(3):262–70. DOI: 10.2174/1567202611666140520122744
47. Ferlini L, Gaspard N. What's New on Septic Encephalopathy? Ten Things You Need to Know. *Minerva Anestesiol.* 2023 Mar;89(3). DOI: 10.23736/S0375-9393.22.16689-7
48. Sekino N, Selim M, Shehadah A. Sepsis-Associated Brain Injury: Underlying Mechanisms and Potential Therapeutic Strategies for Acute and Long-Term Cognitive Impairments. *J Neuroinflammation.* 2022 Dec 29;19(1):101. DOI: 10.1186/s12974-022-02464-4
49. McGrane S, Girard TD, Thompson JL, Shintani AK, Woodworth A, Ely EW, et al. Procalcitonin and C-Reactive Protein Levels at Admission as Predictors of Duration of Acute Brain Dysfunction in Critically Ill Patients. *Crit Care.* 2011;15(2):R78. DOI: 10.1186/cc10070
50. Khan BA, Perkins AJ, Prasad NK, Shekhar A, Campbell NL, Gao S, et al. Biomarkers of Delirium Duration and Delirium Severity in the ICU*. *Crit Care Med.* 2020 Mar;48(3):353–61. DOI: 10.1097/CCM.0000000000004139
51. Ogino Y, Kaneda K, Nakahara T, Todani M, Miyauchi T, Fujita M, Kawamura Y, Oda Y, Tsuruta R. Systemic Inflammation and Delirium in the Peri-Extubation Period of Mechanical Ventilation: An Observational Prospective Study of Intensive Care Unit Patients. *Bull Yamaguchi Med School.* 2015;62:1–10.
52. Girard TD, Ware LB, Bernard GR, Pandharipande PP, Thompson JL, Shintani AK, et al. Associations of Markers of Inflammation and Coagulation with Delirium During Critical Illness. *Intensive Care Med.* 2012 Dec 18;38(12):1965–73. DOI: 10.1007/s00134-012-2678-x
53. Schwalm MT, Pasquali M, Miguel SP, dos Santos JPA, Vuolo F, Comim CM, et al. Acute Brain Inflammation and Oxidative Damage are Related to Long-Term Cognitive Deficits and Markers of

Neurodegeneration in Sepsis-Survivor Rats. *Mol Neurobiol.* 2014 Feb 30;49(1):380–5. DOI: 10.1007/s12035-013-8526-3

54. Tomasiuk R, Mikaszewska-Sokolewicz M, Szlufik S, Rzepecki P, Lazowski T. The Prognostic Value of Concomitant Assessment of NT-proCNP, C-reactive Protein, Procalcitonin, and Inflammatory Cytokines in Septic Patients. *Crit Care.* 2014;18(3):440. DOI: 10.1186/cc13944
55. Vanderheyden M, Bartunek J, Goethals M. Brain and Other Natriuretic Peptides: Molecular Aspects. *Eur J Heart Fail.* 2004 Mar;6(3):261–8. DOI: 10.1016/j.ejheart.2004.01.004
56. Koch A, Voigt S, Sanson E, Dückers H, Horn A, Zimmermann HW, et al. Prognostic Value of Circulating Amino-Terminal Pro-C-type Natriuretic Peptide in Critically Ill Patients. *Crit Care.* 2011;15(1):R45. DOI: 10.1186/cc10007
57. Saller T, Peterss S, Scheiermann P, Eser-Valeri D, Ehler J, Bruegger D, et al. Natriuretic Peptides as a Prognostic Marker for Delirium in Cardiac Surgery—A Pilot Study. *Medicina (B Aires).* 2020 May 27;56(6):258. DOI: 10.3390/medicina56060258
58. Osterbur K, Yu DH, DeClue AE. Interleukin-1β, Tumor Necrosis Factor-α, and Lipopolysaccharide Induce C-type Natriuretic Peptide from Canine Aortic Endothelial Cells. *Res Vet Sci.* 2013 Jun;94(3):478–83. DOI: 10.1016/j.rvsc.2012.10.002
59. Prickett TCR, Doughty RN, Troughton RW, Frampton CM, Whalley GA, Ellis CJ, et al. C-type Natriuretic Peptides in Coronary Disease. *Clin Chem.* 2017 Jan 1;63(1):316–24. DOI: 10.1373/clinchem.2016.257816
60. Bíró É, Tóth G, Telegdy G. Effect of Receptor Blockers on Brain Natriuretic Peptide and C-type Natriuretic Peptide Caused Anxiolytic State in Rats. *Neuropeptides.* 1996 Feb;30(1):59–65. DOI: 10.1016/S0143-4179(96)90056-6
61. Burk AM, Martin M, Flierl MA, Rittirsch D, Helm M, Lampl L, et al. Early Complementopathy After Multiple Injuries in Humans. *Shock.* 2012 Apr;37(4):348–54. DOI: 10.1097/SHK.0b013e3182471795
62. Ward PA. Role of the Complement in Experimental Sepsis. *J Leukoc Biol.* 2008 Mar 1;83(3):467–70. DOI: 10.1189/jlb.0607376.
63. Akrout N, Sharshar T, Annane D. Mechanisms of Brain Signaling During Sepsis. *Curr Neuropharmacol.* 2009 Dec 1;7(4):296–301. DOI: 10.2174/157015909790031175
64. Xu R, Lin F, Bao C, Wang FS. Mechanism of C5a-Induced Immunologic Derangement in Sepsis. *Cell Mol Immunol.* 2017 Sep 7;14(9):792–3. DOI: 10.1038/cmi.2017.68
65. Orhun G, Tuzun E, Ergin Ozcan P, Ulusoy C, Yildirim E, Kucukerden M, et al. Association Between Inflammatory Markers and Cognitive Outcome in Patients with Acute Brain Dysfunction Due to Sepsis. *Arch Neuropsychiatry.* 2018. DOI: 10.1080/00207454.2021.1916489
66. Wang N, Zhong D, Lin J, Ye M, Chen Y, Wang L, et al. MiR-370-3p Aggravates Blood-Brain Barrier Injury and Neuron Apoptosis by Targeting SMURF1 to Activate the TLR4/MyD88/NF-κB Signaling in Sepsis-Associated Encephalopathy. *Mol Cell Toxicol.* 2022 Jul 22. DOI: 10.1017/S031716710005335X
67. Peng LS, Xu Y, Wang QS. YY1 Promotes Microglia M2 Polarization Through the Mir-130A-3P/TREM-2 Axis to Alleviate Sepsis-Associated Encephalopathy. *Shock.* 2022 Aug;58(2):128–36. DOI: 10.1097/SHK.0000000000001914
68. Luo XY, Ying JH, Wang QS. miR-25-3p Ameliorates SAE by Targeting the TLR4/NLRP3 Axis. *Metab Brain Dis.* 2022 Aug 15;37(6):1803–13. DOI: 10.1007/s11011-022-01017-1
69. Guedes J, Cardoso ALC, Pedroso de Lima MC. Involvement of MicroRNA in Microglia-Mediated Immune Response. *Clin Dev Immunol.* 2013;2013:1–11. DOI: 10.1155/2013/186872
70. Vincent JL, Ince C, Pickkers P. Endothelial Dysfunction: A Therapeutic Target in Bacterial Sepsis? *Expert Opin Ther Targets.* 2021 Sep 2;25(9):733–48. DOI: 10.1080/14728222.2021.1988928
71. Hofer S, Bopp C, Hoerner C, Plaschke K, Faden RM, Martin E, et al. Injury of the Blood Brain Barrier and Up-Regulation of ICAM-1 in Polymicrobial Sepsis. *J. Surg. Res.* 2008 May;146(2):276–81. DOI: 10.1016/j.jss.2007.07.021
72. Beltrán-García J, Osca-Verdegal R, Jávega B, Herrera G, O'Connor JE, García-López E, et al. Characterization of Early Peripheral Immune Responses in Patients with Sepsis and Septic Shock. *Biomedicines.* 2022 Feb 23;10(3):525. DOI: 10.3390/biomedicines10030525

73. Hughes CG, Pandharipande PP, Thompson JL, Chandrasekhar R, Ware LB, Ely EW, et al. Endothelial Activation and Blood-Brain Barrier Injury as Risk Factors for Delirium in Critically Ill Patients*. *Crit Care Med.* 2016 Sep;44(9):e809–17. DOI: 10.1097/CCM.0000000000001739
74. Zenaide PV, Gusmao-Flores D. Biomarcadores na encefalopatia séptica: revisão sistemática dos estudos clínicos. *Rev Bras Ter Intensiva.* 2013 Mar;25(1):56–62. DOI: 10.1590/S0103-507X2013000100011
75. Gashilova FF, Zhukova NG. Neuron-Specific Enolase in the Blood Serum as a Diagnostic Marker of Parkinsonism. *Bull Sib Med.* 2005 Sep 30;4(3):28–33. DOI: 10.20538/1682-0363-2005-3-28-33
76. Nguyen DN, Spapen H, Su F, Schiettecatte J, Shi L, Hachimi-Idrissi S, et al. Elevated Serum Levels of S-100β Protein and Neuron-Specific Enolase are Associated with Brain Injury in Patients with Severe Sepsis and Septic Shock*. *Crit Care Med.* 2006 Jul;34(7):1967–74. DOI: 10.1016/j.jcrc.2015.12.021
77. Hsu AA, Fenton K, Weinstein S, Carpenter J, Dalton H, Bell MJ. Neurological Injury Markers in Children with Septic Shock*. *Pediatr Crit Care Med.* 2008 May;9(3):245–51. DOI: 10.1097/PCC.0b013e3181727b22
78. Piazza O, Russo E, Cotena S, Esposito G, Tufano R. Elevated S100B Levels Do Not Correlate with the Severity of Encephalopathy During Sepsis. *Br J Anaesth.* 2007 Oct;99(4):518–21. DOI: 10.1093/bja/aem201
79. Yao B, Zhang LN, Ai YH, Liu ZY, Huang L. Serum S100β Is a Better Biomarker than Neuron-Specific Enolase for Sepsis-Associated Encephalopathy and Determining Its Prognosis: A Prospective and Observational Study. *Neurochem Res.* 2014 Jul 24;39(7):1263–9. DOI: 10.1007/s11064-014-1308-0
80. Sorci G, Riuzzi F, Agneletti AL, Marchetti C, Donato R. S100B Causes Apoptosis in a Myoblast Cell Line in a RAGE-Independent Manner. *J Cell Physiol.* 2004 May;199(2):274–83. DOI: 10.1002/jcp.10462
81. Donato R, Cannon BR, Sorci G, Riuzzi F, Hsu K, Weber DJ, et al. Functions of S100 Proteins. *Curr Mol Med.* 2013 Jan;13(1):24–57. PMID: 22834835
82. Semmler A, Frisch C, Debeir T, Ramanathan M, Okulla T, Klockgether T, et al. Long-Term Cognitive Impairment, Neuronal Loss and Reduced Cortical Cholinergic Innervation after Recovery from Sepsis in a Rodent Model. *Exp Neurol.* 2007 Apr;204(2):733–40. DOI: 10.1016/j.expneurol.2007.01.003
83. Erikson K, Ala-Kokko TI, Koskenkari J, Liisanantti JH, Kamakura R, Herzig KH, et al. Elevated Serum S-100β in Patients with Septic Shock Is Associated with Delirium. *Acta Anaesthesiol Scand.* 2019 Jan;63(1):69–73. DOI: 10.1111/aas.13228
84. Hamed SA, Hamed EA, Abdella MM. Septic Encephalopathy: Relationship to Serum and Cerebrospinal Fluid Levels of Adhesion Molecules, Lipid Peroxides, and S-100B Protein. *Neuropediatrics.* 2009 Apr 6;40(2):66–72. DOI: 10.1055/s-0029-1231054
85. Ely EW, Inouye SK, Bernard GR, Gordon S, Francis J, May L, et al. Delirium in Mechanically Ventilated Patients. *JAMA.* 2001 Dec 5;286(21):2703. DOI: 10.1001/jama.286.21.2703
86. Qin L, Wu X, Block ML, Liu Y, Breese GR, Hong JS, et al. Systemic LPS Causes Chronic Neuroinflammation and Progressive Neurodegeneration. *Glia.* 2007 Apr 1;55(5):453–62. DOI: 10.1002/glia.20467
87. Spronk PE, Riekerk B, Hofhuis J, Rommes JH. The Occurrence of Delirium Is Severely Underestimated in the ICU During Daily Care. *Intensive Care Med.* 2009 Jul 7;35(7):1276–80. DOI: 10.1007/s00134-009-1466-8
88. Henry CJ, Huang Y, Wynne A, Hanke M, Himler J, Bailey MT, et al. Minocycline Attenuates Lipopolysaccharide (LPS)-Induced Neuroinflammation, Sickness Behavior, and Anhedonia. *J Neuroinflammation.* 2008 Dec 13;5(1):15. DOI: 10.1186/1742-2094-5-15
89. Spapen H, Nguyen D, Troubleyn J, Huyghens L, Schiettecatte J. Drotrecogin alfa (Activated) May Attenuate Severe Sepsis-Associated Encephalopathy in Clinical Septic Shock. *Crit Care.* 2010;14(2):R54. DOI: 10.1186/cc8947
90. Piazza O, Cotena S, De Robertis E, Caranci F, Tufano R. Sepsis Associated Encephalopathy Studied by MRI and Cerebral Spinal Fluid S100B Measurement. *Neurochem Res.* 2009 Jul 9;34(7):1289–92. DOI: 10.1007/s11064-008-9907-2

91. van den Boogaard M, Ramakers BP, van Alfen N, van der Werf SP, Fick WF, Hoedemaekers CW, et al. Endotoxemia-Induced Inflammation and Its Effect on the Human Brain. *Crit Care.* 2010;14(3):R81. DOI: 10.1186/cc9001
92. Liao YL, Zhou XY, Ji MH, Qiu LC, Chen XH, Gong CS, et al. S100A9 Upregulation Contributes to Learning and Memory Impairments by Promoting Microglia M1 Polarization in Sepsis Survivor Mice. *Inflammation.* 2021 Feb 12;44(1):307–20. DOI: 10.1007/s10753-020-01334-6
93. Mandelkow EM, Mandelkow E. Biochemistry and Cell Biology of Tau Protein in Neurofibrillary Degeneration. *Cold Spring Harb Perspect Med.* 2012 Jul 1;2(7):a006247–a006247. DOI: 10.1101/cshperspect.a006247
94. Gorlovoy P, Larionov S, Pham TTH, Neumann H. Accumulation of Tau Induced in Neurites by Microglial Proinflammatory Mediators. *The FASEB J.* 2009 Aug 16;23(8):2502–13. DOI: 10.1096/fj.08-123877
95. Pîrşcoveanu DFV, Pirici I, Tudorică V, Bălşeanu TA, Albu VC, Bondari S, et al. Tau Protein in Neurodegenerative Diseases - A Review. *Rom J Morphol Embryol.* 2017;58(4):1141–50. PMID 29556602
96. Esen F, Orhun G, Özcan PE, Brenes Bastos AR, Tüzün E. Diagnosing Acute Brain Dysfunction Due to Sepsis. *Neurol Sci.* 2020 Jan 14;41(1):25–33. DOI: 10.1007/s10072-019-04069-x
97. Petzold A. Neurofilament Phosphoforms: Surrogate Markers for Axonal Injury, Degeneration, and Loss. *J Neurol Sci.* 2005 Jun;233(1–2):183–98. DOI: 10.1016/j.jns.2005.03.015
98. Ehler J, Barrett LK, Taylor V, Groves M, Scaravilli F, Wittstock M, et al. Translational Evidence for Two Distinct Patterns of Neuroaxonal Injury in Sepsis: A Longitudinal, Prospective Translational Study. *Crit Care.* 2017 Dec 23;21(1):262. DOI: 10.1186/s13054-017-1850-7
99. Alirezaei Z, Pourhanifeh MH, Borran S, Nejati M, Mirzaei H, Hamblin MR. Neurofilament Light Chain as a Biomarker, and Correlation with Magnetic Resonance Imaging in Diagnosis of CNS-Related Disorders. *Mol Neurobiol.* 2020 Jan 5;57(1):469–91. DOI: 10.1007/s12035-019-01698-3
100. Sorrells SF, Munhoz CD, Manley NC, Yen S, Sapolsky RM. Glucocorticoids Increase Excitotoxic Injury and Inflammation in the Hippocampus of Adult Male Rats. *Neuroendocrinology.* 2014;100(2–3):129–40. DOI: 10.1159/000367849
101. Hill AR, Spencer-Segal JL. Glucocorticoids and the Brain after Critical Illness. *Endocrinology.* 2021 Mar 1;162(3). DOI: 10.1210/endocr/bqaa242
102. Maxime V, Siami S, Annane D. Metabolism Modulators in Sepsis: The Abnormal Pituitary Response. *Crit Care Med.* 2007 Sep;35(Suppl): S596–601. DOI: 10.1097/01.CCM.0000279097.67263.52
103. Comim CM, Cassol-Jr OJ, Constantino LC, Petronilho F, Constantino LS, Stertz L, et al. Depressive-Like Parameters in Sepsis Survivor Rats. *Neurotox Res.* 2010 Apr 25;17(3):279–86. DOI: 10.1007/s12640-009-9101-6

Chapter 3

The role of microbiota and microbial metabolites in sepsis-associated encephalopathy

Andrey V. Grechko, Corr. Member of the RAS, MD., Ph.D., Irina V. Buyakova, MD., Ph.D., Natalia V. Beloborodova*, MD., Ph.D.

Federal Research and Clinical Center of Intensive Care Medicine and Rehabilitology, Moscow, Russia

Abstract

Brain dysfunction is a major complication of sepsis and is called sepsis-associated encephalopathy (SAE), including delirium, coma, seizure, and focal neurological signs. SAE is undoubtedly associated with bacteria; at the same time it is impossible to name specific etiologically significant bacteria. Sepsis-associated encephalopathy (SAE) is defined as a diffuse brain dysfunction secondary to infection elsewhere in the body without overt CNS infection [1]. From the definition of SAE itself, it follows that the brain is not one of the purulent-inflammatory foci of infection, that is, brain tissues remain sterile, but not intact. It seems obvious that the interaction between microbes and the brain is not carried out directly but at a more subtle molecular level. At the same time, it is still unknown how bacteria participate in SAE, whether their vital activity in the patient's body is related to the development of the neuroinflammatory process, activation of the endothelium, violation of the blood-brain barrier, changes in neurotransmission, and dysfunction of brain cells. The pathogenesis of SAE remains insufficiently studied, and as a result, there are no targeted methods for treating this life-threatening complication. One of the most important problems is the gap in knowledge about the molecules of microbial metabolism, which can cause or, conversely, slow down pathological processes in the brain in sepsis. It is extremely important to understand whether microbial molecules circulating in the blood are signaling and whether they affect the severity and outcome of the septic process in patients with SAE. Intensive search and accumulation of experimental and clinical data on the relationship of encephalopathy with taxonomic and metabolic features of the gut microbiota is underway. Scientific articles of recent years demonstrate how persistently research continues on experimental models of sepsis and SAE, up to the use of germ-free animals, fecal microbiota transplantation (FMT), vagus nerve crossing, etc.

* Corresponding author Natalia V. Beloborodova, Professor, MD., Ph.D.
e-mail address: nvbeloborodova@yandex.ru

Editor: Irina A. Savvina, Natalia V. Beloborodova and Tatyana N. Trofimova
In: Sepsis-Associated Encephalopathy
ISBN: 979-8-89113-178-1

The metabolomic approach makes it possible to study biochemical processes at the intertwining of biochemical pathways of human and microbial metabolism that are potentially involved in the development of SAE and to find new therapeutic targets. In this chapter, we summarize the results of studies, including metabolomic analysis, performed on biological samples from patients and on animal models with SAE. The analysis of the actual data on the interaction of the organism of a critically ill patient with its bacteria through microbial metabolites is an important step toward deciphering the mechanisms of SAE at the molecular level. The authors are convinced that the results obtained along this path will form the basis of fundamentally new approaches to the prevention and treatment of sepsis and SAE.

Keywords: SMOM, SCFA, sepsis-associated microbial metabolites, 4-hydroxyphenyllactic acid, 4-hydroxyphenylacetic acid, aryl hydrocarbon receptor

Abbreviations

4-HPhAA – 4 hydroxyphenylacetic acid
4-HPhLA – 4-hydroxyphenyllactic acid
AHR – aryl hydrocarbon receptor
AMM – aromatic microbial metabolites
BAs – bile acids
BBB – blood-brain barrier
CLP – cecal-ligation and perforation
CNS – central nervous system
FMT – fecal microbiota transplantation
GF – germ-free animals, gnotobionts
Gram (-) – gram-negative bacteria
Gram (+) – gram-positive bacteria
IPA – indolpropinic acid
LPS – lipopolysaccharide of gram-negative bacteria
LTA – lipoteichoic acid
MAMPs – microbial-associated molecular patterns
MCBAs – microbially-conjugated bile acids
PhLA – phenyllactic acid
SAE – sepsis-associated encephalopathy
SCFAs – short-chain fatty acids
SMOM – small molecules originating from microbes
VRE – vancomycin-resistant enterococcus

Introduction

It is known that sepsis is a life-threatening condition associated with bacteria, and in the case of the development of CAE, the probability of death increases. In sepsis, by methods of clinical microbiology gram-positive (*Enterococci* spp., *Staphylococci* spp.) or gram-negative (*Klebsiella pneumonia, Pseudomonas* spp., *Acinetobacter* spp.) species of bacteria are more often isolated from the blood or locus of infection. This does not mean that only a few types of bacteria are involved in the development of sepsis, at least because hundreds of species of bacteria are present and function in the human body as part of it – the microbiota. The list of bacteria – the so-called pathogens – strongly depends on the spectrum of action of the antibiotics used and is often associated with the selection of antibiotic-resistant strains. Previously, microorganisms isolated from blood, liquor, or other sterile media have been cited as the cause or pathogen of sepsis, but in recent years, the theory of the origin of sepsis has undergone major changes, giving way to systemic inflammation, and then multiple organ dysfunction. According to modern international recommendations, the presence of a positive hemoculture is not even included in the list of mandatory signs for the diagnosis of sepsis [2]. This is confirmed by the results of the large-scale studies, for example, the analysis of more than 4000 episodes of severe sepsis did not find a connection between causative organism and bacteremia with mortality [3]. When studying the causes of bacterial-related SAE, more and more attention is being paid to components of microbial cells, especially LPS, which are detected by the innate host immune system throughout the body, including the brain, and are called microbial-associated molecular patterns (MAMPs) [4]. Other small molecules originating from microbes (SMOM) [5] are products of the metabolism of living bacteria, and above all, the microbiota. Today, the search and study of microbial metabolites potentially involved in the mechanisms of brain dysfunction associated with the severity of brain damage and often an unfavorable outcome of SAE are extremely important.

Bacteria and components of their cell walls

SAE is a pathological process based on diffuse cerebral dysfunction caused by an inflammatory reaction of the body to infection, in which microbes do not penetrate the cerebrospinal fluid and brain tissue and cannot directly affect the central nervous system. Published information on the frequency of detection of certain types of bacteria in other tissues or blood of patients with SAE is few and rather contradictory. In sepsis, it is usually possible to isolate from blood and identify the bacterial strains that can survive under the conditions of the use of modern antibiotics. Thus, the strains most often mentioned in publications on the etiology of sepsis are such multi-resistant gram-negative enterobacteria as *Klebsiella pneumonia* and non-fermenting bacteria (*Pseudomonas* sp., *Acinetobacter* sp.), or such gram-positive bacteria (methicillin-resistant *Staphylococcus*, vancomycin-resistant *Enterococcus*). Only in some cases, do the authors note any connection of the isolated bacteria with SAE. For example, in a large-scale study, interesting data were obtained, namely, contrary to generally accepted ideas about the leading role of gram-negative sepsis, the predominance of gram-positive pathogens in CAE was shown. A retrospective analysis of 2,513 patients with sepsis showed that signs of SAE occurred in 53%; among 15 independent risk factors for SAE, the authors indicate *Staphylococcus aureus* bacteremia [6].

It is still unclear how bacteria interact with the brain. It is fair to assume that not whole bacterial cells but their components are participants in the process. The structural components of the bacterial cell wall differ significantly in gram-negative and gram-positive bacteria. The peptidoglycan layer is common to both groups of bacteria, but the fundamental differences are the presence of lipopolysaccharide (LPS) in the outer membrane of gram(-) bacteria, which is also called endotoxin, while gram(+) bacteria do not have an outer membrane, but contain lipoteichoic acids in the cell membrane.

Lipopolysaccharide (LPS). The most studied of the molecular patterns associated with the pathogen can be considered – lipopolysaccharide (LPS). It was found that the reaction of leukocytes (neutrophils/macrophages) to such a pathogen-associated factor as LPS is considered to be the main trigger mechanism for the development of a systemic inflammatory reaction. Leukocytes express receptors such as Toll-like receptors (TLRs) that recognize pathogen patterns, form a complex that enters the bloodstream, and trigger an inflammatory cascade. LPS induces a strong immune response, leading to an increase in the level of pro-inflammatory mediators (e.g., IL-1ß, TNF-α), which affect the brain, induce pathological behavior, and the manifestation of other symptoms of brain dysfunction. LPS is widely used in experimental models of SAE, to study the mechanisms of the inflammatory process in encephalopathy, to compare the effects of different molecules on the brain, etc. [7, 8].

As a complex multicellular structure of the vascular system at the central nervous system (CNS), the blood-brain barrier (BBB) separates the CNS from the system circulation and regulates the influx and efflux of substances to maintain the steady-state environment of the CNS. Lipopolysaccharide (LPS), the cell wall component of gram-negative bacteria, can overcome the BBB and further promote the occurrence and development of sepsis-associated encephalopathy (SAE) [9].

Lipoteichoic acid (LTA). Unlike the effect of TLR4 agonist lipopolysaccharide (LPS), the role of TLR2 agonist lipoteichoic acid from gram-positive bacteria in immune-brain communication has not been sufficiently studied. LTA participates in the activation of peripheral immunity and initiates neuroinflammatory processes in the brain, which are associated with the downregulation of BBB components. The researchers support the need to study the TLR2 agonist LTA as a potential target for therapeutic intervention in acute neuroinflammatory conditions, but further study is required [10–12].

Phospholipid. Among the structural components of the cells of beneficial anaerobic bacteria, special attention has recently been paid to the study of the phospholipid *Akkermansia muciniphila*, which, according to researchers, induces homeostatic immune responses. At the same time, in conclusion, the authors note that the data underlying the model are from in vitro studies, and in vivo studies will be needed to fully validate it [13].

Well-preserved components of microbial cells that are detected by the innate host immune system throughout the body, including the brain, and numerous microbial metabolites are called **microbial-associated molecular patterns**, or for short **MAMPs** [4].

Microbiota as the main source of MAMPs

In patients. In the context of discussing the mechanisms of development of CAE associated with bacteria, it is important to emphasize that violations of the species composition of the microbiota in a seriously ill patient have manifested by profound changes in metabolic processes involving microbiota on the mucous membranes of the digestive tract, respiratory tract, etc. The results of our research allow us to assert that the metabolic dysfunction of the microbiota is not only an obligatory companion of a critical condition but also, quite often, a harbinger predicting the outcome [14–16].

Currently, there are numerous facts in medical practice confirming that the intestinal microbiota of patients in intensive care units (ICU) undergoes many changes due to critical conditions, antibiotics, and other ICU-specific medications [17–19]. It is important to emphasize that deep changes in the microbiota are already present in a critical patient at the time of admission to the ICU, even before the start of antibiotic therapy.

Thus, in a study by Freedberg et al. [20], 301 patients were recruited with an expected long period of treatment in the intensive care unit. Patients were observed for 30 days, during this period 25% had a fatal outcome, and 41% developed a bacterial infection confirmed microbiologically. The association of death and/or infectious complication with the dominance of enterococci in the gut (15%) and with VRE colonization (30%) was established. The author draws attention to the fact that among those patients who were not colonized by the hospital strain of enterococcus (VRE), the very fact of serious dysbiosis with the dominance of enterococcus in the gut microbiota was also associated with an increased risk of death or infection.

At the same time, changes in microbiota metabolism cannot be explained only by the loss of resistance to colonization and the settlement of the patient with multi-resistant hospital pathogens characteristic of the microecology of the intensive care unit. Studies reveal the interindividual diversity and extremely heterogeneous structure of the gut microbiota in critically ill patients. For example, in the study of Lankelma et al. [21], critically ill septic patients show large interpersonal variation in the dysregulation of the gut microbiota. At the same time, the common feature was the disappearance of bacterial genera that performed important functions in the metabolism of the host. The differences in the composition of the microbiota between the healthy control group and all seriously ill patients with sepsis of various genesis (infection of the lungs, abdominal cavity, urinary tract) were very significant, $p = 0.0005$.

In animal experiments. The use of various animal models is a valuable source of information that can significantly expand our understanding of the role of gut microbiota in pathological manifestations of brain functions under the influence of specific factors. The most commonly used experimental model is when neuroinflammation is induced by lipopolysaccharide. The results obtained on rodent models are analyzed in detail in articles of recent years [8, 22, 23]. Of particular interest are experiments that shed light on the mechanisms of behavior change and cognitive functions in animals under the influence of antibiotics. So, in an experiment on mice, it was shown that low-dose penicillin in late pregnancy and early postnatal life induces changes in murine gut microbiota and brain. Penicillin has a long-term effect on the gut microbiota, increases the expression of cytokines in the frontal cortex of the brain, changes the integrity of the blood-brain barrier, and changes behavior. Mice treated with penicillin demonstrate behavioral disorders and show aggression, but some of these changes were prevented by concomitant supplementation with *Lactobacillus rhamnosus* [24].

In another experimental model of autoimmune encephalomyelitis (EAE), the use of antibiotics, on the contrary, led to a positive result. It has been shown that a short three-day course of oral administration to animals of a cocktail of four antibiotics (ampicillin, metronidazole, neomycin, and vancomycin) causes changes in peripheral immune regulation and protects mice from developing signs of EAE [25]. The authors suggested that under the action of chemokines, macrophages are polarized toward the anti-inflammatory phenotype. Thanks to additional data obtained by RT-PCR analysis, it was found that genes associated with anti-inflammatory microglia/macrophages were activated, and pro-inflammatory genes were suppressed. The effect of antibiotics protecting against EAE by increasing regulatory and anti-inflammatory cells can be explained by the fact that antibiotics active against gram (-) bacteria took place in the composition of the drug cocktail. For example, metronidazole is active against gram (-) gut anaerobes, and the aminoglycoside neomycin, which is not absorbed in the intestine, effectively suppresses the growth of gram (-) enterobacteria, which as a result reduced the total amount of LPS. The consequence of the use of such antibiotics was a decrease in the intensity of neuroinflammation induced by LPS, which was regarded as brain protection. And the previous experiment was conducted with penicillin [24]. The spectrum of penicillin activity is limited to gram (+) bacteria, therefore, on the contrary, prerequisites for the dominance of gram (-) bacteria were created in the intestine. Such dysbiosis led to excessive intake of LPS into the bloodstream, and, accordingly, the launch of excessive activation of microglia, cytokine expression in the brain, and the development of cognitive impairment.

These and many other examples show what an important role microbiota changes play in the development of brain dysfunction, especially given the massive antibiotic therapy that is performed in patients with sepsis in the ICU. It is very difficult to interpret correctly the data obtained in the experiment, and even more difficult to try to project the results of experimental studies into the clinic.

Fecal microbiota transplantation (FMT). The method of correction of intestinal microbiota, namely fecal microbiota transplantation (FMT) from healthy donors, now is being actively studied at the experimental level and discussed in the literature. We will limit ourselves to a brief comment, emphasizing that the transfer of microbiota from one individual to another was not accidentally called transplantation, since it is not yet possible to predict the consequences of transplantation of such foreign multicomponent genetic material.

Some authors consider FMT as a future method of modulation of the intestinal microbiota [26]. FMT is usually considered safe, and the common side effects are minor adverse events, including transient diarrhea, abdominal cramps or pain, low-grade fever, bloating, flatulence, and constipation [27]. However, in the course of experimental studies, some undesirable effects were obtained, confirming a high risk of unpredictable dangerous consequences. In the study of Tengeler et al. (2020) young sterile (germ-free) mice were colonized with microbiota from individuals with and without neurodevelopmental (attention-deficit or hyperactivity) disorders, and studied mouse microbiome data, behavior in a behavioral test battery, assessed brain structure and function by magnetic resonance imaging [28]. Authors demonstrate that altered microbial composition could be a driver of altered brain structure and function and concomitant changes in the animals' behavior. Another study by Sharon et al. (2019) also used germ-free mice that had gut microbiota transplanted from donor people with autism spectrum disorders and, for comparison, from healthy donors (control group) [29]. Only in the brains of mice colonized by microbiota from patients with autism, there were changes in genes associated with autism disorder. The authors suggested that the connections between the gut and the brain are involved in the pathophysiology of behavioral abnormalities and modulate the excitability of neurons in the brain and that the gut microbiota regulates behavior through the production of neuroactive metabolites.

Another example is clinical, a randomized, double-blind, placebo-controlled trial, the results of a study on the effectiveness of FMT were published in the *Lancet* in 2022 [30]. According to the study protocol, before starting the FMT procedure, all patients underwent prolonged enteral administration of antibiotics (a cocktail of three drugs: ampicillin + metronidazole + doxycycline), and then orally for 8–56 weeks – lyophilized fecal microbiota. Patients (n=35) were randomized: 15 to receive FMT and 20 to receive a placebo. Adverse events occurred in 10 (67%) patients in the FMT group and 17 (85%) patients in the placebo group during the 8-week induction period and were usually limited to gastrointestinal complaints. Serious side effects included exacerbation of ulcerative colitis (13% in the FMT group, 5% in the placebo group).

Clinical experience of using FMT in various groups of severe patients, including those with mental disorders, is accumulating [30–32]. Comments on the results of the treatment of small groups of patients usually contain positive feedback, while rare publications with data from comparative randomized trials are still inconclusive. We will limit ourselves to a brief comment, emphasizing that the transfer of microbiota from one individual to another had been called transplantation, since it is not yet possible to predict the long-term consequences of transplantation of such foreign multicomponent genetic material as feces.

Microbial metabolites

Attempts to identify patterns of CAE development in patients depending on the bacteria dominating the microbiota, according to the gram-positive/gram-negative ratio principle, did not lead to results. No associations were found between microbiota diversity Firmicutes/Bacteroidetes ratio also. Currently, the metabolomic approach using the technologies of metabolomic analysis is more promising, which will be presented in more detail below.

Emphasizing the diversity and importance of active metabolic processes occurring due to the intestinal microbiota, in the literature the intestine can figuratively call a "metabolic reactor" [33–35]. Intestinal bacteria use food substrates or metabolic products of host organs and tissues entering the intestine from the blood as sources. Some final products of metabolism are formed only by microbial metabolic pathways. Different types of bacteria exchange with each other and transfer the intermediate products of metabolism "along the chain" to other species, implementing a kind of metabolic conveyor [36]. Numerous studies conducted in recent years have shown that several microbial metabolites have a significant effect on the human brain. Some metabolites of intestinal bacteria can affect various brain functions, including those that manifest in encephalopathy associated with sepsis (Fig. 3.1).

Theoretically, for the structural components of cell wall bacteria to be released and get into the internal environment of the body, they must be destroyed (e.g., during phagocytosis) or lysed under the influence of adverse factors (for example, antiseptics). Microbial metabolites differ in that they are products of the metabolism of living bacteria. In patients with sepsis, in the presence of foci of infection in tissues/ organs, the metabolic products of pathogenic bacteria can enter the bloodstream directly.

A feature of SAE is the development of an inflammatory process in brain tissues in the absence of a pathogen in this focus. Consequently, metabolites circulating in the blood, including those originating from the microbiota, can affect the brain. On the contrary, the brain may suffer from a lack of the necessary metabolites when, against the background of massive antimicrobial therapy for sepsis, the microbiota is severely disrupted. The results of experimental studies in the field of gut-brain communication show that a combination of five antibiotics administered to an animal contributes to the development of cognitive disorders caused by antibiotics. Gut dysbiosis was associated with the depletion of metabolites of bacterial origin in the colon, changes in lipid forms, and transformed molecules of microbial origin in plasma [37].

It is important to keep in mind that in a patient with sepsis not only an excess of any microbial metabolites can provoke signs of brain dysfunction but also a lack or absence of metabolites necessary for natural communication of the intestine with the brain. With sepsis, both situations can occur in conditions of depletion of the diversity of the intestinal microbiota.

Short-chain fatty acids (SCFAs). SCFAs are microbial metabolites from dietary fiber, made of complex carbohydrate polysaccharides; they are fermented by gut anaerobes with a

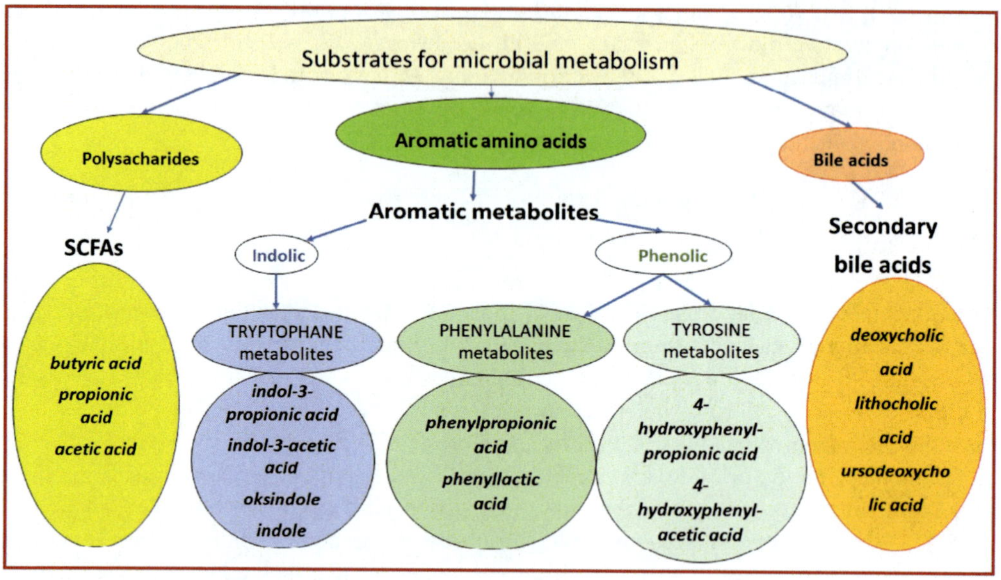

Figure 3.1 Microbial metabolites interacting with the brain.

This Figure shows three groups of substrates for microbial metabolism in the human body, and five groups of microbial metabolites that are potentially involved in interaction with the brain, including in SAE

diverse class of glycoside hydrolases and polysaccharide lyases. In a healthy body with the normal composition of the microbiota, a sufficient amount of SCFAs is produced at millimolar levels. SCFAs are sources of energy nutrition for colonic epithelial cells and thereby provide intestinal barrier function [38].

SCFAs in sepsis have been evaluated using a traditional experimental sepsis model – the method of cecal ligation and perforation (CLP) in adult Wistar rats. On the 10th day after surgery, the content of acetate, propionate, and butyrate in feces significantly ($p<0.05$) decreased in the sepsis group compared to the control (sham) groups. There was no significant difference between isobutyric acid and isovaleric acid between the sepsis and control groups [39].

SCFA can activate anti-inflammatory signaling cascades through interactions with G-protein receptors (GPRs) and modulate intestinal homeostasis. The excess part of SCFAs enters the systemic circulation, and they can penetrate the brain and interact with microglia [40]. The addition of SCFA can have a neuroprotective effect against SAE, preserving or restoring the integrity of the BBB. In particular, in an experiment on a sepsis model, SCFA treatment significantly facilitated behavioral dysfunction and neuroinflammation in mice with SAE, which allowed the researchers to conclude that disorders in the gut microbiota and SCFA metabolites play a key role in SAE [41].

SCFA in sepsis has been evaluated using a traditional experimental sepsis model – the method of cecal ligation and perforation (CLP) in adult Wistar rats. On the 10th day after surgery, the content of acetate, propionate, and butyrate in feces significantly ($p<0.05$)

decreased in the sepsis group compared to the control (sham) groups. There was no significant difference between isobutyric acid and isovaleric acid between the sepsis and control groups [39].

In studies, the greatest attention is paid to butyrate, propionate, and acetate, which perform an important function in the gut.

Butyric acid has received the most attention among SCFAs as a key mediator of anti-inflammatory activity [42]. This metabolite is a potent inhibitor of histone deacetylases (HDAC), which regulate epigenetic signals of gene activation. The potential pharmacological effects of butyrate are widely studied, since in many neurodegenerative diseases there is a violation of histone acetylation. For example, oral administration of butyrate to Alzheimer's mice improved neuroinflammation and cognitive impairment [43]. Some authors, based on their experimental studies, point to the crucial role of the intestinal microbiota in susceptibility to SAE and argue that butyrate, a metabolite of the intestinal microbiota, can have a neuroprotective effect in the process of sepsis [44].

Propionic acid. Propionic acid is produced by bacteria of the genus *Propionibacterium* as the end product of their anaerobic metabolism. Propionic acid has anti-fungicidal and antibacterial effects, so it is used in the food industry. In the human body, it is rapidly oxidized and excreted. In the context of discussing the role of propionic acid as a microbial metabolite in sepsis and CAE, there are conflicting data.

So, in a single-center, prospective study a total of 118 septic patients were enrolled, and was shown, that increased serum level of propionic acid in the early phase of sepsis was associated with mortality. Propionic acid content was also higher in patients with septic shock. The authors concluded that serum propionic acid was a significant predictor of sepsis severity and a prognostic biomarker in sepsis patients along with other inflammation biomarkers [45].

In another clinical study involving about 300 patients (MS) with such an autoimmune and neurodegenerative disease as multiple sclerosis, an initial or initial significant decrease in the level of propionate in both the intestine and blood was confirmed. The violation of the microbiome was revealed involving depletion of some SCFA producers (*Butyricimonas*) and enrichment of some pathobionts (*Flavonifractor* and *Escherichia/Shigella*). After the use of 500 mg sodium-propionate capsules twice daily for 14 days (Flexopharm, Herne, Germany) a steady increase in functionally competent regulatory T cells (Treg) was observed, while the number of Th1 and Th17 cells decreased significantly. The results of the study showed a beneficial effect of sodium-propionate on immunological, neurodegenerative, and clinical indicators, including the frequency of relapses and the progression of disability [46].

Acetic acid. Acetic acid or acetate participates in various metabolic pathways, and is known primarily as an active molecule that easily crosses the BBB, enters the brain, and activates neurons in the hypothalamus. One of the effects of excessive loading with acetate is described as appetite suppression of central origin [47]. Acetate research has been conducted for more than 50 years. Changes in the kinetics of labeled acetate are used to assess the activity of oxidative metabolism of astrocytes in animals and humans; therefore, acetate is called a marker of astrocyte metabolism [48].

The paucity of information about SCFAS in SAE is because the production of this group of metabolites is sharply reduced in sepsis under conditions of suppression of normal anaerobic microflora in the gut.

Amino acid metabolites

Metabolites of tryptophan. Aromatic amino acid tryptophan plays an important role in human endogenous metabolism. The formation of tryptophan derivatives occurs by indole and kynurenine pathways. The indole pathway of tryptophan conversion is conditionally divided into serotonin and microbial, leading to the formation of the neurotransmitter serotonin, melatonin, as well as several other metabolites containing an indole ring, for example, tryptamine, which undergoes further biotransformation to form indolacetic and indolepropionic acids, indole, and indoxyl. The kynurenine pathway is accompanied by the destruction of the indole ring of tryptophan and leads to the formation of L-kynurenine, kynurenic, and quinoline acids or the coenzyme nicotinamide adenine dinucleotide (NAD+). Part of the tryptophan absorbed with food undergoes bacterial biodegradation, resulting in the formation of indole acids (e.g., 3-indole propane) and indole. In modern experimental studies, including the use of gnotobiological (germ-free, GF) animals has been proved that the formation of tryptophan metabolites such as indole-3-acetic acid, indole-3-propionic acid, tryptamine, and indoxyl sulfate is associated with intestinal bacteria [49].

Recently, it has been discovered that several endogenous indole derivatives such as kynurenine participate in AhR activating [50]. The AhR has roles in regulating immunity, stem cell maintenance, and cellular differentiation. Some authors call the aryl hydrocarbon receptor a multifunctional chemical sensor for host defense and homeostatic maintenance. AHR functions in host defense not only via drug metabolism of external chemicals but also by prevention of bacterial infection at multiple steps in the infection process. For example, using tryptophan as an energy source, bacteria in a healthy microbiota produce indole metabolites that serve as AHR ligands; as a result of AHR activation, IL22 expression occurs, antimicrobial proteins are produced and, thus, control over bacterial infection is realized. After a detailed study and analysis of the available facts, the authors concluded "Deeper mechanistic insights into the functional association between commensal microbes and immune cells through AHR activation are expected" [51, 52].

Extremely interesting facts established during the study by a large international team demonstrate that indole, produced by tryptophanase-expressing gut microbes, elicits neurogenic effects in the adult mouse hippocampus. It turned out that the process of neurogenesis is reduced in germ-free (GF) mice and in GF mice mono colonized with a single-gene mutant *Escherichia coli* unable to produce indole, that is, the presence of indole metabolites of microbial origin is necessary for neurogenesis. The results of the experiments showed that the indole-AhR–mediated signaling pathway elevated the expression of three specific genes (*β-catenin*, *Neurog2*, and *VEGF-α genes*), thus identifying a molecular pathway connecting gut microbiota composition and their metabolic function to neurogenesis in the adult hippocampus [53].

Metabolic pathways of microbial biodegradation of tryptophan can lead to the formation of many metabolites, which are presented in great detail [54]. It is not yet possible to determine exactly which of them are AHR ligands.

Indoles. Indoles are metabolites of tryptophan. There is quite a little information about the concentrations of microbial metabolites of the indole structure in the blood. More often it is reported that the level of tryptophan metabolites may be elevated in certain diseases, which we have collected and summarized in the review [55]. The interpretation of data on indole metabolites is rather complicated since it is necessary to take into account the origin of each metabolite (endogenous or microbial) and the significance of changes in its concentration for the body – benefit or harm.

Serotonin is one of the indoles that does not belong to metabolites, but to hormones, however, in this chapter, it is necessary to pay attention to it in connection with some studies that have convincingly shown the connection of serotonin with the metabolism of the microbiota.

Serotonin or 5-hydroxytryptamine is a hormone that performs numerous functions in the central nervous system (CNS) and beyond. At the same time, serotonin is one of the main neurotransmitters and an intercellular mediator. The function of serotonin can be described as contributing to homeostasis by countering disturbances in metabolic cycles, for example, with an excess of arousal, serotonin acts as an inhibitory neurotransmitter. The main sources of serotonin in the body must be enterochromaffin cells and intramural neurons of the intestine. The gut microbiota modulates the serotonin system of the host, which had been confirmed by studies using germ-free animals, or by another way – oral administration of antibiotics to suppress the microbiota. The mechanism of indirect participation of the intestinal microbiota is associated with the production of numerous microbial metabolites, the action of which can affect the serotonergic systems of the body in various ways [56].

It is established that a spore-forming bacteria *Clostridia* spp. from microbiota promote serotonin biosynthesis from colonic enterochromaffin cells [57]. This fact was established in experiments by the colonization of the intestines of germ-free mice, which was accompanied by a significant increase in the concentration of 5-hydroxytryptamine in the intestines and blood of experimental animals. The main amount of serotonin in animals and humans is contained in the mucous membrane and lumen of the intestine, from there it enters the blood and spreads throughout the body by circulating platelets. Elevating luminal concentrations of particular microbial metabolites increases colonic and blood 5-HT, these may influence vagal nerve activity and brain levels of serotonin.

Thus, there are grounds to assert that some microbial metabolites of tryptophan, having an indole structure, are necessary for the normal functioning of the body, and most importantly – for a successful exit from the septic state, including with SAE. At the same time, in conditions of the suppression of biodiversity and disruption of the metabolic function of the microbiota, a shortage of the necessary indole metabolites of microbial origin is inevitable. It can be assumed that in the future this mechanism will be important not only in ensuring the barrier function of the digestive tract mucosa but also in a blood-brain barrier and compensatory correction of the lack of metabolites of the indole structure will be developed to prevent the development of SAE in critical patients.

It is very important to note that the action of indoles depending on the chemical structure can be radically different. The results of experimental studies with individual metabolites are described in the literature. For example, positive neuroprotective effects of indolpropinic acid (IPA) were identified [58, 59], while other microbial metabolites of tryptophan (indole, oxindole, indoxyl sulfate, etc.) harmed the brain (Table 1). According to Elsden SR, 1976, who studied the end products of the metabolism of aromatic amino acids by various *Clostridium* spp., only 4 out of 23 species of *Clostridium* were able to form IPA; moreover, *Clostridium sporogenes* produced IPA in the largest quantities [60].

Metabolites of phenylalanine and tyrosine

In sepsis, among the hundreds of studied metabolites of various groups, it is always such aromatic microbial metabolites (AMM) as phenyl lactic acid (FMC), 4-hydroxyphenyl lactic acid (4-GFMC), and hydroxy-phenylacetic acid (4-GFUC) that significantly increase.

We call these three metabolites "sepsis-associated AMM," the dynamics of their serum concentrations are prognostically significant and closely correlate with the development of septic shock and death [61]. The association with SAE is indicated by such indirect data as multiple increases in the concentration of AMM in the blood serum on the eve of death (one day before death). It is impossible to exclude their direct toxic effects on the brain at high concentrations in the blood, but no such studies have been conducted.

Sepsis-associated AMM are intermediates of the metabolism of aromatic amino acids phenylalanine and tyrosine. By their structure, these are hydroxyphenyl carboxylic acids, they are chemically active compounds capable of reacting rapidly along the hydroxyl group of phenyl. It is important to note that such compounds do not form conjugates, and usually, they are recycled in the human body by anaerobic bacteria, especially by *Bacteroides* spp. [62]. Due to the normal functioning of the microbiota in a healthy body, the level of AMM in the systemic bloodstream is maintained at a constant level, not exceeding a total of 0.2–0.5 mcM. When an excess of AMM appears, the source of which can be any foci of bacterial infection, the bacteria in the intestinal microbiota consume AMM to form the end products of metabolism (e.g., phenylpropionic acid, indolepropionic acid, etc.) [63].

The most detailed participation of AMM in the development of sepsis, septic shock, and the relationship with mortality are summarized in the chapter of Beloborodova N. (2023) [64]. It was shown that for healthy people, the profile of aromatic metabolites of blood serum is characterized by the predominance of phenylpropionic acid (PhPA). And in sepsis, the diagnostic and prognostic value belongs to 4-hydroxyphenyllactic acid (HPhLA), 4-hydroxyphenylacetic (HPhAA), and phenyllactic acid (PhLA). The accumulation of AMM in the blood of patients with sepsis, including SAE development cases, is a consequence of a violation of the mechanisms of homeostasis due to deep microbiota disorders [65]. The following figure shows the results of our microbiological in vitro experiment, the purpose of which was to determine the types of bacteria capable of producing and/or consuming three sepsis-associated AMM in the human body (Fig. 3.2).

We are aware that the results of the cultivation of pure microbial culture in vitro in a rich nutrient medium are very different from the products of the general metabolism of bacteria in the microbiota, where species often function as a conveyor. But even in vitro, when growing pure bacterial cultures, it is noteworthy that the "roles" in metabolism are distributed among different species. For example, *Klebsiella pneumonia* has the most pronounced ability to produce sepsis-associated metabolites from aromatic amino acids, while strict anaerobes *Bacteroides* spp. are actively used of these metabolites for the formation of final (useful) metabolic products. Interestingly, in a clinical study in patients with a diagnosis of severe depressive disorder (n=60), exactly such violations of the proportion of *Prevotella* (this species was previously classified as a *Bacteroids*) and *Klebsiella* in the fecal flora were found, which the authors assess as useful parameters for laboratory diagnosis and treatment [66]. The connection of depression with microbiota metabolites is indicated by many publications in recent years [67, 68].

Confirmation of the participation of AMM, namely HPhAA, is interesting data obtained by a group of researchers from Chongqing Medical University, China [69]. Blood samples from 31 SAE patients and 28 healthy controls were collected, and they were used to detect metabolism changes by gas chromatography-mass spectrometry (GC-MS). The study aimed to determine which metabolites significantly differed between the control and SAE groups. SAE patients were divided into four groups according to the Glasgow Coma Score (GCS). They found a correlation between the concentration of 4-hydroxyphenylacetic acid and the severity of consciousness disorders. The concentration of 4-HPhAA in sepsis patients decreased with a

Type of bacteria	Aromatic microbial metabolites (AMM)					
	PRODUCTION			CONSUMPTION		
AEROBES AND FACULTATIVE ANAEROBES	PhLA	4-HPhLA	4-HPhAA	PhLA	4-HPhLA	4-HPhAA
Staphylococcus aureus	++	++				+
Staphylococcus epidermidis	+	+				+
Enterococcus faecalis	+				+	+
Enterococcus faecium	+				+	+
Escherichia coli	++	++				+
Klebsiella pneumonia	++	++	++			
Acinetobacter baummanii		+	++	+		
Serratia marcescens	+	+				+
Pseudomonas aeruginosa			+			
OBLICATE ANAEROBES						
Bifidobacterium bifidum	++	+				+
Lactobacillus fermentum	++	+				+
Clostridium sporogenes	+	+				+
Clostridium perfringers	+				+	+
Bacteroides fragilis				+	+	+
Bacteroides thetaiotaomicron			+	+	+	
Eubacterium lentum	+	+				+

Figure 3.2 The ability to produce or consume microbial metabolites by some types of bacteria when cultivating a pure culture in vitro.

This figure compares the results of an in vitro experiment: how pure cultures of some types of bacteria produce and/or consume each of the three sepsis-associated aromatic microbial metabolites, (+) in small or (++) large amounts. According to the data presented by Beloborodova N. (2012) and (2023) [64, 65]. Red – clinically significant gram-negative bacteria as the most active producers. Green – representatives of obligate anaerobes (*Bacteroides* spp.) – as the most active consumers. PhLA – phenyllactic acid, HPhLA – 4-hydroxyphenyllactic acid, HPhAA – 4-hydroxyphenylacetic acid

decrease in the GCS. Authors suggest that 4-hydroxyphenylacetic acid may be a potential biomarker for SAE and useful in predicting patient prognosis.

It has also been shown that the level of microbial metabolites in the blood serum changes during antibacterial therapy and depends on the spectrum of antimicrobial activity of drugs [64]. This is very important because SAE develops in the conditions of the current septic condition, and therefore patients need antibacterial therapy. On the other hand, it is precisely the disruption of the connection between the microbiota and the brain that can contribute to the development of encephalopathy, and antibiotics inevitably affect the microbiota. To date, there are no recommendations or algorithms in the intensive care unit for the selection of antibiotics or their combinations, which, along with the antimicrobial effect, would not simultaneously aggravate the metabolic dysfunction of the microbiota. We call this approach to the treatment of sepsis patients the microbiota-oriented therapy strategy [70].

The table below shows examples of several in which certain microbial metabolites are involved, which have been confirmed in experimental or clinical studies (Table 3.1).

Bile acids

Primary bile acids (BA) are mainly produced in hepatocytes from cholesterol with the participation of cytochrome P450 subunits. In the liver, synthesized primary bile acids conjugate with taurine and glycine, which increases the hydrophilicity of atomic groups and gives them a negative charge, which provides a high ability to emulsify and prevents the incorporation of bile acids into cell membranes.

Primary bile acids and their conjugates are excreted with bile into the lumen of the small intestine, then under the influence of the intestinal microbiota, their partial dehydroxylation and deconjugation occur, thus, glycine and taurine are formed by separation with the participation of bacteria [76,77]. Two secondary bases — deoxycholic and lithocholic, are characterized by pronounced hydrophobicity and cytotoxic potential, they are hydrophobic (i.e., lipophilic) and can integrate into the mitochondrial membrane, enhancing the production of reactive oxygen species [78, 79]. At the same time, another metabolite from the group of secondary bile acids, namely ursodeoxycholic acid, is not only recognized as useful but is also used as a drug for many pathological conditions. Bile acid deconjugation is carried out by bacteria (such as *Lactobacilli*, *Bifidobacteria*, *Clostridium*, and *Bacteroides*) with bile salt hydrolase activity. It has been repeatedly shown in experiments that in the absence of bacteria in the gut (as in germ-free animals or mice/rats treated with antibiotics), the pool of bile acids consists mainly of primary conjugated bile acids.

There are bidirectional interactions between gut microbiota and BAs. The BA pool composition depends on gut microbiota producing secondary BAs, whereas BAs significantly influence microbiota composition. Bile acids have pronounced bactericidal activity, so their deficiency negatively affects the gut microbiota. On the other hand, dysbiosis-induced secondary bile acid deficiency promotes intestinal inflammation [80].

Elevation of total bile acid levels has been observed during neuropathological states in humans, such as hepatic encephalopathy, where elevation of bile acids is observed in brain tissue and cerebrospinal fluid. BAs can be transported to the brain from the peripheral circulation. While conjugated BAs require transporters to cross the BBB, unconjugated and lipophilic BAs can cross the BBB by passive diffusion. Many of the therapeutic strategies to treat hepatic encephalopathy, such as lactulose, neomycin, metronidazole, and vancomycin, are targeted at the gut microbiota to reduce ammonia production, but as a secondary effect would influence the conjugation of secondary bile acids. Publications on the significance and mechanisms of the participation of bile acids in brain pathology mainly concern Alzheimer's disease [81, 82]. We have not been able to find studies on secondary bile acids in SAE.

Difficulties in studying BAs are associated with a wide variety of these acids, as well as with the fact that secondary BAs differ in different mammals and in humans, which makes it difficult to experimental study and interpret results.

In 2020, Robert Quinn, Pieter Dorrestein, and colleagues made a breakthrough in our understanding of the gut microbiome and bile acid chemistry: they discovered that gut microbes can conjugate a variety of amino acids to bile acids, generating a diverse set of molecules that had never before been described [79]. Quinn uses his Global Grant for Gut Health to further examine how microbially conjugated bile acids (MCBAs) are generated and how they affect the body. This new finding greatly influences the diversity of bile acids in the mammalian gut, but the effects on host physiology, microbial dynamics, and brain disorders are mostly unknown [83].

Conclusion

Despite the abundance of research and publications on the role of microbiota for health and pathology, as well as on interaction with the brain, there is very little data on specific mechanisms

Table 3.1 Some examples of the involvement of microbial metabolites in the mechanisms and manifestations of encephalopathy in experiments and/or clinic.

Symptoms of encephalopathy	Microbial metabolites			Ref.
	Name of the metabolite	In an experiment or in a clinic	Effect/result	
Neuroinflammation, oxidative stress	Indoxyl sulfate (IS) – tryptophan metabolite	Experiment on mice: injections of indoxyl sulfate 800 mg/kg intraperitoneally	In glial cells, the level of ROS and pro-inflammatory mediators (TNF-α, IL-6, NO, etc.) increases.	Adesso S et al, 2017 [71]
Behavior disorder	Short-chain fatty acids (SCFAs)	During the experiment, rats were given repeated (5–14 days) pulsed intravenous infusions of buffered SCFAs.	Dystonia, behavior disorder, convulsive activity.	MacFabe DF et al, 2015 [72]
Decreased muscle tone and motor activity	Indole – tryptophan metabolite	1) Rats were injected with indole intraperitoneal or intracranial. 2) Germ-free rats were colonized by indole-producing bacterial species.	Immobility, helplessness, increased anxiety, activation of the vagus nerve.	Jaglin M et al, 2018 [73]
Hypotension, reversible coma, reduction of spontaneous motor activity	Oxindole – tryptophan metabolite	Intravenous administration of oxindole 10–100 mg/ kg to rats	Enteral administration of neomycin (an aminoglycoside antibiotic that does not absorb in the intestine) significantly reduced the content of oxindole in the brain.	Carpenedo R, 1998 [74]
Mortality	4-HPhAA, 4-HPhLA –metabolites of tyrosine	In the course of GC-MS monitoring of seriously ill patients with impaired brain function, it was found that in some (n=8) serum concentrations of 4-HPhAA and 4-HPhLA increased by five times.	Negative dynamics of neurological status; the mortality rate was 6 out of 8 (75%) cases.	Grechko AV et al, 2022 [16]

(Continued)

Table 3.1 (Continued)

Symptoms of encephalopathy	Microbial metabolites			Ref.
	Name of the metabolite	In an experiment or in a clinic	Effect/result	
Anxiety, violation of serotonergic neurotransmission	5-hydroxytryptamine and 5-hydroxyindolacetic acid are elevated in the absence of normal microbiota	Experiment on germ-free male mice with subsequent restoration of the microbiota.	Anxiety goes away after the restoration of the intestinal microbiota.	Clarke G et al, 2013 [75]
Neuroprotection	Indolepropionic acid (IPA) – tryptophan metabolite	Some groups of newborn germ-free mice were colonized with different microbial cultures, including *Clostridium sporogenes*, and serum tryptophan metabolites were studied (LC-MS/MS).	The protective role of indolepropionic acid in the brain is shown.	Dodd D et al, 2017 [59]
Oxidative stress prevented	Indolepropionic acid (IPA)	The effect of IPA on b-amyloid neurotoxicity and neuroprotection was tested on rat fetal neurons.	IPA is the most potent naturally occurring scavenger of free radicals. IPA prevented oxidative stress and the death of primary neurons.	Chyan YJ et al, 1999 [58]

associated with microbial metabolites in the development of SAE, on such severe manifestations of encephalopathy as delirium or coma.

Historically, the gut microbiota, microbial metabolites, and brain have been studied independently. Scientists and specialists in the field of microbiome study and neurologists could hardly meet on general scientific forums or pages of scientific journals. The last two decades have been marked by radical changes, the interaction of the microbiome and the brain is currently in the focus of researchers' attention. This trend will undoubtedly allow us to accumulate facts in the coming years, decipher the complex language of communication between the intestine and the brain, and find new opportunities to manage such a severe complication of sepsis as SAE. In conclusion, we would like to quote a phrase from the article by Needham et al. (2020) "As specific effects of microbial molecular messages and their gut-brain signaling routes continue to be uncovered, the potential increases for the development of novel therapeutic principles and modalities" [4]. We hope that soon a targeted modification of the metabolism of the gut microbiota will be developed and implemented, including for the prevention and treatment of SAE.

References

1. Chaudhry N, Duggal AK. Sepsis associated encephalopathy. *Adv Med*. 2014;2014:762320. doi: 10.1155/2014/762320.
2. Singer M, Deutschman CS, Seymour CW, et al. The third international consensus definitions for sepsis and septic shock (sepsis-3). *JAMA*. 2016 Feb 23;315(8):801–810. doi: 10.1001/jama.2016.0287.
3. Zahar JR, Timsit JF, Garrouste-Orgeas M, et al. Outcomes in severe sepsis and patients with septic shock: Pathogen species and infection sites are not associated with mortality. *Crit Care Med*. 2011 Aug;39(8):1886–1895. doi: 10.1097/ccm.0b013e31821b827c.
4. Needham BD, Kaddurah-Daouk R, Mazmanian SK. Gut microbial molecules in behavioral and neurodegenerative conditions. *Nat Rev Neurosci*. 2020;21:717–731. doi: 10.1038/s41583-020-00381-0.
5. Beloborodova NV, Osipov GA. Small molecules originating from microbes (SMOM) and their role in a microbes-host relationship. *Microb Ecol Health Dis*. 2000;12:12–21. doi: 10.1080/089106000435545.
6. Sonneville R, De Montmollin E, Poujade J, et al. Potentially modifiable factors contributing to sepsis-associated encephalopathy. *Intensive Care Med*. 2017;43:1075–1084. doi: 10.1007/s00134-017-4807-z.
7. Jacob A, Hensley LK, Safratowich BD at al. The role of the complement cascade in endotoxin-induced septic encephalopathy. *Lab Invest*. 2007 Dec;87(12):1186–1194. doi: 10.1038/labinvest.3700686.
8. Skrzypczak-Wiercioch A, Sałat K. Lipopolysaccharide-induced model of neuroinflammation: Mechanisms of action, research application and future directions for its use. *Molecules*. 2022 Aug 26;27(17):5481. doi: 10.3390/molecules27175481.
9. Peng X, Luo Z, He S et al. Blood-brain barrier disruption by lipopolysaccharide and sepsis-associated encephalopathy. *Front Cell Infect Microbiol*. 2021 Nov 4;11:768108. doi: 10.3389/fcimb.2021.768108.
10. Boveri M, Kinsner A, Berezowski V, Lenfant AM, Draing C, Cecchelli R, et al. Highly purified lipoteichoic acid from gram-positive bacteria induces *in vitro* blood brain barrier disruption through glia activation: Role of pro-inflammatory cytokines and nitric oxide. *Neuroscience* 2006;137:1193–1209. doi: 10.1016/j.neuroscience.2005.10.011.
11. Mayerhofer R, Fröhlich EE, Reichmann F, et al. Diverse action of lipoteichoic acid and lipopolysaccharide on neuroinflammation, blood-brain barrier disruption, and anxiety in mice. *Brain Behav Immun*. 2017 Feb;60:174–187. doi: 10.1016/j.bbi.2016.10.011.
12. Howe AM, Cosgrave A, Ó'Murchú M, et al. Characterizing lipoteichoic acid as an *in vitro* model of acute neuroinflammation. *Int Immunopharmacol*. 2020;85:106619. doi: 10.1016/j.intimp.2020.106619.
13. Bae M, Cassilly CD, Liu X, et al. *Akkermansia muciniphila* phospholipid induces homeostatic immune responses. *Nature*. 2022;608:168–173. doi: 10.1038/s41586-022-04985-7.

14. Chernevskaya E., Klimenko N. Pautova A, et al. Host-microbiome interactions mediated by phenolic metabolites in chronically critically ill patients. *Metabolites*. 2021;11(2):122. https://doi.org/10.3390/metabo11020122.
15. Beloborodova NV, Grechko AV. Dialogue between the human microbiome and the brain // Chapter 3. In *Human Microbiome*, Eds. Beloborodova NV, Grechko AV. IntechOpen, UK. 2021, pp. 27–66. doi: 10.5772/intechopen.94431.
16. Grechko AV, Buyakova IV, Beloborodova NV. Microbiota dysfunction in patients with brain damage in chronic critical condition. *Russ Neurol J.* 2022;27(1):94–104. https://doi.org/10.30629/2658-7947-2022-27-1-94-104.
17. Yeh A, Rogers MB, Firek B, Neal MD, Zuckerbraun BS, Morowitz MJ. Dysbiosis across multiple body sites in critically ill adult surgical patients. *Shock*. 2016 Dec;46(6):649–654. doi: 10.1097/SHK.0000000000000691.
18. Ruppé É, Lisboa T, Barbier F. The gut microbiota of critically ill patients: First steps in an unexplored world. *Intensive Care Med.* 2018;44:1561–1564. https://doi.org/10.1007/s00134-018-5309-3.
19. Szychowiak P, Villageois-Tran K, Patrier J, et al. The role of the microbiota in the management of intensive care patients. *Ann Intensive Care.* 2022;12:3. https://doi.org/10.1186/s13613-021-00976-5.
20. Freedberg DE, Zhou MJ, Cohen ME, et al. Pathogen colonization of the gastrointestinal microbiome at the intensive care unit admission and risk for subsequent death or infection. *Intensive Care Med.* 2018;44:1203–1211. https://doi.org/10.1007/s00134-018-5268-8.
21. Lankelma JM, van Vught LA, Belzer C, Schultz MJ, van der Poll T, de Vos WM, Wiersinga WJ. Critically ill patients demonstrate large interpersonal variation in intestinal microbiota dysregulation: A pilot study. *Intensive Care Med.* 2017;43(1):59–68. doi: 10.1007/s00134-016-4613-z.
22. Tiwari P, Dwivedi R, Bansal M, Tripathi M, Dada R. Role of gut microbiota in neurological disorders and its therapeutic significance. *J Clin Med.* 2023 Feb 19;12(4):1650. doi: 10.3390/jcm12041650. PMID: 36836185; PMCID: PMC9965848.
23. Ratsika A, Cruz Pereira JS, Lynch CMK, Clarke G, Cryan JF. Microbiota-immune-brain interactions: A lifespan perspective. *Curr Opin Neurobiol.* 2023 Feb;78:102652. doi: 10.1016/j.conb.2022.102652. Epub 2022 Dec 1. PMID: 36463579.
24. Leclercq S, Mian F, Stanisz A et al. Low-dose penicillin in early life induces long-term changes in murine gut microbiota, brain cytokines, and behavior. *Nat Commun.* 2017;8:15062. https://doi.org/10.1038/ncomms15062.
25. Seifert HA, Benedek G, Nguyen H, et al. Antibiotics protect against EAE by increasing regulatory and anti-inflammatory cells. *Metab Brain Dis.* 2018 Oct;33(5):1599–1607. doi: 10.1007/s11011-018-0266-7.
26. Airola C, Severino A, Porcari S, et al. Future modulation of gut microbiota: From eubiotics to FMT, engineered bacteria, and phage therapy. *Antibiotics (Basel).* 2023 May 8;12(5):868. doi: 10.3390/antibiotics12050868.
27. Park SY, Seo GS. Fecal microbiota transplantation: Is it safe? *Clin Endosc.* 2021 Mar;54(2):157–160. doi: 10.5946/ce.2021.072.
28. Tengeler AC, Dam SA, Wiesmann M, et al. Gut microbiota from persons with attention-deficit/hyperactivity disorder affects the brain in mice. *Microbiome.* 2020;8:44. https://doi.org/10.1186/s40168-020-00816-x.
29. Sharon G, Cruz NJ, Kang DW, et al. Human gut microbiota from Autism spectrum disorder promote behavioral symptoms in mice. *Cell.* 2019 May 30;177(6):1600–1618.e17. doi: 10.1016/j.cell.2019.05.004.
30. Haifer C, Paramsothy S, Kaakoush NO, et al. Lyophilized oral faecal microbiota transplantation for ulcerative colitis (LOTUS): A randomized, double-blind, placebo-controlled trial. *Lancet Gastroenterol Hepatol.* 2022 Feb;7(2):141–151. doi: 10.1016/S2468-1253(21)00400-3.
31. Taur Y, Coyte K, Schluter J, et al. Reconstitution of the gut microbiota of antibiotic-treated patients by autologous fecal microbiota transplant. *Sci Transl Med.* 2018. Sep 26;10(460):eaap9489. doi: 10.1126/scitranslmed.aap9489.
32. Borkent J, Ioannou M, Laman JD, et al. Role of the gut microbiome in three major psychiatric disorders. *Psychol Med.* 2022 May;52(7):1222–1242. doi: 10.1017/S0033291722000897.

33. Shenderov BA. Modern condition and prospective host microecology investigations. *Microb Ecol Health Dis.* 2007;19(3):145e9. doi: 10.1080/08910600701520933.
34. Shenderov BA, Midtvedt T. Epigenomic programming: A future way to health. *Microbial Ecol Health Dis.* 2014;25:995. doi: 10.3402/mehd.v25.24145.
35. Oleskin AV, Shenderov BA. Neuromodulatory effects and targets of the SCFAs and gasotransmitters produced by the human symbiotic microbiota. *Microb Ecol Health Dis.* 2016 Jul 5;27:30971. doi: 10.3402/mehd.v27.30971.
36. Beloborodova NV. Interaction of host-microbial metabolism in sepsis. In *Sepsis*, ed. Kumar V. InTechOpen, 2017, pp. 3–19. doi: 10.5772/68046.
37. Fröhlich EE, Farzi A, Mayerhofer R, et al. Cognitive impairment by antibiotic-induced gut dysbiosis: Analysis of. *Brain Behav Immun.* 2016 Aug;56:140–155. doi: 10.1016/j.bbi.2016.02.020.
38. Hoyles L, Snelling T, Umlai UK, et al. Microbiome–host systems interactions: Protective effects of propionate upon the blood-brain barrier. *Microbiome.* 2018;6:55. doi: 10.1186/s40168-018-0439-y.
39. Giridharan VV, Generoso JS, Lence L, et al. A crosstalk between gut and brain in sepsis-induced cognitive decline. *J Neuroinflammation.* 2022 May 23;19(1):114. doi: 10.1186/s12974-022-02472-4.
40. Wenzel TJ, Gates EJ, Ranger AL, et al. Short-chain fatty acids (SCFAs) alone or in combination regulate select immune functions of microglia-like cells. *Mol Cell Neurosci.* 2020 Jun;105:103493. doi: 10.1016/j.mcn.2020.103493.
41. Li Z, Zhang F, Sun M, et al. The modulatory effects of gut microbes and metabolites on blood-brain barrier integrity and brain function in sepsis-associated encephalopathy. *PeerJ.* 2023 Mar 28;11:e15122. doi: 10.7717/peerj.15122.
42. Siddiqui MT, Cresci GAM. The immunomodulatory functions of butyrate. *J Inflamm Res.* 2021 Nov 18;14:6025–6041. doi: 10.2147/JIR.S300989.
43. Wang C, Zheng D, Weng F, et al. Sodium butyrate ameliorates the cognitive impairment of Alzheimer's disease by regulating the metabolism of astrocytes. *Psychopharmacology (Berl).* 2022 Jan;239(1):215–227. doi: 10.1007/s00213-021-06025-0.
44. Zhang H, Xu J, Wu Q, et al. Gut microbiota mediates the susceptibility of mice to sepsis-associated encephalopathy by butyric acid. *J Inflamm Res.* 2022 Mar 30;15:2103–2119. doi: 10.2147/JIR.S350566.
45. Weng J, Wu H, Xu Z, et al. The role of propionic acid at diagnosis predicts mortality in patients with septic shock. *J Crit Care.* 2018 Feb;43:95–101. doi: 10.1016/j.jcrc.2017.08.009.
46. Duscha A, Gisevius B, Hirschberg S, et al. Propionic acid shapes the multiple sclerosis disease course by an immunomodulatory mechanism. *Cell.* 2020 Mar 19;180(6):1067–1080.e16. doi: 10.1016/j.cell.2020.02.035.
47. Frost G, Sleeth ML, Sahuri-Arisoylu M, et al. The short-chain fatty acid acetate reduces appetite via a central homeostatic mechanism. *Nat Commun.* 2014 Apr 29;5:3611. doi: 10.1038/ncomms4611.
48. Wyss MT, Magistretti PJ, Buck A, et al. Labeled acetate as a marker of astrocytic metabolism. *J Cereb Blood Flow Metab.* 2011;31:1668–1674.
49. Palego L, Betti L, Rossi A, et al. Tryptophan biochemistry: Structural, nutritional, metabolic, and medical aspects in humans. *J Amino Acids.* 2016;2016:8952520. doi: 10.1155/2016/8952520.
50. Hubbard TD, Murray IA, Perdew GH. Indole and tryptophan metabolism: Endogenous and dietary routes to Ah receptor activation. *Drug Metab Dispos.* 2015 Oct;43(10):1522–1535. doi: 10.1124/dmd.115.064246.
51. Kawajiri K, Fujii-Kuriyama Y. The aryl hydrocarbon receptor: A multifunctional chemical sensor for host defence and homeostatic maintenance. *Exp Anim.* 2017 May 3;66(2):75–89. doi: 10.1538/expanim.16-0092.
52. Dong F, Hao F, Murray IA, et al. Intestinal microbiota-derived tryptophan metabolites are predictive of Ah receptor activity. *Gut Microbes.* 2020 Nov 9;12(1):1–24. doi: 10.1080/19490976.2020.1788899.
53. Wei GZ, Martin KA, Xing PY, et al. Tryptophan-metabolizing gut microbes regulate adult neurogenesis via the aryl hydrocarbon receptor. *Proc Natl Acad Sci U S A.* 2021 Jul 6;118(27):e2021091118. doi: 10.1073/pnas.2021091118.
54. Beloborodova NV, Grechko AV, Olenin AY. Metabolomic discovery of microbiota dysfunction as the cause of pathology. In *Metabolomics - New Insights into Biology and Medicine.* IntechOpen, 2020. http://doi.org/10.5772/intechopen.87176.

55. Beloborodova NV, Chernevskaya EA, Getsina ML. Indolic structure metabolites as potential biomarkers of non-infectious diseases. *Curr Pharm Des.* 2021;27(2):238–249. doi: 10.2174/13816128 26666201022121653.
56. Legan TB, Lavoie B, Mawe GM. Direct and indirect mechanisms by which the gut microbiota influence host serotonin systems. *Neurogastroenterol Motil.* 2022 Oct;34(10):e14346. doi: 10.1111/ nmo.14346.
57. Yano JM, Yu K, Donaldson GP, Shastri GG, et al. Indigenous bacteria from the gut microbiota regulate host serotonin biosynthesis. *Cell.* 2015 Apr 9;161(2):264–276. doi: 10.1016/j.cell.2015.02.047. Erratum in: *Cell.* 2015 Sep 24;163:258.
58. Chyan YJ, Poeggeler B, Omar RA, et al. Potent neuroprotective properties against the Alzheimer beta-amyloid by an endogenous melatonin-related indole structure, indole-3-propionic acid. *J Biol Chem.* 1999 Jul 30;274(31):21937–21942. doi: 10.1074/jbc.274.31.21937.
59. Dodd D, Spitzer MH, Van Treuren W, et al. A gut bacterial pathway metabolizes aromatic amino acids into nine circulating metabolites. *Nature.* 2017;551:648–652. doi: 10.1038/nature24661.
60. Elsden SR, Hilton MG, Waller JM. The end products of the metabolism of aromatic amino acids by *Clostridia. Arch Microbiol.* 1976 Apr 1;107(3):283–288. doi: 10.1007/BF00425340.
61. Beloborodova NV, Sarshor YN, Bedova AY, et al. Involvement of aromatic metabolites in the pathogenesis of septic shock. *Shock.* 2018 Sep;50(3):273–279. doi: 10.1097/SHK.0000000000001064.
62. Beloborodova NV, Baĭramov IT, Olenin A, et al. Exometabolites of some anaerobic microorganisms of human microflora. *Biomed Khim.* 2011 Jan–Feb;57(1):95–105. doi: 10.18097/pbmc20115701095.
63. Moss CW, Lambert MA, Goldsmith DJ. Production of hydrocinnamic acid by *Clostridia. Appl. Microbiol.* 1970;19:375–378. doi: 10.1128/am.19.2.375-378.1970.
64. Beloborodova NV. Serum aromatic microbial metabolites as biological markers in intensive care. In *Biomarkers in Trauma, Injury and Critical Care. Biomarkers in Disease: Methods, Discoveries, and Applications*, Eds. Rajendram R, Preedy VR, Patel VB, Springer, Cham. 2023. Chapter 13, pp. 245–268. https://doi.org/10.1007/978-3-031-07395-3_64.
65. Beloborodova NV. Integration of metabolism in man and his microbiome in critical conditions. *Gen. Reanimatol.* 2012;8(4):42. https://doi.org/10.15360/1813-9779-2012-4-42.
66. Lin P, Ding B, Feng C, et al. Prevotella and Klebsiella proportions in fecal microbial communities are potential characteristic parameters for patients with major depressive disorder. *J Affect Disord.* 2017 Jan 1;207:300–304. doi: 10.1016/j.jad.2016.09.051.
67. Simpson CA, Diaz-Arteche C, Eliby D, et al. The gut microbiota in anxiety and depression - A systematic review. *Clin Psychol Rev.* 2021;83:101943. DOI https://doi.org/10.1016/j.cpr.2020.101943.
68. Mayneris-Perxachs J, Castells-Nobau A, Arnoriaga-Rodríguez M, et al. Microbiota alterations in proline metabolism impact depression. *Cell Metab.* 2022 May 3;34(5):681–701.e10. doi: 10.1016/j. cmet.2022.04.001.
69. Zhu J, Zhang M, Han T, et al. Exploring the biomarkers of sepsis-associated encephalopathy (SAE): Metabolomics evidence from gas chromatography-mass spectrometry. *Biomed Res Int.* 2019 Nov 12;2019:2612849. doi: 10.1155/2019/2612849.
70. Chernevskaya EA, Beloborodova NV. Microbiota-oriented diagnostic, and therapy in sepsis, utopia or necessity? In *Infectious Process and Sepsis*, Ed. Nery V. IntechOpen, Rijeka, 2019. doi: 10.5772/ intechopen.89187.
71. Adesso S, Magnus T, Cuzzocrea S, et al. Indoxyl sulfate affects glial function increasing oxidative stress and neuroinflammation in chronic kidney disease: Interaction between astrocytes and microglia. *Front Pharmacol.* 2017 Jun 12;8:370. doi: 10.3389/fphar.2017.00370.
72. MacFabe DF. Enteric short-chain fatty acids: Microbial messengers of metabolism, mitochondria, and mind: Implications in Autism spectrum disorders. *Microb Ecol Health Dis.* 2015 May 29;26:28177. doi: 10.3402/mehd.v26.28177.
73. Jaglin M, Rhimi M, Philippe C, et al. Indole, a signaling molecule produced by the gut microbiota, negatively impacts emotional behaviors in rats. *Front Neurosci.* 2018 Apr 9;12:216. doi: 10.3389/ fnins.2018.00216.

74. Carpenedo R., Mannaioni G., Moroni F. Oxindole, a sedative tryptophan metabolite, accumulates in the blood and brain of rats with acute hepatic failure. *J. Neurochem.* 70, 1998–2003. doi: 10.1046/j.1471-4159.1998.70051998.x.
75. Clarke G, Grenham S, Scully P, et al. The microbiome-gut-brain axis during early life regulates the hippocampal serotonergic system in a sex-dependent manner. Mol. Psychiatry. 2013. 18, 666–673. doi: 10.1038/mp.2012.77.
76. Mertens KL, Kalsbeek A, Soeters MR, et al. Bile acid signaling pathways from the enterohepatic circulation to the central nervous system. *Front Neurosci.* 2017 Nov 7;11:617. doi: 10.3389/fnins.2017.00617.
77. Palmela I, Correia L, Silva RF, et al. Hydrophilic bile acids protect human blood-brain barrier endothelial cells from disruption by unconjugated bilirubin: An in vitro study. *Front Neurosci.* 2015;9:80. doi: 10.3389/fnins.2015.0008027.
78. Krähenbühl S, Talos C, Fischer S, et al. Toxicity of bile acids on the electron transport chain of isolated rat liver mitochondria. *Hepatology.* 1994 Feb;19(2):471–479. doi: 10.1002/hep.1840190228.
79. Quinn M, McMillin M, Galindo C, et al. Bile acids permeabilize the blood-brain barrier after bile duct ligation in rats via Rac1-dependent mechanisms. *Dig Liver Dis.* 2014;46(6):527–534. doi: 10.1016/j.dld.2014.01.159.
80. Sinha SR, Haileselassie Y, Nguyen LP, et al. Dysbiosis-induced secondary bile acid deficiency promotes intestinal inflammation. *Cell Host Microbe.* 2020 Apr 8;27(4):659–670.e5. doi: 10.1016/j.chom.2020.01.021.
81. Kowalski K, Mulak A. Brain-gut-microbiota axis in Alzheimer's disease. *J Neurogastroenterol Motil.* 2019 Jan 31;25(1):48–60. doi: 10.5056/jnm18087.
82. Mulak A. Bile acids as key modulators of the brain-gut-microbiota axis in Alzheimer's disease. *J Alzheimers Dis.* 2021;84(2):461–477. doi: 10.3233/JAD-210608.
83. Garcia CJ, Kosek V, Beltrán D, et al. Production of new microbially conjugated bile acids by human gut microbiota. *Biomolecules.* 2022 May 11;12(5):687. doi: 10.3390/biom12050687.

Chapter 4

Clinical assessment of sepsis-associated encephalopathy

Irina A. Savvina[1,2]*, MD., Ph.D., Kristina M. Bykova[1], MD., Eleonora T. Nazaralieva[3], MD., Ph.D.

[1] Department of Anesthesiology and Intensive Care, Almazov National Medical Research Centre of Ministry of Health Care of Russian Federation, Saint Petersburg, Russian Federation

[2] Department of Anesthesiology and Intensive Care named after V.L. Vanevskiy of the North-Western State Medical University named after Ilya I. Mechnikov of the Ministry of Health of Russian Federation, Saint Petersburg, Russian Federation

[3] Department of Pediatric Neurosurgery, Almazov National Medical Research Centre of Ministry of Health Care of Russian Federation, Saint Petersburg, Russian Federation

Abstract

Dysfunction of the central nervous system in sepsis is realized in the form of sepsis-associated encephalopathy (SAE) with various levels of neurological deficit, including delirium and coma. SAE is a heterogeneous condition due to variability in pathogens, pathophysiology, and treatment. Acute cerebral insufficiency remains a frequent complication of sepsis, with chronic consequences in some cases because the brain is an organ that can be severely affected during episodes of infection. Septic encephalopathy, being a risk factor for long-term disorders of consciousness and mortality, has been identified as an independent syndrome and requires further clinical study to develop diagnostic approaches and prognosis.

Keywords: sepsis-associated encephalopathy, delirium, coma, long-term cognitive impairment, polyneuropathy, dysautonomia.

Introduction

Sepsis is still the leading cause of death in critically ill patients. With over 19 million patients worldwide diagnosed with sepsis each year and approximately 5.3 million patients dying from it (Rudd et al. 2020), sepsis is a major health problem worldwide. Neurological complications,

* Corresponding author: Irina A. Savvina, Professor, MD., Ph.D.
e-mail address: irinasavvina@mail.ru

Editor: Irina A. Savvina, Natalia V. Beloborodova and Tatyana N. Trofimova
In: Sepsis-Associated Encephalopathy
ISBN: 979-8-89113-178-1

such as long-term cognitive impairment, delirium, coma, reduced activity and exercise tolerance, weakness, neuropathies, and myopathies, have a strong impact not only on mortality but also on persistent morbidity and reduced quality of life in survivors. It is important to note that cognitive impairment is a common clinical syndrome in patients with sepsis, especially in the elderly. Thus, SAE is a neurological dysfunction of the central nervous system caused by sepsis (Mazeraud, Bozza, and Sharshar 2018).

SAE diagnostics

Two key prerequisites for a diagnosis of SAE are the presence of an extracranial infection and an impaired mental state. The primary clinical sign of SAE is a change in mental state, especially consciousness, and cognition. SAE can manifest itself both at the beginning of sepsis and later in the course of the septic process, as part of multiple organ dysfunction.

The prevalence of septic encephalopathy varies widely from 8 to 70% in critically ill patients (Gofton and Young 2012). Such a wide range can be explained by the nonspecificity of clinical manifestations and the difficulties of making a definite diagnosis. The lack of a unified nomenclature and a clear definition of neurocognitive disorders in sepsis is an additional circumstance that makes it difficult to diagnose SAE, so the use of a unified terminology will be an important first step toward setting a standard (Slooter et al. 2020).

Several conditions must be ruled out before a diagnosis of SAE is made, such as medications, electrolyte disturbances, and direct infections of the central nervous system (meningitis, encephalitis, brain abscess, and septic embolism) (Sharshar, Bozza, and Chrétien 2014).

Tachycardia is a common clinical manifestation caused by fever, hypoxia, and shock. Fever usually indicates a systemic infection and is a hallmark of sepsis. The fever itself can disrupt brain metabolism and lead to neurological damage (Sun et al. 2013). Tachycardia and fever usually indicate a severe course of diseases that are associated with a higher risk of SAE. Tachycardia is associated with cognitive impairment indirectly. According to this interpretation, delirium was accompanied by tachycardia in many patients (Sun et al. 2013).

A thorough examination of the patient, including a complete physical and neurological examination, a history of medication intake, and appropriate instrumental diagnosis in critically ill patients, is the starting point for identifying SAE.

SAE is, in fact, a diagnosis of exclusion, so the focus of clinicians should be on the rapid exclusion of primary CNS pathology. At the same time, sources of non-CNS infection should be identified and properly investigated. The differential diagnosis of SAE may include bacterial or viral meningitis, encephalitis, cerebral abscess, malignancy, major electrolyte disturbances, use of illegal or prescription drugs, traumatic brain injury, or cerebrovascular disease (Carter and Underwood 2022).

The etiology of SAE is multifactorial, with the role and significance of various factors differing between individual patients and clinical contexts. Another key consideration is the degree of pre-existing brain damage and the "cognitive reserve" that patients have (Calsavara et al. 2018).

Clinical neurological screening

SAE is a reflection of a critical illness in the central nervous system. The clinical manifestations of SAE include impaired attention, cognition, and consciousness ranging from delirium (50%) to coma (46%) (Mazeraud, Bozza, and Sharshar 2018).

Because SAE is often the first sign of organ failure in sepsis, clinicians should look for sepsis in any patient who develops delirium (Rasulo et al. 2017).

Clinical neurological screening should be performed using approved scales such as Confusion Assessment Methods for Intensive Care Unit (CAM-ICU) (Appendix 1) (Sharshar et al. 2014), Checklist for screening for delirium in intensive care (Intensive Care Delirium Screening Checklist (ICDSC)) (Appendix 2) (Gusmao-Flores et al. 2012), and Full Outline of UnResponsiveness (FOUR) Score (Appendix 3).

The Glasgow Coma Score is a proven pragmatic way to assess neurological damage in the brain (Sharshar et al. 2014). Most often, SAE is determined based on the Glasgow Coma Scale and diagnosis of delirium (Yang et al. 2020; Chen et al. 2020).

Sepsis-associated delirium

Delirium is an acute disorder of attention and cognitive function in ventilated patients and is associated with worse outcomes (Ely et al. 2004). Delirium is a common and serious problem among acutely ill people. Although associated with higher mortality rates, delirium remains underdiagnosed. The fifth edition of the Diagnostic and Statistical Manual of Mental Disorders (DMS-5) of the American Psychiatric Association revised the diagnostic criteria for delirium (European Delirium Association and American Delirium Society 2014). The Intensive Care Unit Confusion Assessment Method (CAM-ICU) is one of the most validated and reliable tools for monitoring delirium in adult patients in the intensive care unit (Ely et al. 2001).

The etiological triggers of delirium can be divided into two main categories: direct brain damage and secondary in the form of abnormal stress responses (Maclullich et al. 2008). The category of direct cerebral stroke reflects dysfunction or damage to the brain, resulting mainly from indiscriminate influences, such as hypotension, hypoxia, hypercapnia, heart attacks, trauma, and drugs. In contrast, the category of aberrant stress response differs in that it includes the deleterious effects of acute stress and systemic inflammatory responses such as infection, surgical trauma, and anxiety.

While early detection of delirium is important for the eventual diagnosis of SAE, clinicians must remember that delirium and SAE are not synonymous, as SAE is only one of many causes of delirium. Gofton and Young suggest using the Confusion Assessment Method (CAM) to detect delirium in non-ICU patients because of its sensitivity (94–100%) and high positive predictive value (91–94%) (Gofton and Young 2012).

Among ventilated patients with sepsis in the intensive care unit, sepsis-associated delirium was associated with fewer days without mechanical ventilation and longer stays in the intensive care unit. Emergency surgery and additional doses of midazolam and fentanyl may be independent risk factors for sepsis-associated delirium (Yamamoto et al. 2020).

For emergency care, the Months of the Year Backwards (MOTYB) test, which is probably the most reliable one-point bedside test for delirium, is recommended (Hasemann et al. 2021).

MOTYB is a bedside test of cognitive functioning that is very widely used in clinical practice. Its popularity among clinicians is due to its speed of administration, and its availability and acceptability to most patients since it does not require any visual or motor skills other than speech. Patients are first asked to name the months of the year ahead from January to December. They will then be asked to name the months in reverse order from December to January. Patients are considered to have passed this test by reaching July without error. MOTYB has been used to assess several cognitive areas, including attention and concentration (Meagher and Leonard

2008), executive function, working memory (Grober et al. 2011), and central processing speed (James Meagher and Regan 2015).

Current scoring methods for MOTYB are primarily based on accuracy criteria, i.e., either the number of months patients can name without error or using correct/incorrect scores for predefined thresholds such as June, July, or January (Ryan, and et al. 2013). Other methods include analysis of specific response patterns, such as missing two or more months, and repetitions (Cunningham et al. 2015). The time it takes to complete MOTYB is also used as a measure of efficiency.

The 4 A test (4AT) is a bedside rapid delirium screening tool that assesses the main signs of delirium: impaired vigilance, cognition and attention, and abrupt change or fluctuations in symptoms (Appendix 8) (Evensen et al. 2016). 4AT has high sensitivity and specificity for detecting delirium and has been approved for use in patients with acute impairment of consciousness (MacLullich et al. 2019). The use of 4AT turned out to be reasonable and, compared with qSOFA, gave a more detailed characterization of cognitive impairment and signs of delirium (Myrstad et al. 2022). In line with previous studies of critically ill older patients, researchers found that cognitive impairment or delirium symptoms were widespread already at hospital admission (Evensen et al. 2019). In particular, many patients with sepsis had a 4AT score of four or more, indicating delirium. The risk of delayed treatment of sepsis and the high workload in many emergency departments may be counterarguments for the introduction of a new diagnostic tool. However, in patients with cognitive impairment or delirium, rapid screening with the 4AT can provide important additional information. The median time spent on the 4AT assessment was only two minutes, and both nurses and physicians rated delirium screening as helpful in most cases (MacLullich et al. 2019).

SAE is one of the main causes of delirium, but delirium is not the only clinical manifestation of SAE (Zampieri et al. 2011). In addition to delirium, SAE patients often have an abnormal mental state, sleep-wake cycle disturbances, or signs of hallucinations, restlessness, or arousal (Gofton and Young 2012). Other clinical signs of SAE may include tremors, multifocal myoclonus, seizures, paratonic rigidity, and flexor or extensor posture (Sweis, Ortiz, and Biller 2016). Routine use of the CAM-ICU and ICDSC scores is mandatory for assessing delirium in patients with behavioral and mental status changes, although these scores may not be sensitive enough to detect the full spectrum of SAE (Sharshar, Bozza, and Chrétien 2014; Sweis, Ortiz, and Biller 2016). In addition, since sedation is not included in the scales used to assess delirium, it may be a confounding factor in assessing mental status. Therefore, a daily Richmond Agitation and Sedation Scale (RASS) score (Appendix 6) is highly recommended (Gilmore et al. 2015). In addition to the routine assessment of delirium, daily neurological examinations, including arousal level, brainstem function, and motor response, are the basis of neuromonitoring. The Glasgow Coma Scale (GCS) or the FOUR scale is commonly used for this purpose, especially in comatose patients (Gilmore et al. 2015).

Neuroanatomy of functional and neurological disorders in SAE is reflected in Figure 4.1.

Assessment of multiple organ dysfunction

The use of scales of multiple organ failure such as SOFA, SAPS II, allows you to determine the severity of the patient's condition for further solving therapeutic, prognostic, and legal issues. These scales are a clinical tool for assessing a patient's condition to predict the likelihood

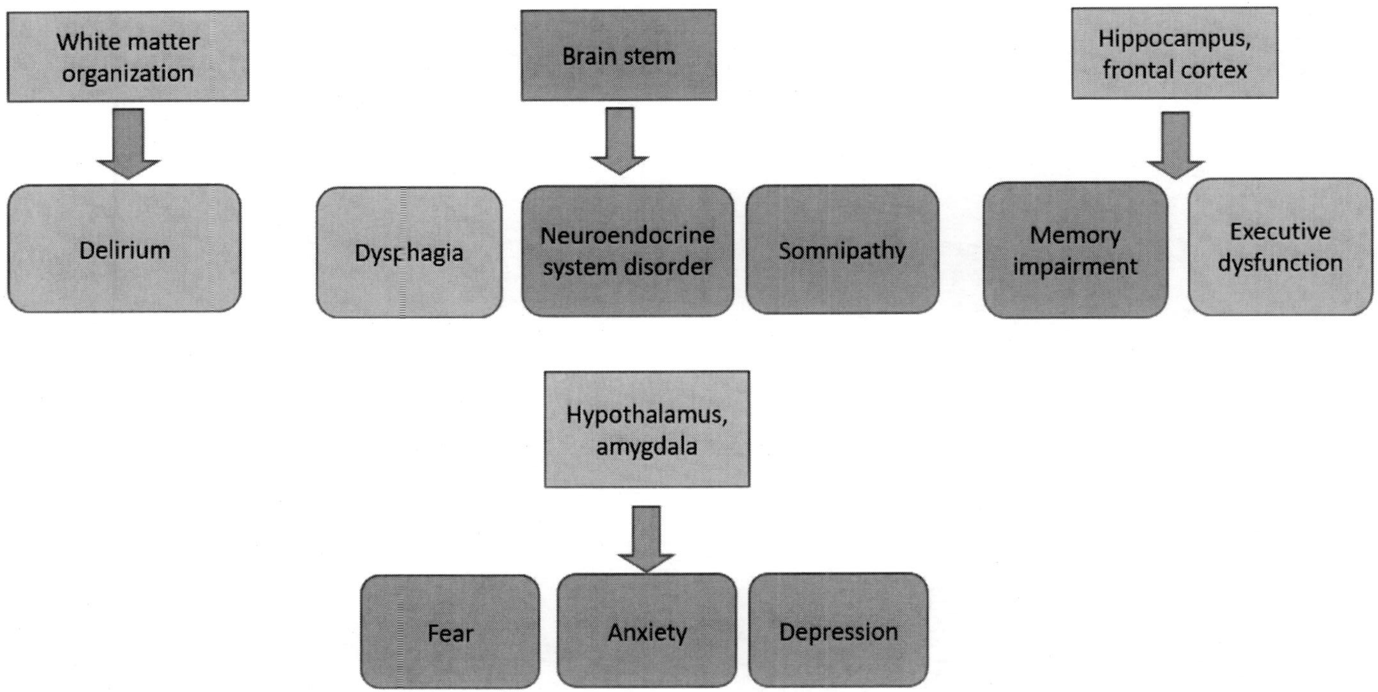

Figure 4.1 Neuroanatomy of functional and neurological disorders in SAE (Yu-Xiao Liu, Yang Yu, Jing-Peng Liu, Wen-Jia Liu, et al., 2022).

of developing a particular outcome, including death, disability, or long-term neurocognitive consequences.

SOFA multiple organ failure score is a classic tool for assessing the severity of sepsis and has good sensitivity and ability to predict outcomes (Appendix 4) (Koch et al. 2020). SOFA is positively correlated with the occurrence of delirium (Liu et al. 2022; Rahimi-Bashar et al. 2021). Delirium in SAE is more often hypoactive than hyperactive. Delirium has been reported to be more common in older ICU patients (Bugiani 2021; Kirfel et al. 2021).

The SAPS II scale is recommended for use to assess the prognosis of patients with SAE (Appendix 5) (L. Zhao et al. 2022). SAPS II is more accurate than APACHE II, a similar intensive care classification score, and is widely used in research to compare morbidity and outcomes across patients. A recent retrospective study suggested that factors such as acute renal failure, hypoglycemia, or hypernatremia, among others, may play a role in the pathophysiology of SAE (Yamaga et al. 2017).

Clinical phenotypes of SAE

Identification of clinical phenotypes in sepsis and the presence of similar biological and prognostic features may lead to more personalized therapy and targeted design of clinical trials.

Recent studies of critically ill patients with heterogeneous diseases have identified phenotypes based on the underlying pathophysiology (Xu et al. 2022; Girard et al. 2018; Peters-Sengers et al. 2022). Xu et al. have identified four clinically definable subphenotypes of sepsis that have provided additional insight into host-pathogen responses (Xu et al. 2022).

From the proposed mechanisms (Girard et al. 2018), four clinical phenotypes of SAE have been identified: ischemic-hypoxic, metabolic, mixed (ischemic-hypoxic and metabolic), and unclassified phenotype. The detailed definitions were as follows:

1. Ischemic-hypoxic SAE

   Hypoxemia or septic shock (hypoxemia was defined as two or more 15-minute intervals during which the lowest SpO_2 was <90%. Septic shock was defined by Sepsis-3 criteria, in combination with any initiation of vasopressors, lactate level > 2 mmol /L, and mean arterial pressure <65 mmHg (Singer et al. 2016)).
2. Metabolic SAE

   Blood urea nitrogen > 17.85 mmol/L or Glucose < 2.5 mmol/L orINR > 2.5 and [aspartate aminotransferase (AST) or alanine transaminase (ALT)] >200 U/L or Sodium < 120 mmol/L or Sodium > 160 mmol/L
3. Mixed SAE

   - Refers to both ischemic-hypoxic and metabolic phenotypes.
4. Unclassified EPS

   None of the above

The four SAE phenotypes had different clinical outcomes. The mixed phenotype had the worst results (Lu et al. 2023). The most significant risk factors for septic encephalopathy were also identified: age, SOFA scores, platelets, Na+, heart rate, respiratory rate, and temperature ($p = 0.05$) (Q. Zhao et al. 2023).

A large prospective cohort study showed that several delirium phenotypes predict different severity of long-term cognitive impairment (Girard et al. 2018). Ischemic-hypoxic SAE phenotypes predicted deterioration in long-term cognitive function, while patients with a metabolic phenotype did not show such an association.

Acute polyneuropathy

Systemic inflammation in sepsis can negatively affect peripheral nerves, skeletal muscles of the extremities, and the diaphragm. ICU-acquired weakness (ICUAW), along with diaphragmatic weakness, is the most common neuromuscular disorder in ICU patients, occurring in 67% of patients with sepsis (Fan et al. 2014); diaphragmatic weakness appears to develop earlier than limb weakness and is more common (Jung et al. 2016). ICUAW is defined as a symmetrical weakness that occurs after the onset of critical illness, affecting all four limbs and respiratory muscles, with the sparing of facial muscles. Muscle tone is reduced, but the deep tendon reflex may or may not be normal. ICUAW arises from varying degrees of overlap between critical illness polyneuropathy (CIP), critical illness myopathy (CIM), and muscle dysfunction atrophy (Latronico and Hermans 2020). The coexistence of CIP and CIM or critical polyneuropathy is the most common condition (Latronico and Bolton 2011). CIP is defined as a sensorimotor axonal polyneuropathy (Figure 4.2), while CIM represents an acute non-denervation primary myopathy.

In awake, cooperating patients, the diagnosis is clinical and is based on a Medical Research Council (MRCs) score, in which the strength of functional limb muscle groups is rated from 0 to 5 (i.e., none, weak, poor, acceptable, good, and normal) (Appendix 7) (Hermans et al. 2012). Scores obtained for the six bilateral muscle groups (wrist flexion, forearm flexion, shoulder abduction, ankle dorsiflexion, knee extension, and hip flexion) can range from 0 (complete paralysis) to 60 (normal muscle strength). Clinically significant ICUAW is defined as an MRC below 48/60, while severe ICUAW is defined as less than 36/60 (Hermans et al. 2012; Vanhoutte et al. 2012). A four-point ordinal scale for MRCs has recently been introduced, but its validation has not yet been completed (Vanhoutte et al. 2012).

Assessment of the functional state of the autonomic nervous system

Assessment of the functional state of the autonomic nervous system is carried out by calculating the Kerdo autonomic index, assessing the severity of pain using the Behavioral Pain Scale (BPS) (Appendix 9); brainstem scores (Pittsburg BrainStem Score (PBSS)) (Appendix 10); trends in the patient's hemodynamic profile with invasive measurement of systemic hemodynamics, assessment of heart rate variability (variable cardiointervalography), thermometry (peripheral and central), photoplethysmographic assessment of the perfusion index, quantitative assessment of muscle strength on the MRC scale; diagnosis of the severity of the syndrome of paroxysmal sympathetic hyperactivity in case of its development with gross dysfunction of the oral parts of the brainstem.

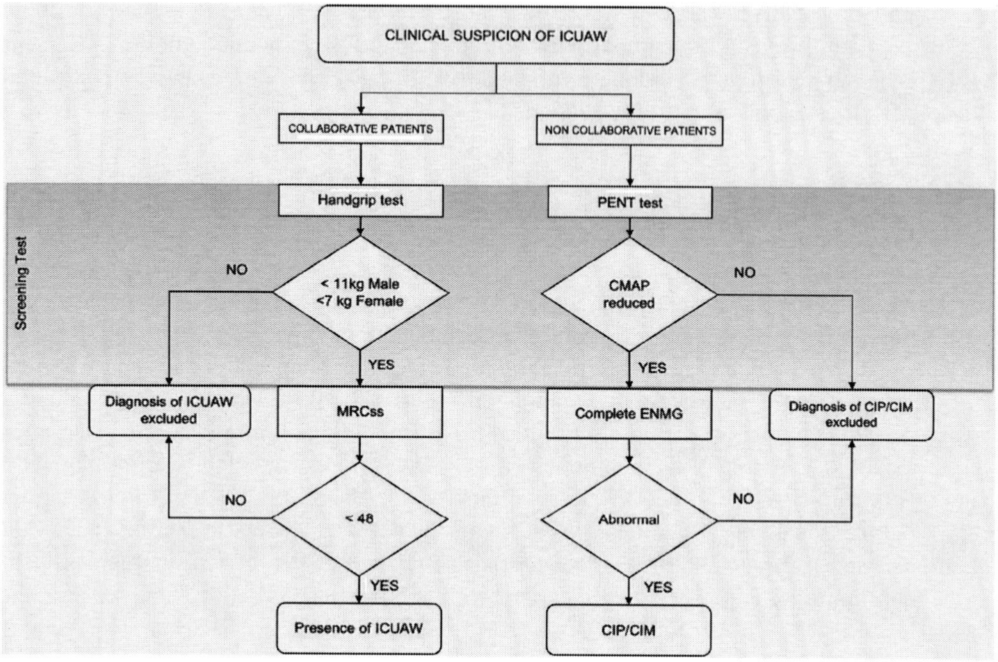

Figure 4.2 Diagnostic flowchart for ICU-acquired weakness (ICUAW), critical illness polyneuropathy, and critical illness myopathy. CMAP, compound muscle action potential; ENMG, electroneuromyography; MRCss, Medical Research Council Sum Score; PENT, peroneal nerve test (Simone Piva, Michele Bertoni, Nicola Gitti, Francesco A. Rasulo, Nicola Latronico, 2023).

Delayed cognitive impairment

Although SAE is a reversible syndrome, mild to moderate residual neuropsychiatric symptoms, including depression, anxiety, or cognitive impairment, may persist in up to 40% of patients up to 1 year after hospital discharge (Barichello et al. 2019).

In a large multicenter prospective cohort study, Pandharipande et al. (2013) studied the general critically ill patient population to quantify the incidence of cognitive impairment at 3 and 12 months after ICU discharge, as well as to investigate any potential risk factors associated with ICU stay. The study found that patients' global cognitive scores were 1.5 below the average for the general population and were similar to those of patients with mild cognitive impairment. In particular, after 3 months, 40% of patients had worse overall cognitive performance than those observed after moderate traumatic brain injury, and 26% had performance similar to those of patients with mild Alzheimer's disease. This impairment was also confirmed after 12 months, meaning that cognitive impairments tend to persist for a long time. In addition, the same study found that cognitive impairment after critical illness was not limited to the elderly and that overall cognitive performance scores were low regardless of the severity of comorbidities. A study by Pandharipande et al. included the general population of ICU patients admitted to the ICU, regardless of their initial diagnosis; however, 30% of patients had an initial diagnosis of sepsis, suggesting that even after an acute event, patients with severe sepsis had long-term functional and cognitive impairment.

Other studies have been conducted to examine sepsis and septic shock as independent variables associated with long-term cognitive impairment. In particular, a prospective cohort study conducted by Iwashyna et al. (2010) included survivors of severe sepsis to determine the change in cognitive impairment and physical functioning compared to their pre-sepsis state, with each patient acting as their control. The authors found that an episode of severe sepsis was associated with clinically significant progression to moderate or severe cognitive impairment and that this outcome was not associated with the presence of pre-existing cognitive impairment. In addition, the long-term negative effects of sepsis were associated not only with cognitive but also with functional outcomes, since patients with initially better physical functioning had worse outcomes. Another important finding by Iwashyna was that changes in functional and cognitive outcomes after severe sepsis were worse than those observed after general hospitalization, suggesting that severe sepsis may be an independent risk factor for long-term cognitive and functional impairment.

The time window for long-term cognitive impairment has been investigated but with conflicting results. Calsavara et al. (2018) evaluated patients with sepsis at discharge from the intensive care unit and 12 months later, reporting early deterioration in the Mini-Mental State Examination (MMSE) and constructive practice immediately after discharge from the intensive care unit with partial improvement after 12 months. In contrast to these results, a prospective study by Wang et al. (2021) showed no drastic cognitive decline after sepsis but showed a faster cognitive decline in the long term. In particular, this study showed that compared with the control population, the cognitive decline accelerated seven times, and the likelihood of cognitive impairment increased by 8% each year after a septic event. Although the two studies have different results regarding the immediate phase of sepsis, both of them confirm the presence of long-term cognitive decline that persists even after 12 months.

All of these studies support an association between an episode of severe sepsis and the development of long-term cognitive and functional impairment.

In summary, neurological and cognitive deficits in lesions of various brain structures in sepsis in patients with SAE are reflected in Figure 4.3.

Conclusion

The scales are a clinical tool for assessing the condition of a severe septic intensive care patient to predict the likelihood of developing a particular outcome, including death, disability, or long-term neurocognitive consequences.

The creation of a universal tool for assessing the severity of encephalopathy and determining the dynamics of recovery of neurocognitive functions in a particular patient will help the practitioner evaluate the effectiveness of therapeutic measures, as well as supplement specific neuroprotective or metabotropic therapy.

Despite significant advances in the treatment of sepsis, SAE is still associated with the development of acute cerebral insufficiency, severe autonomic dysfunction in the form of autonomic distress syndrome, and high mortality due to dystrophic and necrobiotic changes in the autonomic nuclei of the autonomic nervous system, as studies by pathologists have shown.

Conflict of interest: The authors declare that there is no conflict of interest.

Acknowledgments: The authors express their deep gratitude to their teachers – neurologists and neurosurgeons of the Russian Polenov Scientific Research Neurosurgical Institute – the first in the world Institute of the Surgery of the Neurological Diseases founded in 1926 in Petrograd.

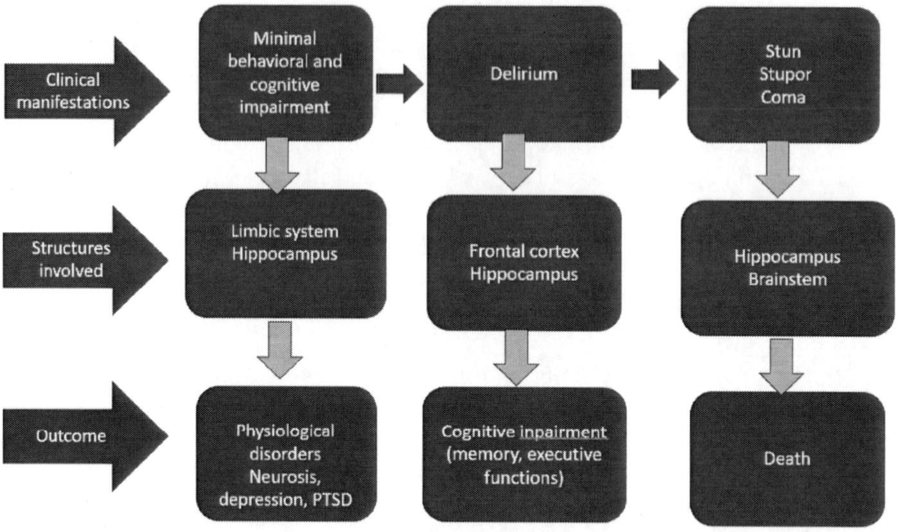

Figure 4.3 Neurological and cognitive deficits in lesions of various brain structures in sepsis in patients with SAE (Aurélien Mazeraud, Cássia Righy, Eleonore Bouchereau, Sarah Benghanem, et al., 2020).

Appendix 1. The Confusion Assessment Method for the Intensive Care Unit (CAM-ICU) Flowsheet (Ely et al. 2001).

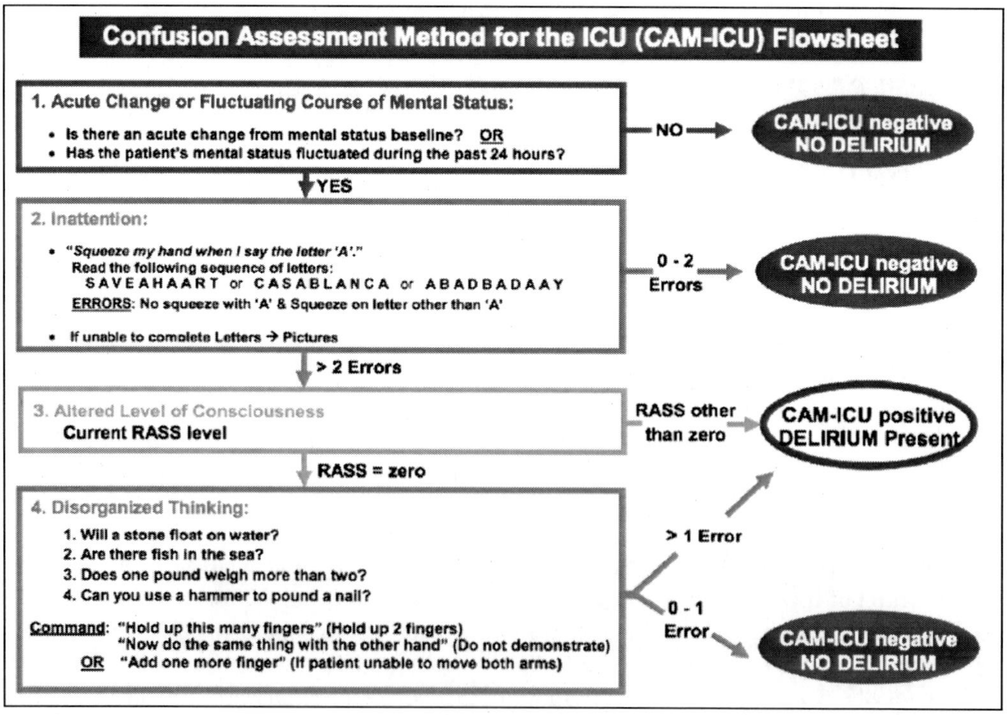

Appendix 2. Intensive Care Delirium Screening Checklist (ICDSC)

Intensive Care Delirium Screening Checklist (ICDSC)

1. Altered level of consciousness. Choose one from A to E

A. Exaggerated response to normal stimulation	SAS = 5, 6, 7 or RASS = +1 to +4	(1 point)
B. Normal wakefulness	SAS = 4 or RASS = 0	(0 points)
C. Response to mild or moderate stimulation (follows commands)	SAS = 3 or RASS = −1 to −3	(1 point)
D. Response only to intense and repeated stimulation (e.g., loud voice and pain)	SAS = 2 or RASS = −4	Stop assessment[a]
E. No response	SAS = 1 or RASS = −5	Stop assessment[a]

2. Inattention (1 point if any present)
   A. Difficulty in following commands or
   B. Easily distracted by external stimuli or
   C. Difficulty in shifting focus
   Does the patient follow you with their eyes?

3. Disorientation (1 point for any abnormality)
   A. Mistake in either time, place, or person
   Does the patient recognize ICU caregivers who have cared for him/her and not recognize those who have not? What kind of place are you in? (list examples)

4. Hallucinations or delusions (1 point for either)
   A. Equivocal evidence of hallucinations or a behavior due to hallucinations (hallucination = perception of something that is not there with no stimulus) or
   B. Delusions or gross impairment of reality testing (delusion = false belief that is fixed/unchanging)
   Any hallucinations now or over past 24 hr? Are you afraid of the people or things around you? (fear that is inappropriate to the clinical situation)

5. Psychomotor agitation or retardation (1 point for either)
   A. Hyperactivity requiring the use of additional sedative drugs or restraints in order to control potential danger (e.g., pulling IV catheters out or hitting staff) or
   B. Hypoactive or clinically noticeable psychomotor slowing or retardation
   Based on documentation and observation over shift by primary caregiver

6. Inappropriate speech or mood (1 point for either)
   A. Inappropriate, disorganized, or incoherent speech or
   B. Inappropriate mood related to events or situation
   Is the patient apathetic to current clinical situation (i.e., lack of emotion)?
   Any gross abnormalities in speech or mood? Is patient inappropriately demanding?

7. Sleep/wake cycle disturbance (1 point for any abnormality)
   A. Sleeping < 4 hr at night or
   B. Waking frequently at night (do not include wakefulness initiated by medical staff or loud environment) or
   C. Sleep ≥ 4 hr during day
   Based on primary caregiver assessment

8. Symptom fluctuation (1 point for any)
   Fluctuation of any of the above items (i.e., 1–7) over 24 hr (e.g., from one shift to another)
   Based on primary caregiver assessment

Total Intensive Care Delirium Screening Checklist score (add 1–8) ____________

[a]Delirium assessment can not be completed in patients who are stuporous or comatose.
SAS = Riker Sedation-Agitation Scale, RASS = Richmond Agitation-Sedation Scale.
Modified from Devlin JW, Marquis F, Riker RR, et al: Combined didactic and scenario-based education improves the ability of intensive care unit staff to recognize delirium at the bedside. *Crit Care* 2008; 12:R19.

Appendix 3. FOUR (Full Outline of UnResponsiveness) Score

1. Eye response Eyelids open or opened, tracking, or blinking to command +4 Eyelids open but not tracking +3 Eyelids closed but open to loud voice +2 Eyelids closed but open to pain +1 Eyelids remain closed with pain 0
2. Motor response (upper extremities) Thumbs-up, fist, or peace sign +4 Localizing to pain +3 Flexion response to pain +2 Extension response to pain +1 No response to pain or generalized myoclonus status 0
3. Brainstem reflexes Pupil and corneal reflexes present +4 One pupil wide and fixed +3 Pupil OR corneal reflex absent +2 Pupil AND corneal reflexes absent +1 Absent pupil, corneal, and cough reflexes 0
4. Respiration pattern Not intubated, regular breathing pattern +4 Not intubated, Cheyne-Stokes breathing pattern +3 Not intubated, irregular breathing +2 Breathes above ventilatory rate +1 Breathes at ventilator rate or apnea 0

Appendix 4. The Sequential Organ Failure Assessment (SOFA) score

SOFA score	1	2	3	4
Respiration PaO_2/ FIO_2 (mm Hg)	<400	<300	<220	<100
Coagulation Platelets $\times 10^3/mm^3$	<150	<100	<50	<20
Liver Bilirubin (mg/dL)	1.2–1.9	2.0–5.9	6.0–11.9	>12.0
Cardiovascular Hypotension (mcg/ kg/min)	MAP <70 mmHg	Dopamine ≤5 or dobutamine (any)	Dopamine>5 or norepinephrine ≤0.1	Dopamine>15 or norepinephrine>0.1
Glasgow Coma Score	13–14	10–12	6–9	<6
Renal Creatinine (μmol/l) or Urine output (mL/ day)	110–170	171–299	300–440 or<500	>440 or <200

Appendix 5. Simplified Acute Physiology Score (SAPS II). Evaluates health status at the start of ICU admission and predict mortality risk

1. Age (years) Below 40 (0 points) 40–59 (7 points) 60–69 (12 points) 70–74 (15 points) 75–79 (16 points) 80 and above (18 points)
2. Type of admission Scheduled surgical (0 points) Medical (6 points) Unscheduled surgical (8 points)
3. Heart rate (bpm) Below 40 (11 points) 40–69 (2 points) 70–119 (0 points) 120–159 (4 points) 160 and above (7 points)
4. Systolic blood pressure (mmHg) Below 70 (13 points) 70–99 (5 points) 100–199 (0 points) 200 and above (2 points)
5. Temperature (C or F) Below 39 °C (0 points) 39 °C and above (3 points) Below 102.2 °F (0 points) 102.2 °F and above (3 points)
6. Glasgow coma score Below 6 (26 points) 6 – 8 (13 points) 9 – 10 (7 points) 11 – 13 (5 points) 14 – 15 (0 points)
7. PaO_2 (mmHg)/FiO_2 (%) if mechanical ventilation or CPAP N/A (0 points) Below 100 (11 points) 100–199 (9 points) 200 and above (6 points)

(Continued)

Appendix 5. (Continued)

8. Urine output (L/24h) Below 0.5 (11 points) 0.5–0.99 (4 points) 1 and above (0 points)
9. Serum Urea (g/L) or BUN (mg/dL) SU: below 0.6 (0 points) SU: 0.6–1.79 (6 points) SU: 1.8 and above (10 points) BUN: below 28 (0 points) BUN: 28–83 (6 points) BUN: 84 and above (10 points)
10. Sodium (mEq/L) Below 125 (5 points) 125–144 (0 points) 145 and above (1 point)
11. Potassium (mEq/L) Below 3 (3 points) 3–4.9 (0 points) 5 and above (3 points)
12. Bicarbonate (mEq/L) Below 15 (6 points) 15–19 (3 points) 20 and above (0 points)
13. Bilirubin (mg/dL) Below 4 (0 points) 4–5.9 (4 points) 6 and above (9 points)
14. White blood cells/mm3 Less than 1,000 (12 points) 1,000–19,000 (0 points) 20,000 and above (3 points)
15. Chronic diseases None (0 points) Metastatic cancer (9 points) Hematologic malignancy (10 points) AIDS (17 points)

Appendix 6. Richmond Agitation Sedation Scale (RASS)

Score Term Description
+4 Combative Overtly combative, violent, immediate danger to staff
+3 Very agitated Pulls or removes tube(s) or catheter(s); aggressive
+2 Agitated Frequent non-purposeful movement, fights ventilator
+1 Restless Anxious but movements not aggressive vigorous
0 Alert and calm
−1 Drowsy Not fully alert, but has sustained awakening (eye-opening/eye contact) to voice (>10 seconds)
−2 Light sedation Briefly awakens with eye contact to voice (<10 seconds)
−3 Moderate sedation Movement or eye-opening to voice (but no eye contact)
−4 Deep sedation No response to voice, but movement or eye opening to physical stimulation
−5 Unarousable No response to voice or physical stimulation

Appendix 7. Medical Research Council (MRC) Scale

Grade 5: Muscle contracts normally against full resistance.
Grade 4: Muscle strength is reduced but muscle contraction can still move the joint against resistance.
Grade 3: Muscle strength is further reduced such that the joint can be moved only against gravity with the examiner's resistance completely removed. As an example, the elbow can be moved from full extension to full flexion starting with the arm hanging down at the side.
Grade 2: Muscles can move only if the resistance of gravity is removed. As an example, the elbow can be fully flexed only if the arm is maintained in a horizontal plane.
Grade 1: Only a trace or flicker of movement is seen or felt in the muscle or fasciculations are observed in the muscle.
Grade 0: No movement is observed.
The muscle scale grades muscle power on a scale of 0 to 5 to the maximum expected for that muscle.

Appendix 8. 4 AT test (Assessment test for delirium and cognitive impairment)

4AT

(label)

Patient name:

Date of birth:

Patient number:

Assessment test for delirium & cognitive impairment

Date: **Time:**

Tester:

CIRCLE

[1] ALERTNESS

This includes patients who may be markedly drowsy (eg. difficult to rouse and/or obviously sleepy during assessment) or agitated/hyperactive. Observe the patient. If asleep, attempt to wake with speech or gentle touch on shoulder. Ask the patient to state their name and address to assist rating.

Normal (fully alert, but not agitated, throughout assessment)	0
Mild sleepiness for <10 seconds after waking, then normal	0
Clearly abnormal	4

[2] AMT4

Age, date of birth, place (name of the hospital or building), current year.

No mistakes	0
1 mistake	1
2 or more mistakes/untestable	2

[3] ATTENTION

Ask the patient: "Please tell me the months of the year in backwards order, starting at December." To assist initial understanding one prompt of "what is the month before December?" is permitted.

Months of the year backwards	Achieves 7 months or more correctly	0
	Starts but scores <7 months / refuses to start	1
	Untestable (cannot start because unwell, drowsy, inattentive)	2

[4] ACUTE CHANGE OR FLUCTUATING COURSE

Evidence of significant change or fluctuation in: alertness, cognition, other mental function (eg. paranoia, hallucinations) arising over the last 2 weeks and still evident in last 24hrs

No	0
Yes	4

4 or above: possible delirium +/- cognitive impairment
1-3: possible cognitive impairment
0: delirium or severe cognitive impairment unlikely (but delirium still possible if [4] information incomplete)

4AT SCORE ☐

GUIDANCE NOTES Version 1.2. Information and download: **www.the4AT.com**

The 4AT is a screening instrument designed for rapid initial assessment of delirium and cognitive impairment. A score of 4 or more *suggests* delirium but is not diagnostic: more detailed assessment of mental status may be required to reach a diagnosis. A score of 1-3 suggests cognitive impairment and more detailed cognitive testing and informant history-taking are required. A score of 0 does not definitively exclude delirium or cognitive impairment: more detailed testing may be required depending on the clinical context. Items 1-3 are rated *solely on observation of the patient at the time of assessment*. Item 4 requires information from one or more source(s), eg. your own knowledge of the patient, other staff who know the patient (eg. ward nurses), GP letter, case notes, carers. The tester should take account of communication difficulties (hearing impairment, dysphasia, lack of common language) when carrying out the test and interpreting the score.

Alertness: Altered level of alertness is very likely to be delirium in general hospital settings. If the patient shows significant altered alertness during the bedside assessment, score 4 for this item. **AMT4 (Abbreviated Mental Test - 4):** This score can be extracted from items in the AMT10 if the latter is done immediately before. **Acute Change or Fluctuating Course:** Fluctuation can occur without delirium in some cases of dementia, but marked fluctuation usually indicates delirium. To help elicit any hallucinations and/or paranoid thoughts ask the patient questions such as, "Are you concerned about anything going on here?"; "Do you feel frightened by anything or anyone?"; "Have you been seeing or hearing anything unusual?"

https://www.the4at.com/

Appendix 9. Behavioral Pain Scale (BPS)

Item	Description	Score
Facial expression	Relaxed	1
	Partially tightened (e.g., brow lowering)	2
	Fully tightened (e.g., eyelid closing)	3
	Grimacing	4
Upper limbs	No movement	1
	Partially bent	2
	Fully bent with finger flexion	3
	Permanently retracted	4
Compliance with ventilation	Tolerating movement	1
	Coughing but tolerating ventilation for most of the time	2
	Fighting ventilator	3
	Unable to control ventilation	4

Appendix 10. Pittsburgh Brainstem Score (PBSS)

Brain stem reflex	Finding	Points
Lash reflex	Present either side	2
	Absent both sides	1
Corneal reflex	Present either side	2
	Absent both sides	1
Doll's eye and/or ice water calorics	Present either side	2
	Absent both sides	1
Right pupil reaction to light	Present	2
	Absent	1
Left pupil reaction to light	Present	2
	Absent	1
Gag and/or cough reflex	Present	2
	Absent	1

References

Barichello, Tatiana, Pavani Sayana, Vijayasree V. Giridharan, Anithachristy S. Arumanayagam, Boomadevi Narendran, Amanda Della Giustina, Fabricia Petronilho, João Quevedo, and Felipe Dal-Pizzol. 2019. «Long-Term Cognitive Outcomes After Sepsis: A Translational Systematic Review». *Molecular Neurobiology* 56 (1): 186–251. https://doi.org/10.1007/s12035-018-1048-2.

Bugiani, Orso. 2021. «Why Is Delirium More Frequent in the Elderly?» *Neurological Sciences: Official Journal of the Italian Neurological Society and the Italian Society of Clinical Neurophysiology* 42 (8): 3491–3503. https://doi.org/10.1007/s10072-021-05339-3.

Calsavara, Allan J. C., Priscila A. Costa, Vandack Nobre, and Antonio L. Teixeira. 2018. «Factors Associated With Short and Long Term Cognitive Changes in Patients with Sepsis». *Scientific Reports* 8 (1): 4509. https://doi.org/10.1038/s41598-018-22754-3.

Carter, Bethan L., and Jonathan Underwood. 2022. «Sepsis and the Brain: A Review for Acute and General Physicians». *Clinical Medicine* 22 (5): 392–95. https://doi.org/10.7861/clinmed.2022-0346.

Chen, Jiayi, Xiaobei Shi, Mengyuan Diao, Guangyong Jin, Ying Zhu, Wei Hu, and Shaosong Xi. 2020. «A Retrospective Study of Sepsis-Associated Encephalopathy: Epidemiology, Clinical Features, and Adverse Outcomes». *BMC Emergency Medicine* 20 (1): 77. https://doi.org/10.1186/s12873-020-00374-3.

Cunningham, E. L., A. P. Passmore, D. F. McAuley, and B. McGuinness. 2015. «Reciting the Months of the Year Backwards: What Is a "normal" Score?» *Age and Ageing* 44 (3): 537–38. https://doi.org/10.1093/ageing/afv056.

Della Giovampaola, Maria, Irene Cavalli, and Luciana Mascia. 2022. «Neuropsychological Outcome of Critically Ill Patients with Severe Infection». *Biomedicines* 10 (3): 526. https://doi.org/10.3390/biomedicines10030526.

Ely, E. W., R. Margolin, J. Francis, L. May, B. Truman, R. Dittus, T. Speroff, S. Gautam, G. R. Bernard, and S. K. Inouye. 2001. «Evaluation of Delirium in Critically Ill Patients: Validation of the Confusion Assessment Method for the Intensive Care Unit (CAM-ICU)». *Critical Care Medicine* 29 (7): 1370–79. https://doi.org/10.1097/00003246-200107000-00012.

Ely, E. Wesley, Ayumi Shintani, Brenda Truman, Theodore Speroff, Sharon M. Gordon, Frank E. Harrell, Sharon K. Inouye, Gordon R. Bernard, and Robert S. Dittus. 2004. «Delirium as a Predictor of Mortality in Mechanically Ventilated Patients in the Intensive Care Unit». *JAMA* 291 (14): 1753–62. https://doi.org/10.1001/jama.291.14.1753.

European Delirium Association and American Delirium Society. 2014. «The DSM-5 Criteria, Level of Arousal and Delirium Diagnosis: Inclusiveness Is Safer». *BMC Medicine* 12 (October): 141. https://doi.org/10.1186/s12916-014-0141-2.

Evensen, Sigurd, Thea Forr, Ahmad Al-Fattal, Cathrine de Groot, Greger Lønne, Edith Roth Gjevjon, Geir V. Berg, and Sverre Bergh. 2016. «Nytt verktøy for å oppdage delirium og kognitiv svikt». *Tidsskrift for Den norske legeforening*, February. https://doi.org/10.4045/tidsskr.15.1334.

Evensen, Sigurd, Ingvild Saltvedt, Anette Hylen Ranhoff, Marius Myrstad, Christian Myrstad, Marte Mellingsæter, Marte Sofie Wang-Hansen, and Bjørn Erik Neerland. 2019. «Delirium og kognitiv svikt blant eldre i norske akuttmottak». *Tidsskrift for Den norske legeforening*, March. https://doi.org/10.4045/tidsskr.18.0578.

Fan, Eddy, Fern Cheek, Linda Chlan, Rik Gosselink, Nicholas Hart, Margaret S. Herridge, Ramona O. Hopkins, et al. 2014. «An Official American Thoracic Society Clinical Practice Guideline: The Diagnosis of Intensive Care Unit-Acquired Weakness in Adults». *American Journal of Respiratory and Critical Care Medicine* 190 (12): 1437–46. https://doi.org/10.1164/rccm.201411-2011ST.

Gilmore, Emily J., Nicolas Gaspard, Huimahn A. Choi, Emily Cohen, Kristin M. Burkart, David H. Chong, Jan Claassen, and Lawrence J. Hirsch. 2015. «Acute Brain Failure in Severe Sepsis: A Prospective Study in the Medical Intensive Care Unit Utilizing Continuous EEG Monitoring». *Intensive Care Medicine* 41 (4): 686–94. https://doi.org/10.1007/s00134-015-3709-1.

Girard, Timothy D., Jennifer L. Thompson, Pratik P. Pandharipande, Nathan E. Brummel, James C. Jackson, Mayur B. Patel, Christopher G. Hughes, et al. 2018. «Clinical Phenotypes of Delirium during Critical Illness and Severity of Subsequent Long-Term Cognitive Impairment: A Prospective Cohort Study». *The Lancet: Respiratory Medicine* 6 (3): 213–22. https://doi.org/10.1016/S2213-2600(18)30062-6.

Gofton, Teneille E., and G. Bryan Young. 2012. «Sepsis-Associated Encephalopathy». *Nature Reviews: Neurology* 8 (10): 557–66. https://doi.org/10.1038/nrneurol.2012.183.

Grober, Ellen, Charles B. Hall, Steven R. Hahn, and Richard B. Lipton. 2011. «Memory Impairment and Executive Dysfunction Are Associated with Inadequately Controlled Diabetes in Older Adults». *Journal of Primary Care & Community Health* 2 (4): 229–33. https://doi.org/10.1177/2150131911409945.

Gusmao-Flores, Dimitri, Jorge Ibrain Figueira Salluh, Ricardo Ávila Chalhub, and Lucas C. Quarantini. 2012. «The Confusion Assessment Method for the Intensive Care Unit (CAM-ICU) and Intensive Care Delirium Screening Checklist (ICDSC) for the Diagnosis of Delirium: A Systematic Review and Meta-Analysis of Clinical Studies». *Critical Care (London, England)* 16 (4): R115. https://doi.org/10.1186/cc11407.

Hasemann, Wolfgang, Nikki Duncan, Caoimhe Clarke, Eva Nouzova, Lisa-Marie Süßenbach, Catriona Keerie, Valentina Assi, et al. 2021. «Comparing Performance on the Months of the Year Backwards Test in Hospitalised Patients with Delirium, Dementia, and No Cognitive Impairment: An Exploratory Study». *European Geriatric Medicine* 12 (6): 1257–65. https://doi.org/10.1007/s41999-021-00521-4.

Hermans, Greet, Beatrickx Clerckx, Tine Vanhullebusch, Johan Segers, Goele Vanpee, Christophe Robbeets, Michael Paul Casaer, Pieter Wouters, Rik Gosselink, and Greet Van Den Berghe. 2012. «Interobserver Agreement of Medical Research Council Sum-Score and Handgrip Strength in the Intensive Care Unit». *Muscle & Nerve* 45 (1): 18–25. https://doi.org/10.1002/mus.22219.

Iwashyna, Theodore J., E. Wesley Ely, Dylan M. Smith, and Kenneth M. Langa. 2010. «Long-Term Cognitive Impairment and Functional Disability among Survivors of Severe Sepsis». *JAMA* 304 (16): 1787–94. https://doi.org/10.1001/jama.2010.1553.

James Meagher, Maeve Leonard, and Suzanne Timmons Regan. 2015. «Months Backward Test: A Review of Its Use in Clinical Studies». *World Journal of Psychiatry* 5 (3): 305–14. https://doi.org/10.5498/wjp.v5.i3.305.

Jung, Boris, Pierre Henri Moury, Martin Mahul, Audrey de Jong, Fabrice Galia, Albert Prades, Pierre Albaladejo, Gerald Chanques, Nicolas Molinari, and Samir Jaber. 2016. «Diaphragmatic Dysfunction in Patients with ICU-Acquired Weakness and Its Impact on Extubation Failure». *Intensive Care Medicine* 42 (5): 853–61. https://doi.org/10.1007/s00134-015-4125-2.

Kirfel, Andrea, Jan Menzenbach, Vera Guttenthaler, Johanna Feggeler, Andreas Mayr, Mark Coburn, and Maria Wittmann. 2021. «Postoperative Delirium after Cardiac Surgery of Elderly Patients as an Independent Risk Factor for Prolonged Length of Stay in Intensive Care Unit and in Hospital». *Aging Clinical and Experimental Research* 33 (11): 3047–56. https://doi.org/10.1007/s40520-021-01842-x.

Koch, Christian, Fabian Edinger, Tobias Fischer, Florian Brenck, Andreas Hecker, Christian Katzer, Melanie Markmann, Michael Sander, and Emmanuel Schneck. 2020. «Comparison of QSOFA Score, SOFA Score, and SIRS Criteria for the Prediction of Infection and Mortality among Surgical Intermediate and Intensive Care Patients». *World Journal of Emergency Surgery: WJES* 15 (1): 63. https://doi.org/10.1186/s13017-020-00343-y.

Latronico, Nicola, and Charles F. Bolton. 2011. «Critical Illness Polyneuropathy and Myopathy: A Major Cause of Muscle Weakness and Paralysis». *The Lancet: Neurology* 10 (10): 931–41. https://doi.org/10.1016/S1474-4422(11)70178-8.

Latronico, Nicola, and Greet Hermans. 2020. «Critical Illness Neuromyopathy: Clinical, Electrophysiological, and Histological Diagnosis». In: *Post-Intensive Care Syndrome* Edit. by Jean-Charles Preiser, Margaret Herridge, and Elie Azoulay, 43–59. Lessons from the ICU. Cham: Springer International Publishing. https://doi.org/10.1007/978-3-030-24250-3_4.

Liu, Hui, Qing Zhao, Xiaoli Liu, Xin Hu, Li Wang, and Feihu Zhou. 2022. «Incidence and Interaction Factors of Delirium as an Independent Risk of Mortality in Elderly Patients in the Intensive Units: A Retrospective Analysis from MIMIC-IV Database». *Aging Clinical and Experimental Research* 34 (11): 2865–72. https://doi.org/10.1007/s40520-022-02215-8.

Lu, Xin, Mubing Qin, Joseph Harold Walline, Yanxia Gao, Shiyuan Yu, Zengzheng Ge, Chao Gong, Huadong Zhu, Djillali Annane, and Yi Li. 2023. «Clinical Phenotypes of Sepsis-Associated Encephalopathy: A Retrospective Cohort Study». *Shock*. https://doi.org/10.1097/SHK.0000000000002092.

Maclullich, Alasdair M. J., Karen J. Ferguson, Thomas Miller, Sophia E. J. A. de Rooij, and Colm Cunningham. 2008. «Unravelling the Pathophysiology of Delirium: A Focus on the Role of Aberrant Stress Responses». *Journal of Psychosomatic Research* 65 (3): 229–38. https://doi.org/10.1016/j.jpsychores.2008.05.019.

MacLullich, Alasdair M. J., Susan D. Shenkin, Steve Goodacre, Mary Godfrey, Janet Hanley, Antaine Stíobhairt, Elizabeth Lavender, et al. 2019. «The 4 'A's Test for Detecting Delirium in Acute Medical Patients: A Diagnostic Accuracy Study». *Health Technology Assessment (Winchester, England)* 23 (40): 1–194. https://doi.org/10.3310/hta23400.

Mazeraud, Aurélien, Fernando A. Bozza, and Tarek Sharshar. 2018. «Sepsis-Associated Encephalopathy Is Septic». *American Journal of Respiratory and Critical Care Medicine* 197 (6): 698–99. https://doi.org/10.1164/rccm.201712-2593ED.

Meagher, David, and Maeve Leonard. 2008. «The Active Management of Delirium: Improving Detection and Treatment». *Advances in Psychiatric Treatment* 14 (4): 292–301. https://doi.org/10.1192/apt.bp.107.003723.

Myrstad, Marius, Kanika Kuwelker, Sigurd Haakonsen, Therese Valebjørg, Nina Langeland, Bård Reiakvam Kittang, Guri Hagberg, Bjørn Erik Neerland, and Marit Stordal Bakken. 2022. «Delirium Screening with 4AT in Patients Aged 65 Years and Older Admitted to the Emergency Department with Suspected Sepsis: A Prospective Cohort Study». *European Geriatric Medicine* 13 (1): 155–62. https://doi.org/10.1007/s41999-021-00558-5.

Pandharipande, P. P., T. D. Girard, J. C. Jackson, A. Morandi, J. L. Thompson, B. T. Pun, N. E. Brummel, et al. 2013. «Long-Term Cognitive Impairment after Critical Illness». *The New England Journal of Medicine* 369 (14): 1306–16. https://doi.org/10.1056/NEJMoa1301372.

Peters-Sengers, Hessel, Joe M. Butler, Fabrice Uhel, Marcus J. Schultz, Marc J. Bonten, Olaf L. Cremer, Brendon P. Scicluna, Lonneke A. van Vught, Tom van der Poll, and MARS Consortium. 2022. «Source-Specific Host Response and Outcomes in Critically Ill Patients with Sepsis: A Prospective Cohort Study». *Intensive Care Medicine* 48 (1): 92–102. https://doi.org/10.1007/s00134-021-06574-0.

Rahimi-Bashar, Farshid, Ghazal Abolhasani, Nahid Manouchehrian, Nasrin Jiryaee, Amir Vahedian-Azimi, and Amirhossein Sahebkar. 2021. «Incidence and Risk Factors of Delirium in the Intensive Care Unit: A Prospective Cohort». *BioMed Research International* 2021: 6219678. https://doi.org/10.1155/2021/6219678.

Rasulo, Frank Anthony, Giuseppe Bellelli, Eugene Wesley Ely, Alessandro Morandi, Pratik Pandharipande, and Nicola Latronico. 2017. «Are You Ernest Shackleton, the Polar Explorer? Refining the Criteria for Delirium and Brain Dysfunction in Sepsis». *Journal of Intensive Care* 5 (1): 23. https://doi.org/10.1186/s40560-017-0218-z.

Rudd, Kristina E., Sarah Charlotte Johnson, Kareha M. Agesa, Katya Anne Shackelford, Derrick Tsoi, Daniel Rhodes Kievlan, Danny V. Colombara, et al. 2020. «Global, Regional, and National Sepsis Incidence and Mortality, 1990–2017: Analysis for the Global Burden of Disease Study». *Lancet (London, England)* 395 (10219): 200–211. https://doi.org/10.1016/S0140-6736(19)32989-7.

Ryan, Daniel James, Niamh Annmarie O'Regan, Ronán Ó. Caoimh, Josie Clare, Marie O'Connor, Maeve Leonard, John McFarland, et al. 2013. «Delirium in an Adult Acute Hospital Population: Predictors, Prevalence and Detection». *BMJ Open* 3 (1): e001772. https://doi.org/10.1136/bmjopen-2012-001772.

Sharshar, Tarek, Fernando Bozza, and Fabrice Chrétien. 2014. «Neuropathological Processes in Sepsis». *The Lancet Neurology* 13 (6): 534–36. https://doi.org/10.1016/S1474-4422(14)70064-X.

Sharshar, Tarek, Giuseppe Citerio, Peter J. D. Andrews, Arturo Chieregato, Nicola Latronico, David K. Menon, Louis Puybasset, Claudio Sandroni, and Robert D. Stevens. 2014. «Neurological Examination of Critically Ill Patients: A Pragmatic Approach. Report of an ESICM Expert Panel». *Intensive Care Medicine* 40 (4): 484–95. https://doi.org/10.1007/s00134-014-3214-y.

Simone Piva, Michele Bertoni, Gitti, Nicola Gitti, Francesco A. Rasulo, Nicola Latronico. 2023. Neurological Complications of Sepsis. *Current Opinion in Critical Care* 29 (2): 75–84. https://doi.org/10.1097/MCC.0000000000001022.

Singer, Mervyn, Clifford S. Deutschman, Christopher Warren Seymour, Manu Shankar-Hari, Djillali Annane, Michael Bauer, Rinaldo Bellomo, et al. 2016. «The Third International Consensus Definitions for Sepsis and Septic Shock (Sepsis-3)». *JAMA* 315 (8): 801–10. https://doi.org/10.1001/jama.2016.0287.

Slooter, Arjen J. C., Wim M. Otte, John W. Devlin, Rakesh C. Arora, Thomas P. Bleck, Jan Claassen, Matthew S. Duprey, et al. 2020. «Updated Nomenclature of Delirium and Acute Encephalopathy: Statement of Ten Societies». *Intensive Care Medicine* 46 (5): 1020–22. https://doi.org/10.1007/s00134-019-05907-4.

Sun, Gang, Shaowen Qian, Qingjun Jiang, Kai Liu, Bo Li, Min Li, Lun Zhao, Zhenyu Zhou, Karen M. von Deneen, and Yijun Liu. 2013. «Hyperthermia-Induced Disruption of Functional Connectivity in the Human Brain Network». *PloS One* 8 (4): e61157. https://doi.org/10.1371/journal.pone.0061157.

Sweis, Rochelle, Jorge Ortiz, and José Biller. 2016. «Neurology of Sepsis». *Current Neurology and Neuroscience Reports* 16 (3): 21. https://doi.org/10.1007/s11910-016-0623-z.

Vanhoutte, Els Karla, Catharina Gerritdina Faber, Sonja Ingrid van Nes, Bart Casper Jacobs, Pieter Antoon van Doorn, Rinske van Koningsveld, David Reid Cornblath, et al. 2012. «Modifying the Medical Research Council Grading System through Rasch Analyses». *Brain: A Journal of Neurology* 135 (Pt 5): 1639–49. https://doi.org/10.1093/brain/awr318.

Wang, Henry E., Mohammed M. Kabeto, Marquita Gray, Virginia G. Wadley, Paul Muntner, Suzanne E. Judd, Monika M. Safford, Jordan Kempker, and Deborah A. Levine. 2021. «Trajectory of Cognitive Decline After Sepsis». *Critical Care Medicine* 49 (7): 1083–94. https://doi.org/10.1097/CCM.0000000000004897.

Xu, Zhenxing, Chengsheng Mao, Chang Su, Hao Zhang, Ilias Siempos, Lisa K. Torres, Di Pan, Yuan Luo, Edward J. Schenck, and Fei Wang. 2022. «Sepsis Subphenotyping Based on Organ Dysfunction Trajectory». *Critical Care (London, England)* 26 (1): 197. https://doi.org/10.1186/s13054-022-04071-4.

Yamaga, Satoshi, Nobuaki Shime, Romain Sonneville, Etienne de Montmollin, and Jean-François Timsit. 2017. «Risk Factors for Sepsis-Associated Encephalopathy». *Intensive Care Medicine* 43 (10): 1548–49. https://doi.org/10.1007/s00134-017-4875-0.

Yamamoto, Tomonori, Yasumitsu Mizobata, Yu Kawazoe, Kyohei Miyamoto, Yoshinori Ohta, Takeshi Morimoto, and Hitoshi Yamamura. 2020. «Incidence, Risk Factors, and Outcomes for Sepsis-Associated Delirium in Patients with Mechanical Ventilation: A Sub-Analysis of a Multicenter Randomized Controlled Trial». *Journal of Critical Care* 56 (April): 140–44. https://doi.org/10.1016/j.jcrc.2019.12.018.

Yang, Jin, Yuanjie Li, Qingqing Liu, Li Li, Aozi Feng, Tianyi Wang, Shuai Zheng, Anding Xu, and Jun Lyu. 2020. «Brief Introduction of Medical Database and Data Mining Technology in Big Data Era». *Journal of Evidence-Based Medicine* 13 (1): 57–69. https://doi.org/10.1111/jebm.12373.

Yu-Xiao Liu, Yang Yu, Jing-Peng Liu, Wen-Jia Liu, Yang Cao, Run-Min Yan, Yong-Ming Yao. 2022. Neuroimmune Regulation in Sepsis-Associated Encephalopathy: The Interaction Between the Brain and Peripheral Immunity. *Front Neurol.* 13: 892480. https://doi.org/10.3389/fneur.2022.892480

Zampieri, Fernando Godinho, Marcelo Park, Fabio Santana Machado, and Luciano Cesar Pontes Azevedo. 2011. «Sepsis-Associated Encephalopathy: Not Just Delirium». *Clinics* 66 (10): 1825–31. https://doi.org/10.1590/S1807-59322011001000024.

Zhao, Lina, Shaowei Hou, Risu Na, Bin Liu, Zhiwei Wang, Yun Li, and Keliang Xie. 2022. «Prognostic Role of Serum Ammonia in Patients with Sepsis-Associated Encephalopathy Without Hepatic Failure». *Frontiers in Public Health* 10: 1016931. https://doi.org/10.3389/fpubh.2022.1016931.

Zhao, Qing, Jianguo Xiao, Xiaoli Liu, and Hui Liu. 2023. «The Nomogram to Predict the Occurrence of Sepsis-Associated Encephalopathy in Elderly Patients in the Intensive Care Units: A Retrospective Cohort Study». *Frontiers in Neurology* 14. https://www.frontiersin.org/articles/10.3389/fneur.2023.1084868.

Chapter 5

Neurophysiological assessment of sepsis-associated encephalopathy

Elena N. Zharova[1]*, MD., Ph.D., Irina A. Savvina[2,3], MD., Ph.D., Konstantin E. Lebedev[4], MD., Ph.D., Kristina M. Bykova[2], MD

[1] Department of Restorative Treatment and Medical Rehabilitation, Russian Polenov Scientific Research Neurosurgical Institute – the branch of the Almazov National Medical Research Centre of Ministry of Health Care of Russian Federation, Saint Petersburg, Russian Federation

[2] Department of Anesthesiology and Intensive Care, Almazov National Medical Research Centre of Ministry of Health Care of Russian Federation, Saint Petersburg, Russian Federation

[3] Department of Anesthesiology and Intensive Care named after V.L. Vanevskiy of the North-Western State Medical University named after Ilya I. Mechnikov of the Ministry of Health of Russian Federation, Saint Petersburg, Russian Federation

[4] Department of Functional Diagnostics, Almazov National Medical Research Centre of Ministry of Health Care of Russian Federation, Saint Petersburg, Russian Federation

Abstract

Neurophysiological monitoring is an important diagnostic option to complement clinical, laboratory, and instrumental methods for objectifying acute brain injury.

In particular, the registration of multimodal evoked potentials (EPs) is a neurophysiological diagnostic method used to verify damage to anatomical pathways and central nervous system (CNS) structures caused by various neurological and metabolic disorders (Madl et al. 1993, 2000; Zauner et al. 2000).

Electroencephalography is an important diagnostic tool to detect changes in the bioelectrical activity of the brain against the background of critical conditions and systemic infections. Bedside neurophysiological EEG and EP monitoring in the ICU enables clinicians to make the right decisions about the management of the resuscitated patient – prolongation of sedation, transition to the diagnostic window, change in the structure of neurovegetative blockade, etc.

* Corresponding author: Elena N. Zharova, MD., Ph.D.
e-mail: garlen@inbox.ru

Editor: Irina A. Savvina, Natalia V. Beloborodova and Tatyana N. Trofimova
In: Sepsis-Associated Encephalopathy
ISBN: 979-8-89113-178-1

This chapter assesses the diagnostic value of EEG and multimodal EPs at the first signs of SAE to make recommendations for the early diagnosis of SAE. Acute cerebral damage in the form of SAE is observed more frequently in patients with sepsis in the early stages of the disease than is usually assumed.

Keywords: multimodal (somatosensory, visual, auditory brainstem) evoked potentials, electroencephalography, sepsis-associated encephalopathy, sepsis.

Abbreviations

BAEPs – brainstem auditory-evoked potentials
BESS – non-convulsive status epilepticus
BSEG – bispectral electroencephalogram
ECEG – electrocorticoencephalography
EPs – evoked potentials
ICU – intensive care unit
PES – intermittent epileptiform discharges
SAE – sepsis-associated encephalopathy
SABD – sepsis-associated brain dysfunction
SSEPs – somatosensory-evoked potentials
TV – triphasic wave
VEPs – visual-evoked potentials

Introduction

Sepsis-associated encephalopathy (SAE) is common in critically ill patients in intensive care. Given the importance of early diagnosis of CNS damage in sepsis for timely correction of cerebral abnormalities, it is advisable to consider some types of neurophysiological monitoring that objectify acute cerebral damage.

Evoked potentials (EPs) of the brain are an objective and non-invasive neurophysiological method for studying the conduction function of the nervous system. EPs are recorded by averaging low-amplitude CNS signals in response to various stimulations.

Visual, auditory, somatosensory, motor, and cognitive EPs are distinguished, which are used to assess the corresponding conduction pathways. The method makes it possible to assess the functional state and the extent of damage to nerve structures as well as the prognosis for recovery or deterioration in the course of treatment in dynamics.

Recording of multimodal evoked potentials (VP_s) is used to check damage to anatomical pathways and CNS structures caused by various neurological and metabolic disorders (Madl et al. 1993, 2000; Zauner et al. 2000). EPs are recorded by averaging low-amplitude CNS signals in response to different stimulations.

The prognostic value of each modality varies according to the etiology of the disease. A distinction should be made between tests whose abnormalities indicate a poor prognosis (bilateral absence of N20 in SSEP studies in an anoxic coma or signs of midbrain lesions according to AEPs in traumatic brain injury) and those whose relative normality indicates a good prognosis (the integrity of boot conduction in TBI, presence of P300 cognitive evoked potentials – regardless of the etiology of coma).

The information obtained from the EP study is extremely important for the assessment of neurological status. The multimodal EP is used in neurology, neurosurgery, psychology, and psychiatry.

Together with EPs, EEG is widely used in intensive care units as continuous neuromonitoring for early detection of non-convulsive seizures in adults and neonates (Procaccio et al. 2001).

It is important to note that both EEG and EPs along with electroneuromyography (ENMG) recording is an option for non-invasive bedside neurophysiological monitoring of critically ill patients in the ICU to assess cerebral dysfunction of various etiologies, which should greatly improve the individual management of patients in the ICU (Guerit et al. 2009, 2010).

The role of neurophysiological assessment in ICU patients with sepsis and sepsis-associated encephalopathy

EEG monitoring at the bedside

Electroencephalography (EEG) allows online recording of brain bioelectrical activity patterns, providing rapid electrophysiological measurements of brain dysfunction at the bedside to complement clinical and imaging assessment of patients with encephalopathy.

Seizures and periodic discharges (a variant of abnormal EEG) are known to be common non-specific signs in critically ill patients requiring EEG monitoring and are associated with an unfavorable outcome. Both the progressive slowing of background EEG activity with increasing cerebral insufficiency and the decline in EEG reactivity to external stimuli provide important diagnostic and prognostic information (Sutter et al. 2013).

Abnormal EEG occurs earlier in severe infections and at the onset of sepsis. Thus, studies (Sutter et al. 2013; Bricolo et al. 1987) found that transient encephalopathic EEG changes can occur in humans. One hour after manifestation, diffuse slow-wave activity (θ-wave, δ-wave) is a common manifestation of SAE on the EEG.

The diagnosis of SAE may precede neurological changes in patients who have undergone EEG monitoring (Oddo et al. 2009). In two-thirds of cases, abnormal rearrangements in the EEG did not produce clinical manifestations (Guérit et al. 2009).

Sepsis with multiple organ failure may present with abnormal EEG manifestations. Diffuse or multifocal EEG abnormalities were found in the majority of patients with SAE deaths.

EEG monitoring in patients with severe infection contributes to the early detection of encephalopathy and is characterized by the appearance of diffuse slow waves, triphasic waves, and EEG suppression. EEG monitoring data for patients with sepsis from a clinical trial conducted at the Almazov National Medical Research Centre of the Ministry of Health Care of the Russian Federation for sepsis-associated encephalopathy are shown in Figures 5.1, 5.2, 5.3, and 5.4A and B.

EEG can certainly be used as a sensitive tool for the diagnosis of SAE, especially at an early stage. The EEG of patients with SAE shows the progressive delay of consciousness by theta, delta, or triphasic waves (TV), suppressed bundles, and periodic epileptiform discharges (PES) or non-convulsive status epilepticus (BESS) (Eidelman et al. 1996; Sutter et al. 2013). The mortality rate of patients with SAE correlates with the severity of abnormalities produced by EEG

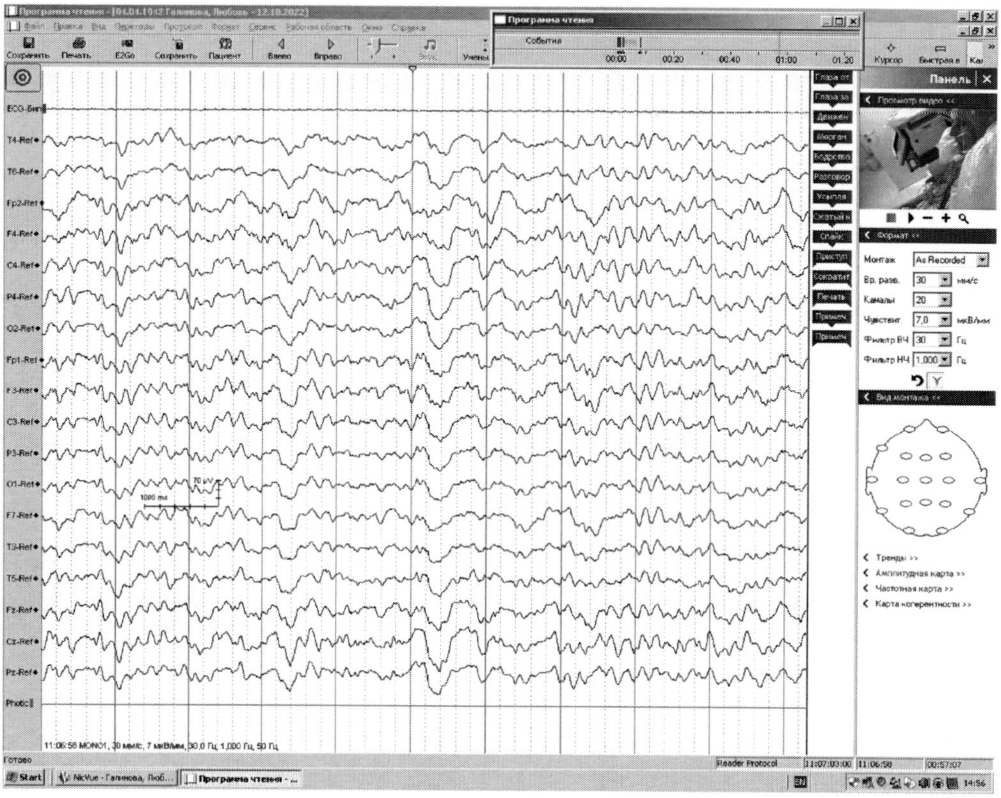

Figure 5.1 EEG of patient G., 80-year-old, on the 2nd day after sepsis diagnosis. The primary focus is on peritonitis. The patient is under the condition of a propofol infusion of 2 mg/kg/h.

On the EEG, the main rhythm is practically absent. The recording shows polymorphic activity with a predominance of the slow-wave theta band with moderate amplitude (40 μV). No interhemispheric asymmetry or paroxysmal activity was recorded. The EEG data indicate widespread changes of a diffuse nature. BIPAP-assisted ventilation: BP 14 per minute; 97% saturation with FiO_2 0.5. Inotropic support: dopamine 2.0 μg/kg/min, norepinephrine 0.15 μg/kg/min. Scale values: SOFA 9, SAPS 40, RASS −4 under sedation, FOUR 12. Discharge from the hospital on day 20.

recording (Eidelman et al. 1996; Sutter et al. 2013). The absence of EEG reactivity on the first day of sepsis is associated with mortality one year after sepsis (Chong et al. 2005).

Abnormal EEG in sepsis is more often dominated by diffuse slow waves (θ-wave, δ-wave) (Young classification) (Young et al. 1990; Zhou et al. 2022). The Young EEG is divided into four stages: Stage 0 – normal EEG, Stage 1 – the predominance of θ-waves, Stage 2 – δ-waves, Stage 3 – low amplitude EEG, θ- and δ-waves, Stage 4 – multiple triphasic waves, suppressed EEG.

EEG changes in SAE can be divided into five categories: normal EEG, θ-waveform, δ-waveform, triphasic waveform, and EEG suppression (Zhou et al. 2022).

The prognosis for SAE worsens with increasing EEG abnormalities and severity of encephalopathy. According to the Synek classification, the EEG is divided into benign (0 to 2), indeterminate (3), or malignant (4 and 5) bioelectrical activity (Synek grade). Synek grade > 3 is more

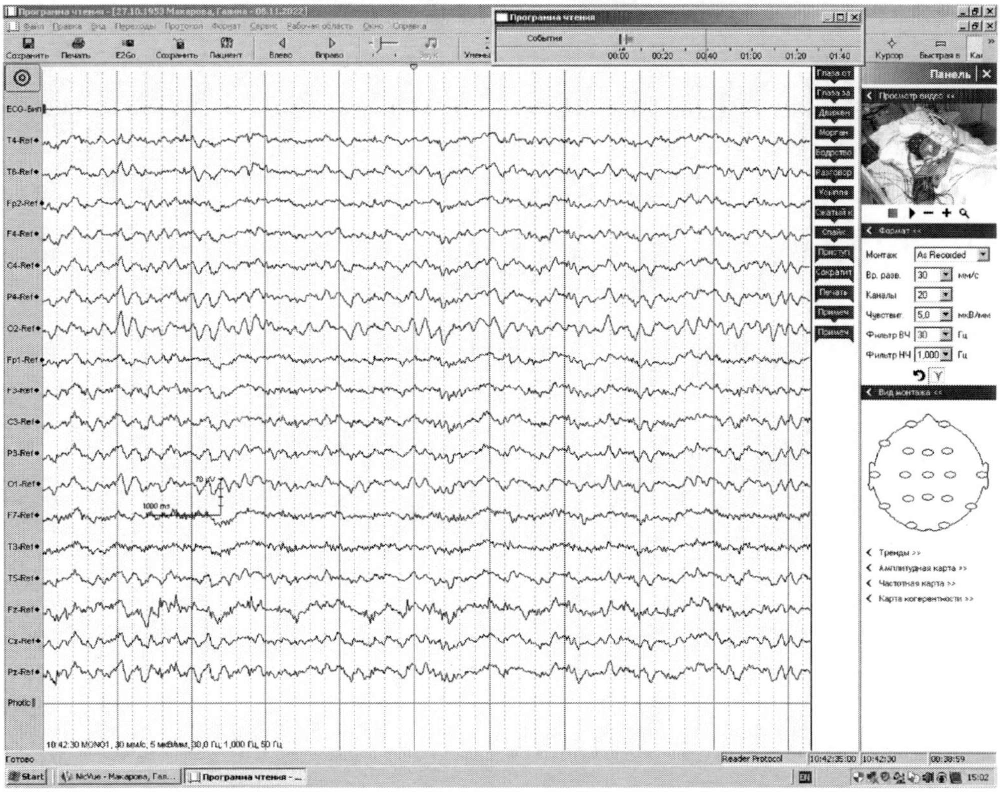

Figure 5.2 EEG of patient M., 69-year-old. The 13th day after the diagnosis of sepsis. The primary focus is on pneumonia. EEG recording with residual sedation. On the EEG the main rhythm is deformed.

The recording shows polymorphic activity dominated by a slow-wave theta region with reduced amplitude. No interhemispheric asymmetry or paroxysmal activity was recorded.
The EEG data showed widespread changes of a diffuse nature.
Compared to the EEG data of the previous study, there was some positive dynamic.
Vasopressor support with norepinephrine up to 0.2 μg/kg/min.
Scale values: SOFA 18, SAPS 51, RASS −2 under residual sedation, FOUR 11. Died on day 18.

common in the clinic. Some early EEG changes are associated with increased mortality and frequency of delirium (Ebersoldt et al. 2007; Yamanashi et al. 2022). In particular, loss of EEG response with Synek's grade ≥3 and Young's grade > 1 were risk factors for mortality on admission to the ICU. In the population with SAEs, the proportion of patients with non-convulsive status epilepticus was 17.7%. Delta waves, triphasic waves, EEG suppression, and recurrent EEG manifestations indicated an unfavorable prognosis of SAE. According to Shinozaki et al., the abnormal EEG features were potentially reversible. About 21.1% of CAE survivors after discharge and about 42.8% of CAE survivors had normal EEG after 3 months (Shinozaki et al. 2019).

Thus, the absence of an EEG response and delta waves are not only unfavorable prognostic factors in the population of patients with SAE but also risk factors for an unfavorable prognosis in other ORITs. While these signs do not provide a basis for identifying SAE, they can reliably reflect an unfavorable prognosis (Zhou et al. 2022).

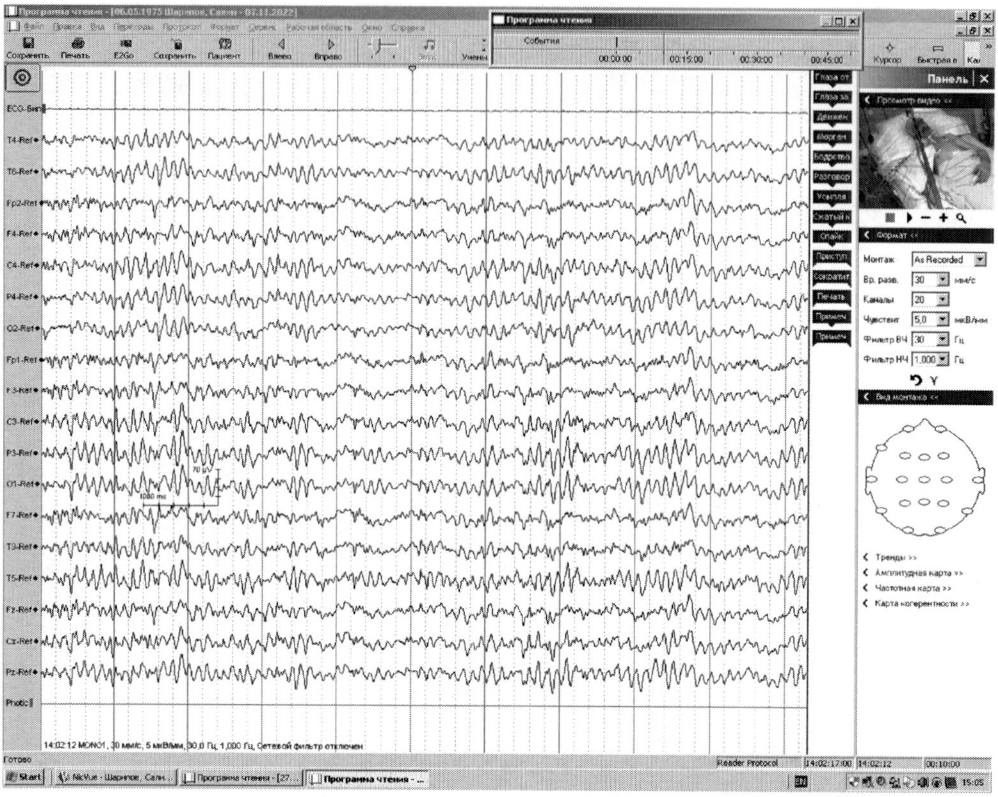

Figure 5.3 EEG of patient Sh., 47-year-old, on the 2nd day after sepsis diagnosis. The primary focus was on peritonitis. The main rhythm of the EEG is regular. Alpha activity dominates all leads. Zonal differences are not present. Against this background, episodic brief bilateral flashes of alpha waves are registered. There are no abnormalities during functional stress. The EEG data indicate moderate general changes with the involvement of the boot formations of the diencephalic level.

His condition is severe, he is conscious, adequately, spatially, and temporally oriented and has a personality of his own. Inotropic support: dopamine 2 μg/kg/min.
SOFA 7, SAPS 36, RASS 0 without sedation, no CAM-ICU delirium.
Discharge from the hospital on day 16.

Bispectral index monitoring uses frontal sensors to collect frontal EEG data and a proprietary algorithm to transform the raw EEG (Shinozaki et al. 2019). Mortality was highest in patients with sepsis with a high BSEEG score (Yamanashi et al. 2022). The bispectral electroencephalography score can predict mortality among elderly patients in general, and even among dementia patients, as soon as 30 days (Saito et al.2021). Even after adjustment for covariates, a high BSEEG score remains an important predictor of death in patients with sepsis. The BSEEG can help assess and diagnose SAE with delirium, and a high BSEEG score is a risk factor for poor prognosis of sepsis (Yamanashi, et al. 2021).

The absence of EEG reactivity predicts mortality but not functional outcomes (Sutter et al. 2013).

The responsiveness of the EEG to external simulations depends on the preservation of brainstem structures such as the ascending reticular formation but does not necessarily reflect the activity of the higher brain (Moruzzi et al. 1949). These findings highlight the importance

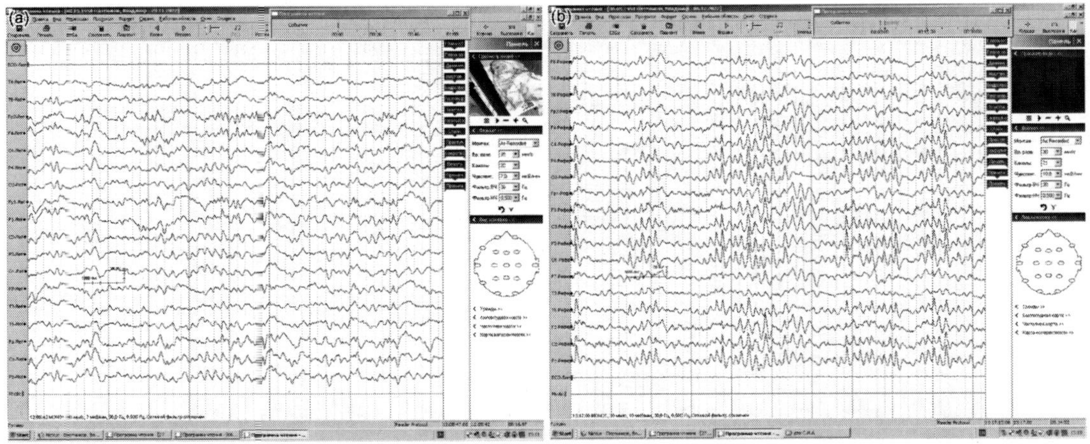

Figure 5.4A, B EEG of patient P., 64-year-old. The primary focus of infection – peritonitis.

A – EEG on the 2nd day after the diagnosis of sepsis under the condition of propofol sedation of 2 mg/kg/h.

There is practically no main rhythm on the EEG. The recording is polymorphic with a predominance of the slow-wave theta region. Against this background, episodic short bursts of paroxysmal activity are recorded as "sharp-slow waves" with subsequent desynchronization of the rhythm. The EEG data indicate widespread changes with disruption of cortical-subcortical interactions.

Out of sedation clear consciousness. Executes simple commands. Breathing: assisted lung ventilation in BIPAP mode: respiratory rate 14 per minute; Saturation 98% against the background of FiO_2 0.4. Hemodynamics against the background of inotropic support: dopamine 2 mcg/kg/min, norepinephrine 0.05 µg/kg/min.

Scale score: SOFA 11, SAPS 43, RASS −3 on the background of sedation, FOUR 10, CAM-ICU no delirium.

B-EEG on the 9th day after sepsis diagnostics without any sedation.

On the EEG, the main rhythm is practically absent.

The record is represented by polymorphic activity with a predominance of slow-wave theta range of moderate amplitude.

Interhemispheric asymmetry and paroxysmal activity were not registered.

EEG data indicate gross widespread changes of a diffuse nature.

Scale score: SOFA 8, SAPS 40, RASS −1 without sedation, FOUR 14, GCS 11.

Inotropic support: dopamine 3 mcg/kg/min. Respiration: assisted ventilation in BIPAP mode: respiratory rate 14 per minute; Saturation 95% against the background of FiO_2 0.5.

The patient died on the 38th day of stay in ICU.

of secondary brain dysfunction and perhaps specifically brainstem dysfunction in critical states. The researchers also found that sedation was associated with a reduction in non-convulsive seizures or intermittent discharges and a lack of EEG reactivity. The sedative effect may impair the reactivity test during EEG. However, as observed in some studies (Shehabi et al. 2010), continuous sedation is associated with increased mortality.

In summary, EEG monitoring offers an excellent opportunity to improve our ability to predict and prevent seizures and thus to predict and potentially prevent neuronal damage (Chong et al. 2005) in SAE.

The SSEPs in sepsis and sepsis-associated encephalopathy

Somatosensory-evoked potential (SSEP) recording, an objective non-invasive method of neuromonitoring at the bedside of the critical patient, is a sensitive technique for detecting and quantifying CNS dysfunction caused by various metabolic disturbances, as confirmed by studies of several authors (Zauner et al. 2000; Madl et al. 2000).

SSEPs record stimulus conduction along sensory pathways from afferent fibers of peripheral nerves along the posterior horns of the spinal cord, then cross second-order neurons after leaving the nuclei of the dorsal column and project to third-order neurons in the ventral posterior nucleus of the thalamus. Third-order neurons from the thalamus project to the somatosensory cortex and various other areas involved in sensory processing (Cruccu et al. 2008) (Figure 5.5).

Registration of SSEPs is an important method for monitoring and quantifying patients with sepsis (especially when sedation techniques are used). As sedation is one of the most commonly used treatments in the ICU, the use of SSEPs to assess SAE in the ICU has certain advantages. When recording SSEPs in patients with sepsis, an increase in latency was observed in the subcortical and cortical pathways, and the significance of the changes correlated completely with the severity of the disease. Assessment of SSEP changes in patients with SAE suggests impaired subcortical and cortical relationships.

According to Zauner, Gendo, and Kramer, the latencies of significant peaks were significantly prolonged in patients with multiple organ failure and encephalopathy (Zauner et al. 2002). Further analysis showed that peak latencies of SSEPs with and without sepsis showed no difference in incubation time (Zauner et al. 2000), suggesting that SSEPs should not be used in patient groups with multiple organ failure.

In conclusion, recording peak SSEP latencies and inter-peak SSEP intervals that increase peak SSEP latency is a reliable method for assessing the severity of metabolic encephalopathy in sepsis (Zauner et al. 2000, 2002).

Short-latency SSEPs characterize the functional state of the pathways between the cervical thickening of the spinal cord and the sensory cortex (Bricolo et al. 1987; Gnezditsky 2003).

Short-latency SSEPs occurring 13–20 ms after a stimulus and produced by subcortical pathways between the cervical spinal cord thickening and the cerebral bridge were altered in 34% of cases in a 2008 Italian study by Rinaldi et al.

The study of short-latency SSEPs reflects functional and structural brain lesions between the N13 cervical spinal cord segments and the N20 cortical peaks (subcortical SSEPs pathway). The N13 peak is generated in structures caudal to the bridge, between the spinal roots of the cervical thickening and the bridge, and in the nuclei of the dorsal column. The N20 peak is formed in the sensory cortex. In our study, nerve conduction and the size of the subcortical SSEP pathway were prolonged in 80% of our patients. The N20 peak latency and the value of the N13–N20

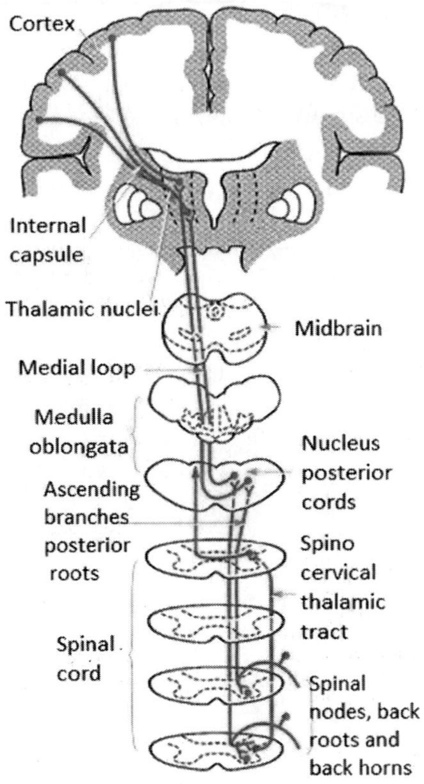

Figure 5.5 Anatomy of the conducting pathways of the SSEPs.

inter-peak interval increased in 9 out of 10 patients. Because peak SSEP latencies provide a more sensitive electrophysiological assessment compared to other methods (e.g., physical examination, neurological scales), SSEPs appear to be a more reliable method for diagnosing septic encephalopathy. The alteration in the subcortical SSEP pathway seen in the patients in our study could be due to decreased blood flow or impaired microcirculation in the brain. Furthermore, patients in septic shock suffer from oxygen deficiency and require a higher oxygen supply. Consequently, local tissue hypoxia could be responsible for the increased subcortical SSEP pathway. Furthermore, other studies have shown that continuous sedation of patients did not affect peak latency and prognostic significance of SSEPs (Zhou et al. 2022; Zauner et al. 2000; Madl et al. 2000). Peak latencies and amplitudes of short-latency SSEPs illustrating clinical neurological examinations remain unchanged during sedation (Zhou et al. 2022).

The most common region for detecting cerebral focal lesions is the subcortical pathway – between the dorsal column nucleus and the sensory cortex. A variety of central nervous system lesions may be seen in sepsis. Multiple microabscesses, small ischemic foci, hippocampal or watershed infarcts, astrocyte, and microglial proliferation, multiple small white matter hemorrhages, and central bridging myelinolysis have been described. Specific brain regions such as the insula and cingulate cortex are prone to neuronal loss in sepsis-induced brain dysfunction (Orhun et al. 2019, 2020). One or even a combination of these neuropathological processes may be responsible for the subtle focal changes in the subcortical somatosensory pathways seen in our patients in the SSEP study.

There is now a consensus that the bilateral absence of the N20 somatosensory potential during median nerve stimulation is the most reliable predictor of adverse patient outcome (death or transition to a vegetative state) in postanoxic coma (Zandbergen et al. 2006; Wijdicks et al. 2006). A recent functional MRI study has confirmed a link between this observation and blood oxygenation-dependent signaling in the primary somatosensory cortex (Gue'rit et al. 2009).

One problem is the waiting time that must elapse before the bilateral absence of N20 is considered a sufficient argument for refusing further resuscitative measures. Indeed, reversible bilateral disappearance of N20 after brief systemic hypoperfusion is common during surgical monitoring. All participants in the consensus study (Gue'rit et al. 2009) consider that a period of 24 hours is sufficient and that this period can be reduced to 12 hours if there are other clinical symptoms (5 Glasgow Coma Scale score in the absence of sedation) and/or (long-term circulatory arrest, age of the patient) arguments for the severity of cerebral anoxia.

Another question was whether these criteria remain reliable. The data are confirmed in a study of the effects of therapeutic mild hypothermia (34 to 32°C), after which survival and neurological outcome improved following cardiac arrest (Arrich et al. 2009; Oddo et al. 2014). For any degree of neuronal dysfunction, the prognosis is better with hypothermia than with normothermia, and the amplitude of SSEPs is not reduced (Gue'rit et al. 2009). However, the bilateral absence of cortical SSEPs still indicates a life-threatening prognosis for hypothermic patients (Tiainen et al. 2005).

Changes in electrogenesis during metabolic and/or toxic coma may either correspond to the response of the normal brain in a state of the abnormal biochemical environment, and the changes may always be reversible regardless of their intensity, or secondary, potentially irreversible lesions may occur due to a primary metabolic disorder (e.g., hemorrhages due to hypo coagulation).

The International Society for Hepatic Encephalopathy and Nitrogen Metabolism (ISHEN) guidelines for neurophysiological studies of hepatic encephalopathy recently published three major findings (Gue'rit et al. 2009). First, clinical neurophysiological testing can be used to monitor hepatic encephalopathy; the choice of the exact technique depends on the expected degree of encephalopathy (EEG for mild degrees, SSEPs for increasing severity). Second, although EEG monitoring is justified for identifying patients with non-convulsive epilepsy, EEG, BAEP, and SSEPs can also complement the neurologic picture, including intracranial pressure (ICP) monitoring. Third, even if there is a bilateral absence of N20 in the SSEPs study, this is not enough to rule out transplantation surgery and it would be ethically unacceptable to perform liver transplantation in such a patient without further evaluation to rule out irreversible changes in brain activity. An Italian study also presents a practical way to combine EEG and SSEP recordings in patients with severe brain damage (Amantini et al. 2009).

An overview of the current use of neurophysiological assessment in the ICU

Several studies have reported abnormal electroencephalography (EEG) or altered evoked potentials (EPs) in sepsis. However, the role of these tests in the diagnosis and prognostic evaluation of sepsis-associated encephalopathy remains unclear.

A systematic review was conducted that included articles published in the PubMed database between 1 January 1966 and 31 December 2013. Two prospective case-control studies reported EP changes with different results (Rosengarten et al. 2012; Zauner et al. 2002). In a study of visual-evoked potentials (VEPs), the amplitude of spikes in patients with sepsis did not differ from that of healthy controls, whereas SSEP latencies were significantly increased in patients with sepsis (Zauner et al. 2002). These SSEP changes were proportional to the severity of sepsis and unaffected by sedation, which is a major advantage compared to the changes in EEG examination.

There are data on the association and prognostic significance of changes in evoked potentials in encephalopathy. Acute brain dysfunction was characterized by impaired mental status, usually occurring during sepsis, and develops quite early (Taccone et al. 2013; Iacobone et al. 2009), often before functional changes in other organs (Eidelman et al. 1996; Bolton et al. 1993). The pathophysiology of SAE is multifactorial and appears to be related to the effects of systemic inflammation on cerebral perfusion and neuronal activity, without direct CNS infection (Hughes et al. 2012; Gofton et al. 2012). Hypoperfusion and cerebral ischemia contributing to systemic hypotension, loss of cerebral autoregulation (Terborg et al. 2001), and impaired microcirculation (Hughes et al. 2012; Taccone et al. 2014) are the main causes of encephalopathy. In addition to these processes, there are disturbances in neurotransmission and neuronal function. A higher severity of this encephalopathy is associated with a worse outcome of the disease, especially multi-organ failure (Ely et al. 2004; Adam et al. 2013).

BAEPs record the conduction of stimuli along the auditory pathway. The peripheral end of the auditory analyzer is the organ of Corti, located in the cochlea of the inner ear. Its receptor cells are connected to the dendrites of the spiral node. The axons of this node form the auditory nerve (VIII pair), which runs through the internal auditory canal to the cerebellopontine angle. The axons of the first neuron terminate at the cochlear nuclei, which transmit impulses via the nuclei of the trapezoid body and the olive complex to the nuclei of the lateral loop to the inferior tubercles of the quadriplegia and the medial cranial bodies. From them, the auditory impulses in the auditory radiation reach the fields of the primary auditory cortex (gyrus Geschl) – fields 42, 41 (Gnezditsky 2003).

VEPs record the conduction of stimuli along the visual pathway. The peripheral part of the visual system includes the eyeball with the lens and the retina, from which the optic nerve is derived. In the chiasm, the optic nerve crosses, and information from the right side of the visual field reaches the left hemisphere and vice versa. At the level of the thalamus, the large bundle branches off into the optic nerve head. The optic afferent orientation then meanders through the lateral patellar body along the optic radiation fibers and reaches areas of information processing – the 17th, 18th, and 19th fields according to Brodmann (Gnezditsky 2003).

We studied SSEPs, BAEPs, and VEPs in 25 patients with sepsis-associated encephalopathy. We studied brief latent SSEPs by alternately stimulating the median nerve in both hands and placing recording electrodes at the projection of CervC6/7-Fpz (N13, N18, P18 peaks were recorded) and at the projection of Cp3/4-Fpz (N20, P23 peaks were recorded). The latency of the N20 peak and the inter-peak interval N13-N20 increased from 60% to 150% on both sides ($p<0.05$) (Figure 5.6, 5.7; Table 5.1, 5.2, 5.3, 5.4, 5.5, 5.6).

The data shown in Figure 5.7 indicate that the latency of spikes N13, and N20 increased during stimulation on both sides of D > S, the inter-peak interval N13–N20 corresponding to conduction at the spinothalamic-cortical level increased, the amplitude of spike N20 decreased by 70–80% on both sides, suggesting inhibition of conduction at this level.

SSEP parameters were moderately altered in 3 of 10 patients (in one patient, N20 latency was increased by 16–17%, interpeak interval N13–N20 was increased by 50% on both sides, and she subsequently survived). In two patients, SSEP parameters were moderately altered,

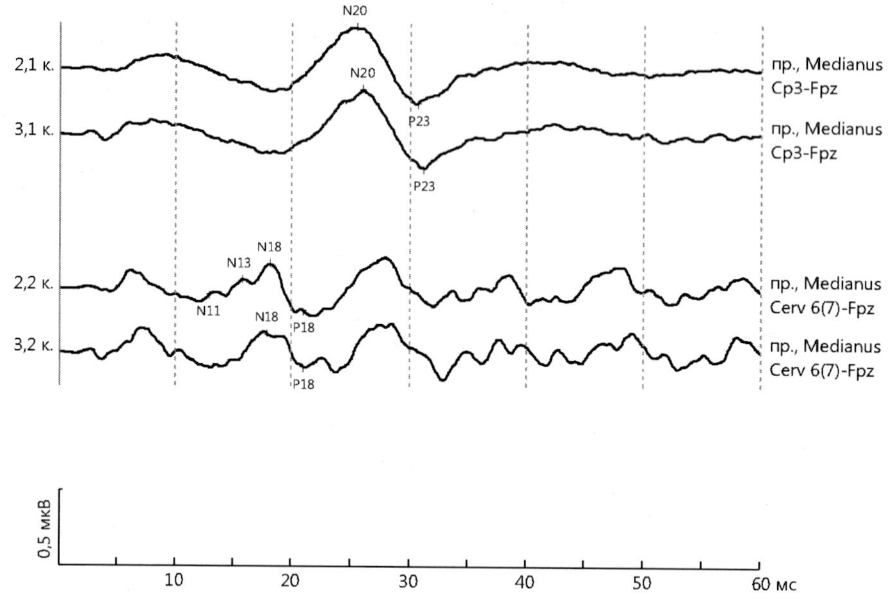

Figure 5.6 SSEPs with short latency during stimulation of the n. medianus dex., Cp4-Fpz, Cerv6-Fpz. Patient M., 74-year-old. Registered on the 2nd day after the onset of sepsis.

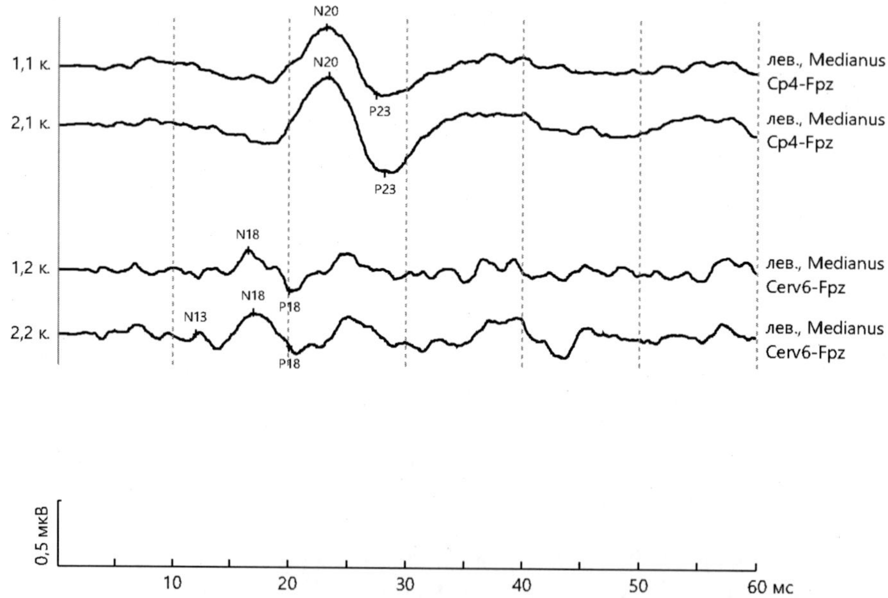

Figure 5.7 Short-latency SSEPs with n. medianus sin. stimulation, Cp4-Fpz, Cerv6-Fpz. Patient M., 74-year-old. Registration is on the 2nd day after sepsis starts.

Table 5.1 Latencies of short-latency SSEPs on the right side of patient M, 74-year-old, diagnosed with sepsis.

N	Directions	Component	Latency, ms	Norm, ms	Deviation, %	Stimulation side	Stimulus	Stimulus duration
2.1 channel	Cp3-Fpz	N20	25.4	20.1	+26.4	Right	23.0 MA	0.1 ms
2.2 ch.	Cerv 6(7)-Fpz	N11	13.0			Right	23.0 MA	0.1 ms
		N13	15.8	13.2	+19.3			
3.1 ch.	Cp3-Fpz	N20	26.1	20.1	+29.7	Right	23.0 MA	0.1 ms

Table 5.2 Intervals of short-latency SSEPs on the right side of patient M, 74-year-old, diagnosed with sepsis.

N	Directions	Component	Latency, ms	Norm, ms	Deviation, %	Stimulation side	Stimulus	Stimulus duration
2.2 ch., 2.1 ch.	Cerv 6(7)-Fpz, Cp3-Fpz	N13–N20	9.66	5.8	+66.5	Right	23.0 MA	0.1 ms
		N11–N13	2.78					

Table 5.3 Amplitudes of short-latency SSEPs on the right side of patient M, 74-year-old, diagnosed with sepsis.

N	Directions	Component	Latency, ms	Norm, ms	Deviation, %	Stimulation side	Stimulus	Stimulus duration
2.1 ch.	Cp3-Fpz	N20-P23	0.491	2.8	-82.5	Right	23.0 MA	0.1 ms
3.1 ch.	Cp3-Fpz	N20-P23	0.511	2.8	-81.8	Right	23.0 MA	0.1 ms

Table 5.4 Latencies of short-latency SSEPs on the left side of patient M, 74-year-old, diagnosed with sepsis.

N	Directions	Component	Latency, ms	Norm, ms	Deviation, %	Stimulation side	Stimulus	Stimulus duration
1.1 ch.	Cp4-Fpz	N20	23.2	20.1	+15.2	Left	26.0 MA	0.1
2.1 ch.	Cp4-Fpz	N20	23.3	20.1	+15.9	Left	26.0 MA	0.1 ms
2.2 ch.	Cerv6-Fpz	N13	12.0	13.2	-8.7	Left	26.0 MA	0.1 ms

Table 5.5 Intervals of short-latency SSEPs on the left side of patient M, 74-year-old, diagnosed with sepsis.

N	Directions	Component	Latency, ms	Norm, ms	Deviation, %	Stimulation side	Stimulus	Stimulus duration
2.2 ch., 2.1 ch.	Cerv6-Fpz, Cp4-Fpz	N13–N20	11.2	5.8	+93.9	Left	26.0 uA	0.1 ms

Table 5.6 Amplitudes of short-latency SSEPs on the left side of patient M, 74-year-old, diagnosed with sepsis.

N	Directions	Component	Latency, ms	Norm, ms	Deviation, %	Stimulation side	Stimulus	Stimulus duration
1.1 ch.	Cp4-Fpz	N20-P23	0.498	2.8	-82.2	Left	26.0 uA	0.1 ms
2.1 ch.	Cp4-Fpz	N20-P23	0.702	2.8	-74.9	Left	26.0 uA	0.1 ms

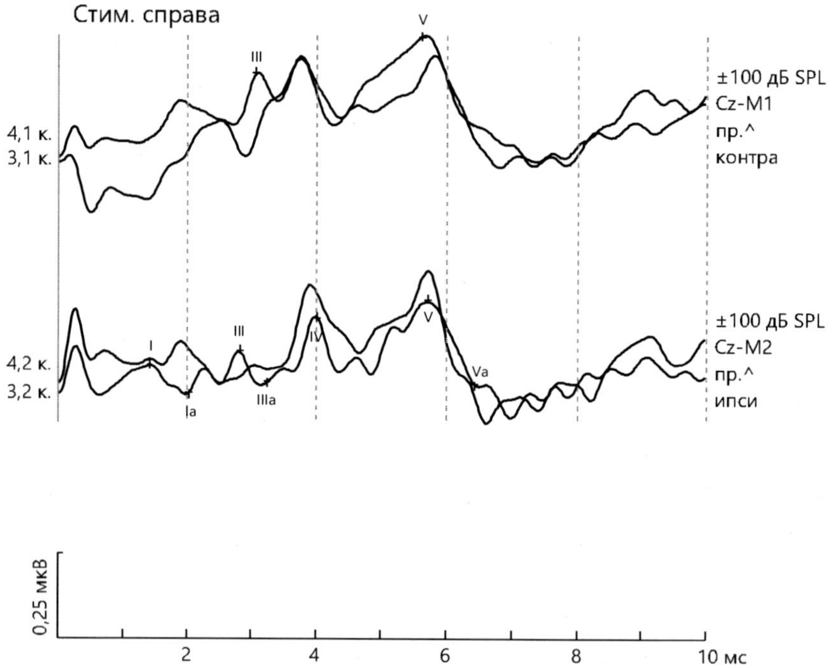

Figure 5.8 Parameters of short-latency BAEPs (right stimulation) in patient P., 64-year-old, with sepsis.

but on BAEP examination, the potentials were of low amplitude, poorly visible, and showed impaired conduction along the brainstem. These two patients subsequently died.

In the BAEPs study, the standard protocol was used – recording electrodes were placed in Cz-M1/M2 and monoauricular stimulation was performed. In 3 out of 10 patients, there were changes in the values of the interpeak intervals I–III, III–V without an increase in the main interval I–V (Figure 5.8, 5.9; Table 5.7, 5.8, 5.9, 5.10).

In 50% of patients, there were low-amplitude EPs that were difficult to reproduce, in one case no BAEPs were recorded at all. Eight out of 25 patients survived – with moderate changes in SSEPs and BAEPs parameters and normal VEPs.

During the VEPs study, we performed monocular stimulation by light flashes using LED glasses. Recording electrodes were placed in the O1/O2-Fz projection. The potential parameters were normal in 8 out of 25 patients (Figure 5.10).

One patient had increased latencies of all peaks during stimulation of the right eye (probably after a stroke in the right hemisphere of the brain from 2022), two patients had increased

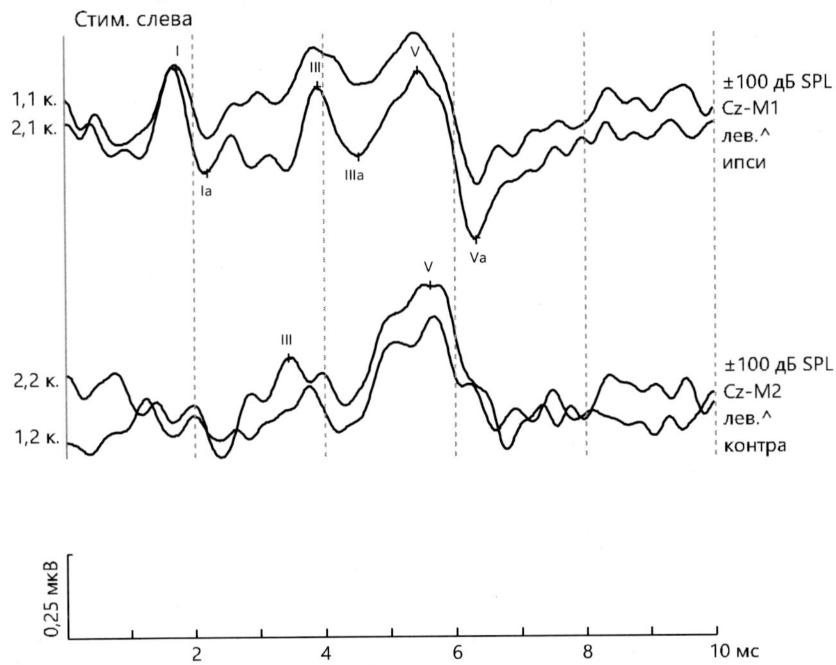

Figure 5.9 Parameters of short-latency BAEPs (left stimulation) in patient P., 64-year-old, with sepsis.

Table 5.7 Latencies of short-latency BAEPs of patient P., 64-year-old, diagnosed with sepsis.

N	Directions	Component	Latency, ms	Norm, ms	Deviation, %	Stimulation side	Stimulus	Stimulus duration
2,1 ch.	Cz-M1	I	1,74	1,7	(N)	Left	±100 dB SPL	0,1 ms
		III	3,91	3,9	(N)			
		V	5,44	5,7	(N)			
2,2 ch.	Cz-M2	III	3,46	3,9	-11,4	Left	±100 dB SPL	0,1 ms
		V	5,63	5,7	(N)	Left		
2,1 ch. 2,2 ch.	Cz-M1 Cz-M2	III	0,45			Left	±100 dB SPL	0,1 ms
		V	0,19					
3,2 ch.	Cz-M2	I	1,41	1,7	(N)	Right	±100 dB SPL	0,1 ms
		III	2,82	3,9	-27,7			
		IV	4,0	5,1	-21,5			
		V	5,7	5,7	(N)			
4,1 ch.	Cz-M1	III	3,08	3,9	-21,1	Left	±100 dB SPL	0,1 ms
		V	5,62	5,7	(N)			

Table 5.8 Intervals of short-latency BAEPs of patient P., 64-year-old, diagnosed with sepsis.

N	Directions	Component	Latency, ms	Norm, ms	Deviation, %	Stimulation side	Stimulus	Stimulus duration
2,1 ch.	Cz-M1	I–III	2,17	2,1	(N)	Left	±100 dB SPL	0,1 ms
		III–V	1,53	1,9	-19,5			
		I–V	3,7	4,0	(N)			
2,2 ch.	Cz-M2	III–V	2,17	1,9	(N)	Left	±100 dB SPL	0,1 ms
3,2 ch.	Cz-M2	I–III	1,41	2,1	-33,0	Right	±100 dB SPL	0,1 ms
		III–V	2,88	1,9	+51,5			
		I–V	4,29	4,0	(N)			
4,1 ch.	Cz-M1	III–V	2,54	1,9	+33,7	Right	±100 dB SPL	0,1 ms

Table 5.9 Amplitudes of short-latency BAEPs of patient P., 64-year-old, diagnosed with sepsis.

N	Directions	Component	Latency, ms	Norm, ms	Deviation, %	Stimulation side	Stimulus	Stimulus duration
2,1 ch.	Cz-M1	I	0,302	0,28	(N)	Left	±100 dB SPL	0,1 ms
		III	0,202	0,23	(N)			
		V	0,494	0,43	(N)			
3,2 ch.	Cz-M2	I	0,082	0,28	-70,8	Right	±100 dB SPL	0,1 ms
		III	0,092	0,23	-59,8			
		IIIa-IV	0,195	0,25	(N)			
		IV-V	0,044					
		V	0,244	0,43	-43,3			

Table 5.10 Amplitudes ratio of short-latency BAEPs of patient P., 64-year-old, diagnosed with sepsis.

N	Directions	Component	Latency, ms	Norm, ms	Deviation, %	Stimulation side	Stimulus	Stimulus duration
2,1 ch.	Cz-M1	I/III	1,5			Left	±100 dB SPL	0,1 ms
		I/V	0,612	0,73	(N)			
		III/V	0,409	0,50	(N)			
3,2 ch.	Cz-M2	I/III	0,883			Right	±100 dB SPL	0,1 ms
		I/V	0,335	0,73	(N)			
		III/V	0,379	0,50	(N)			

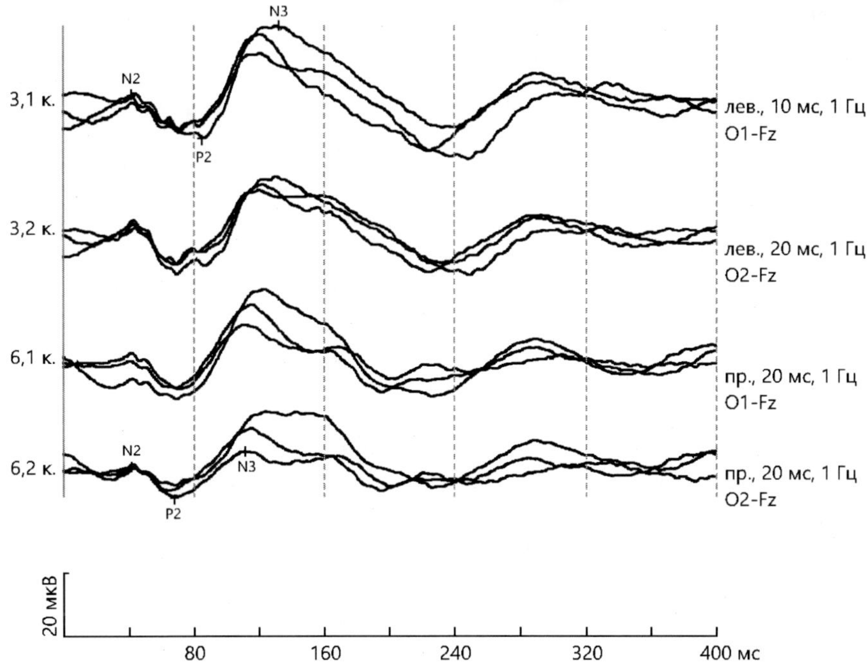

Figure 5.10 Flash VEP parameters in patient P., 64-year-old, diagnosed with sepsis.

Table 5.11 Latencies of flash VEPs, patient P., 64-year-old, diagnosed with sepsis.

N	Directions	Component	Latency, ms	Norm, ms	Deviation, %	Stimulation side	Stimulus	Stimulus duration
1,1 ch.	O1-Fz	N2	41,9	73,0	-42,7	Left		10 ms
		P2	85,3	103	-17,2			
		N3	133	128	(N)			
6,2 ch.	O2-Fz	N2	40,8	73,0	-44,1	Right		20 ms
		P2	67,3	103	-34,7			
		N3	111	128	(N)			

Table 5.12 Amplitudes of flash VEPs, patient P., 64-year-old, diagnosed with sepsis.

N	Directions	Component	Latency, ms	Norm, ms	Deviation, %	Stimulation side	Stimulus	Stimulus duration
1,1 ch.	O1-Fz	N2-P2	13,3	6,6	+102	Left		10 ms
6,2 ch.	O2-Fz	N2-P2	9,55	6,6	(N)	Right		20 ms

latencies of both eyes, and one had decreased amplitude of peaks on both sides with normal latencies. Eight surviving patients had normal VEP parameters.

Conclusion

The diagnosis of SAE requires the identification of brain dysfunction, which depends mainly on the study of clinical electrophysiological and biochemical parameters (Ying Huang et al. 2021).

A national study in Germany shows that clinical assessment is an important and most commonly used tool for monitoring neurological function and that EEG (quantitative, bispectral (BIS), SSEPs, multimodal EPs are used to assess or diagnose functional impairment SAE (Zhou et al. 2022).

Abnormal EEG is more common in sepsis and is dominated by diffuse slow waves (θ-spike, δ-spike) (Young grade).

Measurement of neurophysiological indices provides additional information on the functional status of the brain and allows a reliable assessment of the severity of septic encephalopathy in critically ill patients.

The progressive deceleration of background EEG activity with an increase in cerebral insufficiency and a decrease in EEG reactivity to external stimuli provide important diagnostic and prognostic information.

In the patients who had lesions of the subcortical and cortical pathways, the SSEPs study had a significantly worse prognosis for recovery, and with additional changes in BAEPs, the prognosis for survival was unfavorable, which was related to the severity of the disease (Zauner 2002).

The frequency of subcortical and cortical lesions of SSEPs suggests that this subclinical brain dysfunction is more widespread than commonly thought. The observation of normal SSEPs and BAEPs parameters is a favorable sign, with a prognostic value of awakening in the order of 90% and a probability of a good outcome in the order of 75–80%.

On the contrary, severe changes in BAEP parameters indicative of brainstem disorders were associated with death or coma vigil in more than 90% of cases. In general, signs of brainstem conduction abnormalities are a much more powerful prognostic indicator.

VEP examination provides information about conduction along the visual pathway, which may be impaired even before the onset of SAE due to other causes. SAE is usually observed in patients with systemic diseases. In general, increased latency may also confirm a deterioration in the functional state of the brain.

Clinical neurophysiology provides a functional assessment of the nervous system. It is therefore a method that complements imaging and clinical examination. Neurophysiological examination methods have two major advantages over neurological ones: they can be performed on patients under sedation. As a result, they significantly improve the treatment of individual patients in the ICU.

Further research in this direction is needed.

Conflict of Interest: The authors declare no conflict of interest

Acknowledgments: The authors would like to thank St. Petersburg State Paediatric Medical University, North-Western State Medical University named after I.I. Mechnikov, and Russian Polenov Scientific Research Neurosurgical Institute for knowledge that enriched the author's clinical practice.

References

Adam N, Kandelman S, Mantz J, Chrétien F, Sharshar T. Sepsis-induced brain dysfunction. *Expert Rev Anti Infect Ther.* 2013;11(2):211–221. doi:10.1586/eri.12.159

Amantini A, Fossi S, Grippo A, et al. Continuous EEG-SEP monitoring in severe brain injury. *Neurophysiol Clin.* 2009;39(2):85–93. doi:10.1016/j.neucli.2009.01.006

Angus DC, van der Poll T. Severe sepsis and septic shock [published correction appears in N Engl J Med. 2013 Nov 21;369(21):2069]. *N Engl J Med.* 2013;369(9):840–851. doi:10.1056/NEJMra1208623

Arrich J, Holzer M, Herkner H, Müllner M. Hypothermia for neuroprotection in adults after cardiopulmonary resuscitation. *Cochrane Database Syst Rev.* 2009;(4): CD004128. Published 2009 Oct 7. doi:10.1002/14651858.CD004128.pub2

Bolton CF, Young GB, Zochodne DW. The neurological complications of sepsis. *Ann Neurol.* 1993;33(1):94–100. doi:10.1002/ana.410330115

Bozzani A, Arici V, Ticozzelli G, et al. Intraoperative cerebral monitoring during carotid surgery: A narrative review. *Ann Vasc Surg.* 2022;78:36–44. doi:10.1016/j.avsg.2021.06.044

Bricolo A, Faccioli F, Grosslercher JC, Pasut ML, Pinna GP, Turazzi S. Electrophysiological monitoring in the intensive care unit. *Electroencephalogr Clin Neurophysiol.* Suppl. 1987;39:255–263.

Chong DJ, Hirsch LJ. Which EEG patterns warrant treatment in the critically ill? Reviewing the evidence for treatment of periodic epileptiform discharges and related patterns. *J Clin Neurophysiol.* 2005;22(2):79–91. doi:10.1097/01.wnp.0000158699.78529.af

Cruccu G, Aminoff MJ, Curio G, et al. Recommendations for the clinical use of somatosensory-evoked potentials. *Clin Neurophysiol.* 2008;119(8):1705–1719. doi:10.1016/j.clinph.2008.03.016

Ebersoldt M, Sharshar T, Annane D. Sepsis-associated delirium. *Intensive Care Med.* 2007;33(6):941–950. doi:10.1007/s00134-007-0622-2

Eidelman LA, Putterman D, Putterman C, Sprung CL. The spectrum of septic encephalopathy: Definitions, etiologies, and mortalities. *JAMA.* 1996;275(6):470–473.

Ely EW, Shintani A, Truman B, et al. Delirium as a predictor of mortality in mechanically ventilated patients in the intensive care unit. *JAMA.* 2004;291(14):1753–1762. doi:10.1001/jama.291.14.1753

Gnezditsky VV. *Evoked Brain Potentials in Clinical Practice.* Moscow: MED Press-Inform; 2003.

Gofton TE, Young GB. Sepsis-associated encephalopathy. *Nat Rev Neurol.* 2012;8(10):557–566. doi:10.1038/nrneurol.2012.183

Guérit JM, Amantini A, Amodio P, et al. Consensus on the use of neurophysiological tests in the intensive care unit (ICU): Electroencephalogram (EEG), evoked potentials (EP), and electroneuromyography (ENMG). *Neurophysiol Clin.* 2009;39(2):71–83. doi:10.1016/j.neucli.2009.03.002

Guérit JM, Amantini A, Fischer C, et al. Neurophysiological investigations of hepatic encephalopathy: ISHEN practice guidelines. *Liver Int.* 2009;29(6):789–796. doi:10.1111/j.1478-3231.2009.02030.x

Guérit JM. Neurophysiological testing in neurocritical care. *Curr Opin Crit Care.* 2010;16(2):98–104. doi:10.1097/MCC.0b013e328337541a

Huang Y, Chen R, Jiang L, Li S, Xue Y. Basic research and clinical progress of sepsis-associated encephalopathy. *J Intensive Med.* 2021;1(2):90–95. Published 2021 Sep 24. doi:10.1016/j.jointm.2021.08.002

Hughes CG, Patel MB, Pandharipande PP. Pathophysiology of acute brain dysfunction: What's the cause of all this confusion? *Curr Opin Crit Care.* 2012;18(5):518–526. doi:10.1097/MCC.0b013e328357effa

Iacobone E, Bailly-Salin J, Polito A, Friedman D, Stevens RD, Sharshar T. Sepsis-associated encephalopathy and its differential diagnosis. *Crit Care Med.* 2009;37(10 Suppl): S331–S336. doi:10.1097/CCM.0b013e3181b6ed58

Madl C, Grimm G, Kramer L, et al. Early prediction of individual outcome after cardiopulmonary resuscitation. *Lancet.* 1993;341(8849):855–858. doi:10.1016/0140-6736(93)93061-5

Madl C, Kramer L, Domanovits H, et al. Improved outcome prediction in unconscious cardiac arrest survivors with sensory evoked potentials compared with clinical assessment. *Crit Care Med.* 2000;28(3):721–726. doi:10.1097/00003246-200003000-00020

Moruzzi G, Magoun HW. Brain stem reticular formation and activation of the EEG. *Electroencephalogr Clin Neurophysiol.* 1949;1(4):455–473.

Oddo M, Carrera E, Claassen J, Mayer SA, Hirsch LJ. Continuous electroencephalography in the medical intensive care unit. *Crit Care Med.* 2009;37(6):2051–2056. doi:10.1097/CCM.0b013e3181a00604

Oddo M, Rossetti AO. Early multimodal outcome prediction after cardiac arrest in patients treated with hypothermia. *Crit Care Med.* 2014;42(6):1340–1347. doi:10.1097/CCM.0000000000000211

Orhun G, Esen F, Özcan PE, et al. Neuroimaging findings in sepsis-induced brain dysfunction: Association with clinical and laboratory findings. *Neurocrit Care.* 2019;30(1):106–117. doi:10.1007/s12028-018-0581-1

Orhun G, Tüzün E, Bilgiç B, et al. Brain volume changes in patients with acute brain dysfunction due to sepsis. *Neurocrit Care.* 2020;32(2):459–468. doi:10.1007/s12028-019-00759-8

Procaccio F, Polo A, Lanteri P, Sala F. Electrophysiologic monitoring in neurointensive care. *Curr Opin Crit Care.* 2001;7(2):74–80. doi:10.1097/00075198-200104000-00004

Rosengarten B, Krekel D, Kuhnert S, Schulz R. Early neurovascular uncoupling in the brain during community-acquired pneumonia. *Crit Care.* 2012;16(2):R64. Published 2012 Dec 12. doi:10.1186/cc11310

Saito T, Malicoat JR, Leyden LR, et al. Mortality prediction by bispectral electroencephalography among 502 patients: Its role in dementia. *Brain Commun.* 2021;3(2):fcab037. Published 2021 Mar 13. doi:10.1093/brain-comms/fcab037

Shehabi Y, Riker RR, Bokesch PM, et al. Delirium duration and mortality in lightly sedated, mechanically ventilated intensive care patients. *Crit Care Med.* 2010;38(12):2311–2318. doi:10.1097/CCM.0b013e3181f85759

Shinozaki G, Bormann NL, Chan AC, et al. Identification of patients with high mortality risk and prediction of outcomes in delirium by bispectral EEG. *J Clin Psychiatry.* 2019;80(5):19m12749.

Sutter R, Stevens RD, Kaplan PW. Significance of triphasic waves in patients with acute encephalopathy: A nine-year cohort study. *Clin Neurophysiol.* 2013;124(10):1952–1958. doi:10.1016/j.clinph.2013.03.031

Sutter R, Kaplan PW. Clinical and electroencephalographic correlates of acute encephalopathy. *J Clin Neurophysiol.* 2013;30(5):443–453. doi:10.1097/WNP.0b013e3182a73bc2

Taccone FS, Su F, Pierrakos C, et al. Cerebral microcirculation is impaired during sepsis: an experimental study. *Crit Care.* 2010;14(4):R140. doi:10.1186/cc9205

Taccone FS, Scolletta S, Franchi F, Donadello K, Oddo M. Brain perfusion in sepsis. *Curr Vasc Pharmacol.* 2013;11(2):170–186. doi:10.2174/1570161111311020007

Taccone FS, Su F, De Deyne C, et al. Sepsis is associated with altered cerebral microcirculation and tissue hypoxia in experimental peritonitis. *Crit Care Med.* 2014;42(2):e114–e122. doi:10.1097/CCM.0b013e3182a641b8

Terborg C, Schummer W, Albrecht M, Reinhart K, Weiller C, Röther J. Dysfunction of vasomotor reactivity in severe sepsis and septic shock. *Intensive Care Med.* 2001;27(7):1231–1234. doi:10.1007/s001340101005

Tiainen M, Kovala TT, Takkunen OS, Roine RO. Somatosensory and brainstem auditory evoked potentials in cardiac arrest patients treated with hypothermia. *Crit Care Med.* 2005;33(8):1736–1740. doi:10.1097/01.ccm.0000171536.63641.d9

Wijdicks EF, Hijdra A, Young GB, Bassetti CL, Wiebe S; Quality Standards Subcommittee of the American Academy of Neurology. Practice parameter: prediction of outcome in comatose survivors after cardiopulmonary resuscitation (an evidence-based review): Report of the Quality Standards Subcommittee of the American Academy of Neurology. *Neurology.* 2006;67(2):203–210. doi:10.1212/01.wnl.0000227183.21314.cd

Yamanashi, T., Marra, P.S., Crutchley, K.J. et al. Mortality among patients with sepsis associated with a bispectral electroencephalography (BSEEG) score. *Sci Rep.* 2021;11:14211. https://doi.org/10.1038/s41598-021-93588-9

Yamanashi T., Crutchley K.J., Wahba N.E., et al. Evaluation of point-of-care thumb-size bispectral electroencephalography device to quantify delirium severity and predict mortality. *The British Journal of Psychiatry.* 2022;220:322–329. doi: 10.1192/bjp.2021.101

Young GB, Bolton CF, Austin TW, Archibald YM, Gonder J, Wells GA. The encephalopathy associated with septic illness. *Clin Invest Med.* 1990;13(6):297–304.

Zandbergen EG, Hijdra A, Koelman JH, et al. Prediction of poor outcome within the first 3 days of post-anoxic coma [published correction appears in Neurology. 2006 Apr 11;66(7):1133]. *Neurology.* 2006;66(1):62–68. doi:10.1212/01.wnl.0000191308.22233.88

Zhang LN, Wang XT, Ai YH, et al. Epidemiological features and risk factors of sepsis-associated encephalopathy in intensive care unit patients: 2008–2011. *Chin Med J (Engl).* 2012;125(5):828–831.

Zauner C, Gendo A, Kramer L, Kranz A, Grimm G, Madl C. Metabolic encephalopathy in critically ill patients suffering from septic or nonseptic multiple organ failure. *Crit Care Med.* 2000;28(5):1310–1315. doi:10.1097/00003246-200005000-00009

Zauner C, Gendo A, Kramer L, et al. Impaired subcortical and cortical sensory evoked potential pathways in septic patients. *Crit Care Med.* 2002;30(5):1136–1139. doi:10.1097/00003246-200205000-00030

Zhou ML, Jin GY, Xi SS, Chen JY, Liang DC. Research progress in clinical electrophysiological assessment of patients with sepsis-associated encephalopathy. *Zhongguo Yi Xue Ke Xue Yuan Xue Bao.* 2022;44(5):876–884. doi:10.3881/j.issn.1000-503X.14994

Chapter 6

Neuroradiology of sepsis-associated encephalopathy

Tatyana N. Trofimova[1]*, Corr. Member of the RAS, MD., Ph.D., Polina L. Andropova[1], MD., Rustam S. Talybov[2], MD., Konstantin I. Sebelev[3], MD., Ph.D., Elena G. Potemkina[3], MD., Ph.D., Anton V. Ryzhkov[4], MD.

[1] Department of Neuroradiology, The Human Brain State Institute named after Natalya P. Bekhtereva of the Russian Academy of Science, Saint Petersburg, Russian Federation

[2] Department of Radiology, The Regional Clinical Hospital #2, Tyumen, Russian Federation

[3] Department of Radiation Diagnostics, Russian Polenov Scientific Research Neurosurgical Institute – branch of the Almazov National Medical Research Centre of Ministry of Health Care of Russian Federation, Saint Petersburg, Russian Federation

[4] Department of MRI-diagnostics of Almazov National Medical Research Centre of Ministry of Health Care of Russian Federation, Saint Petersburg, Russian Federation

Abstract

Sepsis-associated encephalopathy (SAE) is a diffuse brain dysfunction due to a systemic inflammatory response syndrome. SAE remains a difficult-to-diagnose complication of sepsis because the symptoms are nonspecific and assessment of cognitive dysfunction is complicated by the frequent use of sedation in critically ill patients. The current practice of clinical laboratory and neurophysiological studies does not answer the question of the presence of morpho-structural changes. The use of neuroimaging methods seems to be very promising, but studying patients with sepsis is difficult, so the number of observations and, as a result, publications is relatively small. In addition, neuroimaging provides invaluable assistance in the exclusion of other diseases that cause brain dysfunction. Although the etiology, clinical manifestations, and pathophysiology of sepsis are heterogeneous, the diagnostic imaging of SAE itself represents a fairly universal neuroradiologic finding. The chapter discusses imaging patterns associated with vasogenic and cytotoxic edema, vasculopathy, sepsis-associated hemorrhages, posterior reversible encephalopathy syndrome, and other neuroradiological findings that are the most common in SAE.

---

* Corresponding author: Tatyana N. Trofimova, Correspondent Member of Russian Academy of Sciences, Professor, MD., Ph.D.
e-mail address: ttrofimova@groupmmc.ru

Editor: Irina A. Savvina, Natalia V. Beloborodova and Tatyana N. Trofimova
In: Sepsis-Associated Encephalopathy
ISBN: 979-8-89113-178-1

Keywords: sepsis-associated encephalopathy, blood-brain barrier damage, cerebral edema, vasculopathy, hypoperfusion, cerebral ischemia, brain hemorrhage, PRES, cerebral microabscess.

Introduction

Currently, sepsis is a major cause of mortality in ICU patients, despite invasive and multi-component noninvasive monitoring systems, the use of modern antibiotics, and high-tech medical care. One of the most common neurologic complications of sepsis is sepsis-associated encephalopathy (SAE), a diffuse cerebral dysfunction primarily due to a systemic inflammatory response syndrome (SIRS). The incidence of SAE in patients with sepsis is approximately 50–70% (Young et al., 1990; Sprung et al., 1990) and is associated with mental status deterioration and increased mortality (in severe SAE cases, it is more than 50% and is usually caused by simultaneous dysfunction of multiple organs).

The pathophysiology of SAE is a complex of interwoven mechanisms that include direct damage to brain tissue by circulating overexpressed inflammatory mediators in sepsis, metabolic disorders, cellular hypoxia, blood-brain barrier (BBB) disruption, neurotransmitter imbalance, dysregulation, and interruption of brain perfusion. The consequence of this combination of neuroinflammatory and ischemic processes is the degeneration of neurons and cell death (apoptosis). The classic clinical presentation of SAE is characterized by impaired consciousness, reversal of circadian rhythms, thought disorder, hallucinations, developing delirium to coma, and seizures (Iwashyna et al., 2009; Iacobone et al., 2009).

The underlying problem remains that the assessment of cognitive dysfunction is complicated by the lack of specific symptoms, effective methods for early diagnosis, and the frequent use of sedation in critically ill patients. Therefore, the diagnosis of SAE remains a diagnosis of exclusion that can be made after other causes of brain dysfunction have been ruled out (Eidelman et al., 1996). Typically, only 28.1% of SAE patients survive for one year after diagnosis (Barichello et al., 2005; Sasse et al., 1995; Mo et al., 2023). Clinical, instrumental, and laboratory evaluation of patients with SAE includes analysis of putative serum markers (Piazza et al., 2007; Piazza et al., 2009), electroencephalographic (EEG) changes (Young et al., 1992), neurophysiological monitoring, and possible imaging biomarkers (Zauner et al., 2002; Chaudhry et al., 2014).

Despite all the advantages offered by EEG (EEG monitoring in sedated patients and a proven correlation of EEG abnormalities with the severity of SAE), this method does not allow the determination of morpho-structural and metabolic changes in the brain (Young et al., 2013; Hosokawa et al., 2014). Neuroimaging methods provide the answer to these questions.

Neuroradiology of sepsis-associated encephalopathy

Even though the etiology, clinical manifestations, and pathophysiology of sepsis are heterogeneous, the diagnostic imaging of SAE itself represents a fairly universal neuroradiologic finding. Primarily, it is vasogenic edema resulting from microcirculation disorders with disruption of the blood-brain barrier. In addition, endothelial activation occurs, leading to the destruction of endothelial cells and the development of cytotoxic edema. As a result, microinfarcts and microabscesses may form in the damaged areas. CT head scans do not provide definitive information about brain abnormalities in the early stages of SAE (Piazza et al., 2009). MRI is the imaging modality of choice for early manifestations of cerebral edema and has high sensitivity and specificity. Advanced stages present as brain abnormalities in the cortex, white matter, and subcortical structures.

Stubbs et al. (2013) systematized the major neuroradiological patterns of SAE (Fig. 6.1) and compared them with ongoing pathophysiological processes:

- Cortical and/or subcortical localization of focal lesions consistent with vasogenic edema;
- Parenchymal brain lesions associated with cytotoxic edema (with further transformation to vasogenic edema);
- Posterior reversible encephalopathy syndrome (occipitoparietal vasogenic edema, leptomeningeal contrast enhancement on MRI, vasospasm, and 'vessel pruning' on MRI/CT angiography);
- Neuroradiological (CT and MRI) abnormalities showing ring enhancement;
- Focal hemorrhages of both cortical and subcortical distributions;
- White matter necrosis (cerebral, cerebellum, brainstem) resulting from severe tissue hypoxia, with impaired diffusion in the basal ganglia, subcortical white matter, and chronic persistent edema;
- Progressive diffuse cortical atrophy.

Imaging findings associated with vasogenic edema

Vasogenic edema is characterized by white matter lesions in periventricular and/or subcortical areas where the blood-brain barrier is disrupted. Piazza et al. (2009) presented four cases of patients with SAE. Clinical and instrumental examination allowed the exclusion of acute ischemic stroke and infectious diseases of the central nervous system. On Day 20, an MRI of the brain (Fig. 6.2) of one of the patients showed small hyperintense areas in the frontal region (cortically and subcortically localized, more evident in the right cerebral hemisphere) on T2-weighted and FLAIR imaging.

In another patient, similar findings were present, localized in the periventricular areas, which might suggest vasogenic edema (probably related to cerebrovascular autoregulation dysfunction rather than BBB dysfunction). Cytotoxic edema was excluded by the diffusion images

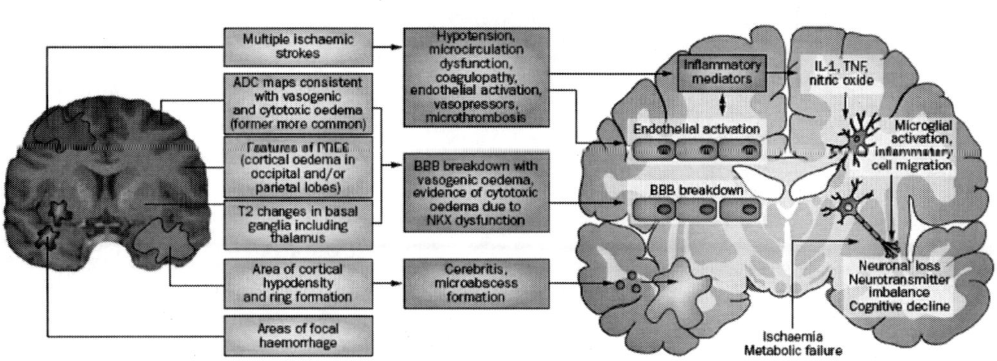

Figure 6.1 Pathophysiological mechanisms of SAE (Stubbs et al., 2013).

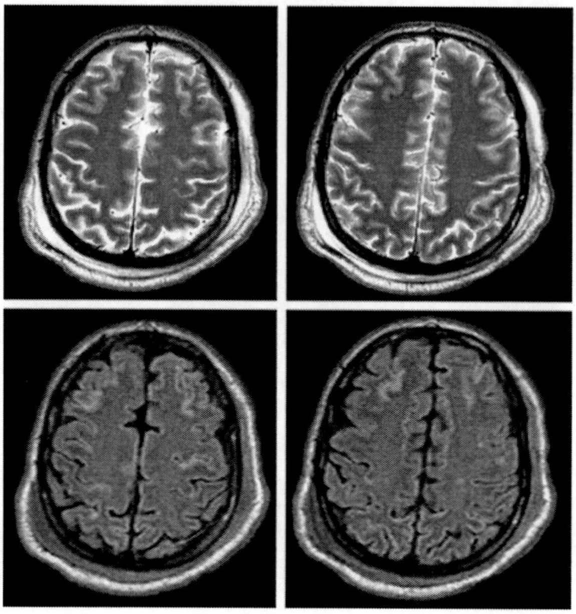

Figure 6.2 A 51-year-old man with severe descending necrotizing mediastinitis. Axial T2-weighted and FLAIR imaging show linear lesions in cortical and subcortical areas, more prominent in the right cerebral hemisphere (Piazza et al., 2009).

The authors did not assume BBB breakdown in the presented cases because S100B did not increase the CSF in patients, which according to some investigators was due to minor blood-brain barrier damage (Heizmann et al., 2004; Larsson et al., 2005). According to Piazza et al. (2009), blood-brain barrier damage is an important factor in SAE, although initial vasogenic edema may evolve into cytotoxic edema (Piazza et al., 2009).

Imaging findings associated with cytotoxic edema

Ahmed et al. (2011) described the case of a 17-year-old female who presented to the emergency department with a Glasgow Coma Scale (GCS) score of 13/15. On examination, the patient was febrile, sleepy, and disoriented. MRI of the brain (on Day 7 of her hospitalization) showed bilateral diffuse symmetric hyperintense signals on FLAIR, hypointense on T1-weighted images in the periventricular, semioval, and deep white matter, and an area in the splenium of the corpus callosum corresponding to a central area of diffusion restriction in the centrum semiovale on DWI and ADC (Fig. 6.3). T1-weighted post-gadolinium imaging shows no enhancement in the hypointense areas listed. The MRI findings were interpreted by the authors as manifestations of cytotoxic edema. The patient died on the 13th day of her hospitalization.

In turn, Abe et al. (2008) describe a case of SAE in a 2-month-old girl with biliary atresia. *Pseudomonas aeruginosa* was isolated from her blood, and the child's altered mental status, intractable seizures, and hemiplegia were suggestive of cerebral dysfunction. CT showed areas of low density in the right cerebral hemisphere (Fig. 6.4). The patient was diagnosed with SAE. The seizures stopped 2 days after the start of treatment, and the child regained consciousness after another 4 days.

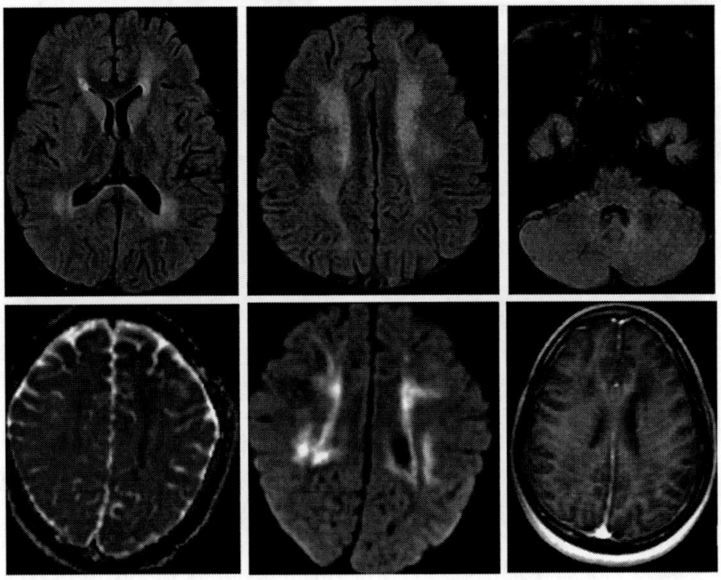

Figure 6.3 A 17-year-old female with sepsis. Axial FLAIR images show areas of hyperintense signals in the centrum semiovale, periventricular, and deep white matter, splenium of the corpus callosum, and lesions of mild hyperintensity in the deep white matter of both cerebellar hemispheres. These areas correspond to the abnormalities on the DWI image. The axial ADC map shows a central area of diffusion restriction in the centrum semiovale. The axial T1-weighted post-contrast image shows no enhancement in the hypointense areas (Ahmed et al., 2011).

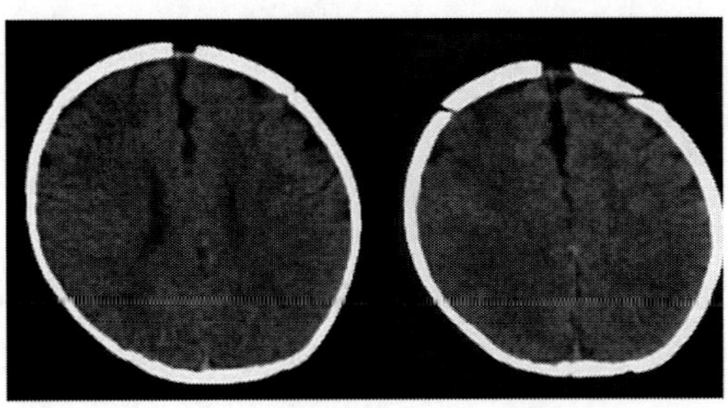

Figure 6.4 Axial imaging of the brain CT showed areas of low density in the right frontal and occipital regions (Abe et al., 2008).

MRI showed areas of hyperintensity in the right cerebral hemisphere on T2-weighted and diffusion-weighted images. Lesions of abnormal intensity were located in the subcortical white matter of the frontal and occipital regions and were hypointense on T1-weighted images and of the high intensity on T2- and diffusion-weighted images. MR angiography revealed no abnormal findings. MRI 4 weeks after the onset of SAE showed moderate atrophic changes in the cortex of the right cerebral hemisphere with preserved areas of the high intensity on T2-WI and reversal of pathological changes on DWI in the same regions. The right hemisphere gyrus also showed high intensity, probably due to residual changes (Fig. 6.5).

Her neurological deficit regressed markedly by the time of the last follow-up examination at 19 months of age. The authors note that the outstanding features of this case were positive bacterial blood cultures and clinical-radiologically confirmed encephalopathy, with no evidence of direct central nervous system infection (CSF analysis was within the normal range and bacterial culture was negative).

According to Hotchkiss et al. (1989), bacterial toxins can directly cause brain dysfunction but do not penetrate the BBB, indicating the important role of bacteremia-induced inflammatory mediators and cytokines in the development of SAE (Sharshar et al., 2004; Papadopoulos et al., 2000; Abe et al., 2008). These factors contribute to the development of cytotoxic edema due to endotheliopathy, as evidenced by the restriction of diffusion in the DWI.

Wu et al. (2018) analyzed the neuroradiological findings of eight children diagnosed with SAE. Brain CT examinations were performed in all patients. CT of five patients showed no pathological changes, two had brain edema, and one had areas of lower density of periventricular white matter of the frontal and parietal lobes (Fig. 6.6).

Four patients were examined by MRI. One patient showed moderate expansion of the external cerebrospinal fluid spaces. Another patient showed hyperintensities in the white matter of the bilateral occipital lobes on T2-weighted imaging (edema) with gyriform enhancement after contrast administration (Fig. 6.7).

The third patient showed not only diffuse abnormal symmetrical signals in the white matter of the cerebral hemispheres and basal ganglia but also lesions with abnormal signals in the cortex of both frontoparietal lobes (Fig. 6.8).

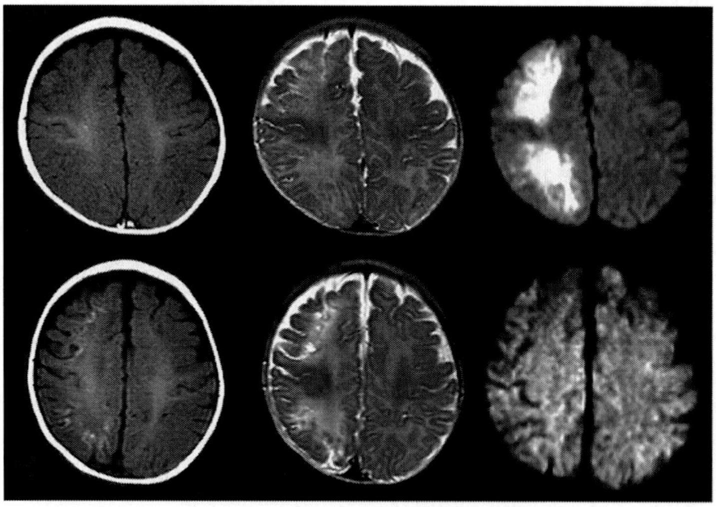

Figure 6.5 Brain MRI on the day after onset (top row) shows abnormal low intensity areas on T1-weighted images in subcortical white matter in the frontal and occipital lobes of the right cerebral hemisphere. T2-weighted and diffusion-weighted images revealed abnormally high intensities in the same regions. Brain MRI at 4 weeks (bottom row) after onset revealed a mild atrophic change with patchy high intensities in the deep gyri on T1-weighted images. Abnormal high-intensity areas were not recognized on diffusion-weighted images but revealed on T2-weighted images (Abe et al., 2008).

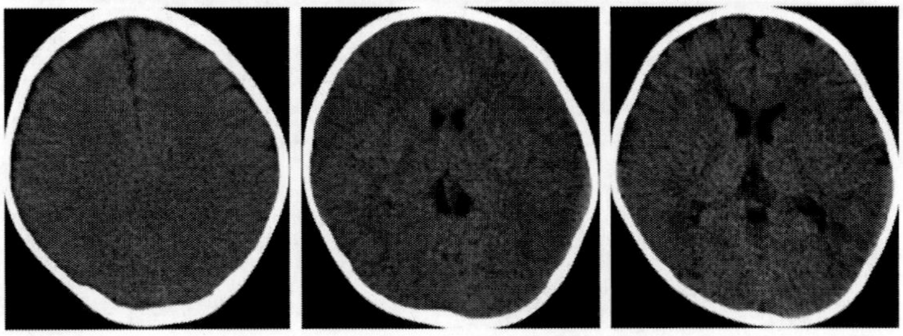

Figure 6.6 CT of three patients showed cerebral edema (in two cases) and areas of lower density of periventricular white matter of the frontal and parietal regions (in one case) (Wu et al., 2018).

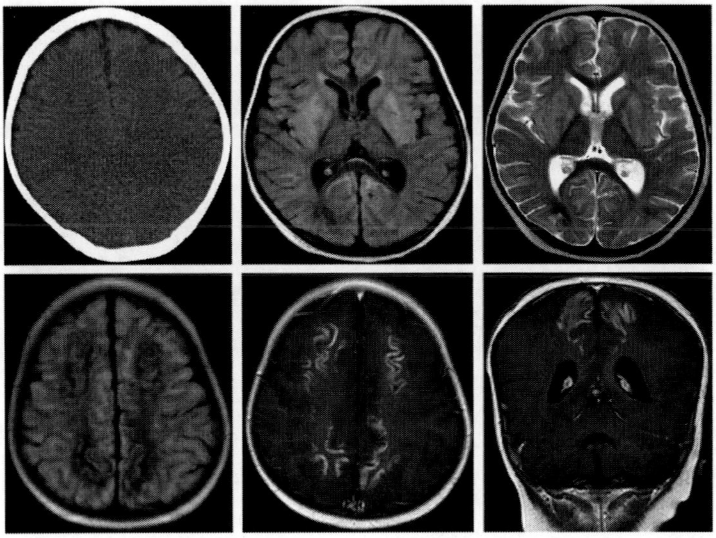

Figure 6.7 A 5-month-old male patient. CT shows diffuse areas of cerebral edema, the disappearance of brain sulci, and blurred edges of gray and white matter. MRI at 16 days shows symmetric areas of high signal in the basal ganglia on T2WI and FLAIR. In the subcortical areas of the frontoparietal lobe, intensity is low on T2WI and FLAIR. Postcontrast T1-WI shows gyriform enhancement of the cortex (Wu et al., 2018).

MRI of the fourth patient showed a diffuse area of abnormal signals consistent with edema in the white matter of both cerebral hemispheres, basal ganglia, and cerebellar hemisphere, and marked gyriform enhancement after contrast (Fig. 6.9).

The authors note that the neurologic deficit persisted in patients with MRI and CT abnormalities. Wu et al. point out that CT has low specificity in the early stages of SAE diagnosis. The findings mainly show diffuse cerebral edema and hypodense areas in the white matter of the cerebral hemispheres. MRI shows changes caused by a combination of vasogenic and cytotoxic edema, mainly in the brain stems, basal ganglia, and semioval centers in a symmetrical distribution.

PRES

Posterior reversible encephalopathy syndrome (PRES) belongs to the spectrum of SAE –associated disorders. There are several theories regarding the pathophysiology of PRES. The most

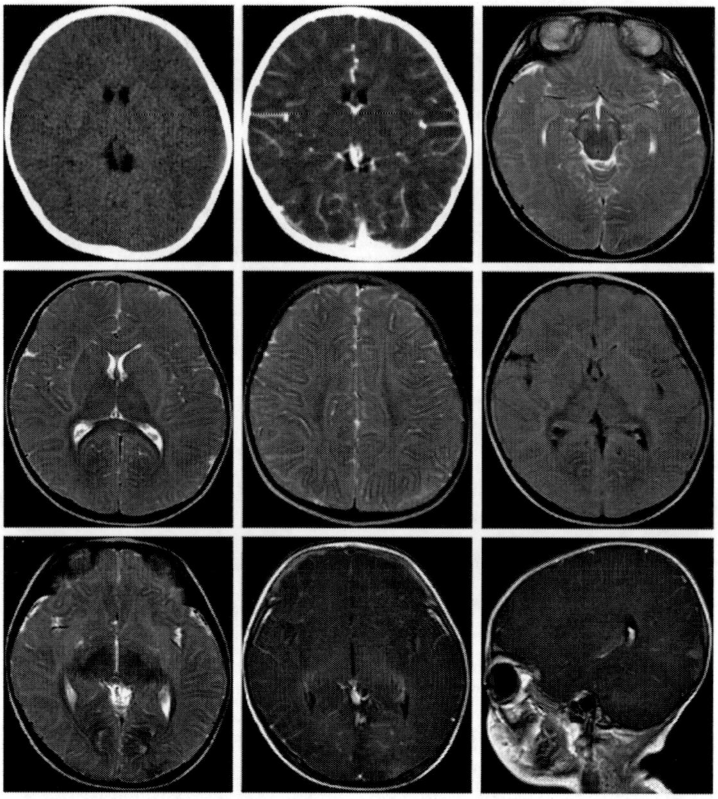

Figure 6.8 An 11-month-old male patient. Brain CT with and without contrast is normal. MRI at 6 days, T2WI shows diffuse and symmetrical high signals in the peduncles, basal ganglia, and semioval areas. FLAIR shows symmetrical areas of high signals in the basal ganglia and white matter. T2WI shows patchy weak signals in bilateral occipital lobes with abnormal enhancement (Wu et al., 2018).

widely accepted theory is that rapidly developing hypertension leads to impaired cerebral autoregulation, particularly in the posterior head. Hyperperfusion is accompanied by extravasation of proteins and fluid, resulting in local vasogenic edema (Hinchey et al., 1996; Primavera et al., 2001; Schwartz et al., 1992). An alternative theory implies endothelial dysfunction (Dekker et al., 1998, Aird, 2003). The third theory suggests that vasospasm followed by ischemia may be responsible (Trommer et al., 1988; Ito et al., 1995; Lin et al., 2003).

Because the second theory is consistent with the presumed pathophysiology of SAE, probably in the presence of sepsis, the posterior reversible encephalopathy syndrome can be considered an integral component of SAE, including its neuroradiological presentation. Studies have shown that PRES is more common in Gram-positive sepsis associated with a marked systemic inflammatory response.

Fugate et al. (2010), after analyzing neuroimaging data from patients with PRES of different etiologies in 109 patients, concluded that cortical involvement was more common in patients with sepsis than in patients without infection. In all patients with sepsis, the changes were mainly localized in the parietooccipital regions. Other researchers have noted that in PRES

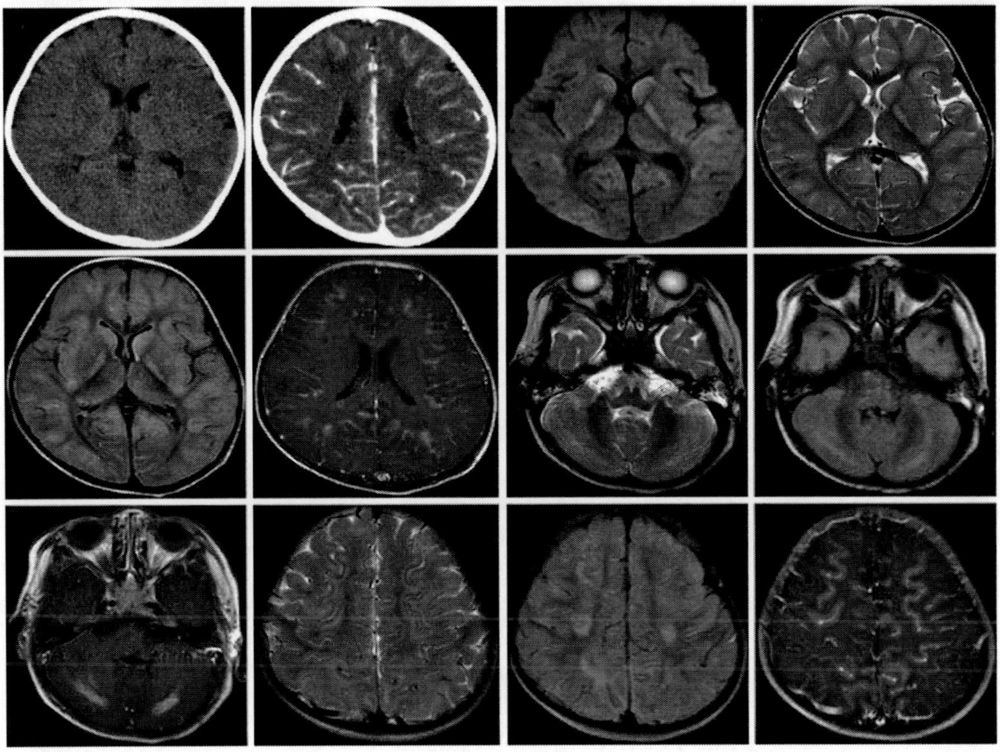

Figure 6.9 A 22-month-old male patient. Plain and contrast CT scans with suspicion of low signal in the bilateral frontal lobe without enhancement. MRI at 6 days, DWI shows diffuse cerebral edema, while T2WI and FLAIR show high signals in bilateral ganglia and white matter areas. T1WI shows gyriform enhancement with positive contrast. On T2WI (G) and FLAIR (H), a small punctate or patchy high signal with marked enhancement is also seen in the cerebellum. T2WI shows a streaky low signal in the bilateral parietooccipital lobes, which show no enhancement on T1WI (Wu et al., 2018).

abnormal findings on MRI are rarely localized only in the white matter of the parietal-occipital regions of the cerebral hemispheres, but frequently involve the cortex, frontal lobes, basal ganglia, and brainstem (Lee et al., 2008; Bartynski et al., 2007).

Fugate et al. (2010) sought to determine the relationship between clinical manifestations and neuroradiological signs of PRES. According to the researchers, there is no convincing evidence of a clear correlation between clinical features and brain imaging at PRES. This is also emphasized by other authors (Mueller-Mang et al., 2009). However, this is in contradiction with other reports suggesting that the extent of vasogenic edema is inversely related to blood pressure, the increase of which, moreover, undoubtedly contributes to the development of PRES. Moreover, some researchers suggest a relationship between the massiveness of the spread of vasogenic edema and the normal blood pressure of patients (Bartynski et al., 2006).

Chacqueneau et al. (2013) described the case of a 4-year-old female patient who presented to the emergency department with fever, aphasia, abdominal pain, and cerebellar syndrome. Sepsis developed as a result of appendicitis peritonitis. After 48 hours, the patient fell into a coma (Glasgow score at 9). MRI showed edema in the white matter of the cerebral and cerebellar hemispheres and in the basal ganglia on T2-weighted and FLAIR imaging (Fig. 6.10). No MRI abnormalities suggestive of cytotoxic edema were found in DWI.

Neuroimaging data were considered manifestations of PRES and SAE. Subsequent follow-up showed positive dynamics of MRI findings, with subtle MRI abnormalities preserved in the cerebellar hemispheres, which was associated with regression of the neurological deficit.

Bartynski et al. (2006) presented 25 cases of PRES with sepsis. This study included 106 patients with PRES of various etiologies, with sepsis accounting for 23.6%. MRI of the brain was performed in all patients. Using the data obtained, the authors evaluated the extent and severity of edema in the affected regions on a 5-point scale:

Grade 1: is characterized by cortex edema, limited subcortical white matter edema, or both. The affected regions are not confluent, and there is also a mild local cortex mass effect or distortion due to the edema (Fig. 6.11).

Grade 2: is characterized by white matter edema that is slightly thicker than cortex edema. The subcortical white matter edema extends into the deep white matter (mainly without much medial to lateral extension). Some affected regions are occasionally confluent. A local cortical mass effect or distortion due to the edema may be seen (Fig. 6.12).

Grade 3: is characterized by white matter edema much thicker than cortex edema. In addition, limited and focal extension to the ventricular surface was noted (development of a broad medial-lateral extension). The affected regions are partially confluent with a moderate local cortex mass effect/distortion due to the edema (Fig. 6.13).

Grade 4: is characterized by white matter edema much more severe than cortex edema. The affected regions essentially extend to the ventricular surface (diffuse broad medial to lateral extension). In addition, the affected regions are almost completely confluent, with no ventricular distortion due to the edema.

Grade 5: White matter edema is severe and dominates the cortex edema. The affected regions are completely confluent and continuous with diffuse, broad medial-to-lateral extension. The MRI abnormalities extend completely to the ventricular surface with ventricular deformity due to the edema (Fig. 6.14).

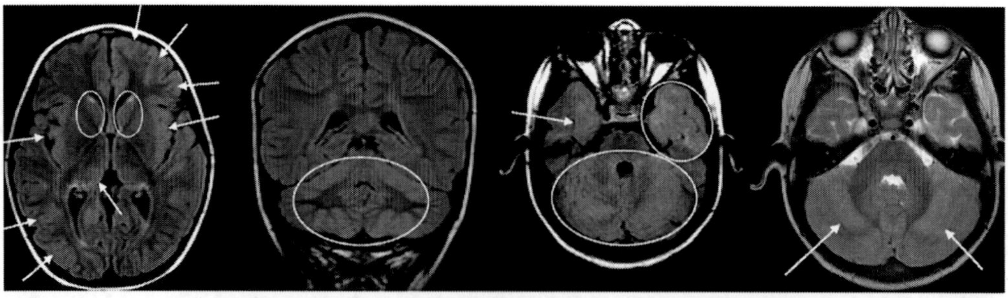

Figure 6.10 A 4-year-old female patient with sepsis secondary to appendicitis peritonitis. T2-weighted and FLAIR images show mild edema in the basal ganglia and white matter of the cerebral and cerebellar hemispheres on both sides (Chacqueneau et al., 2013).

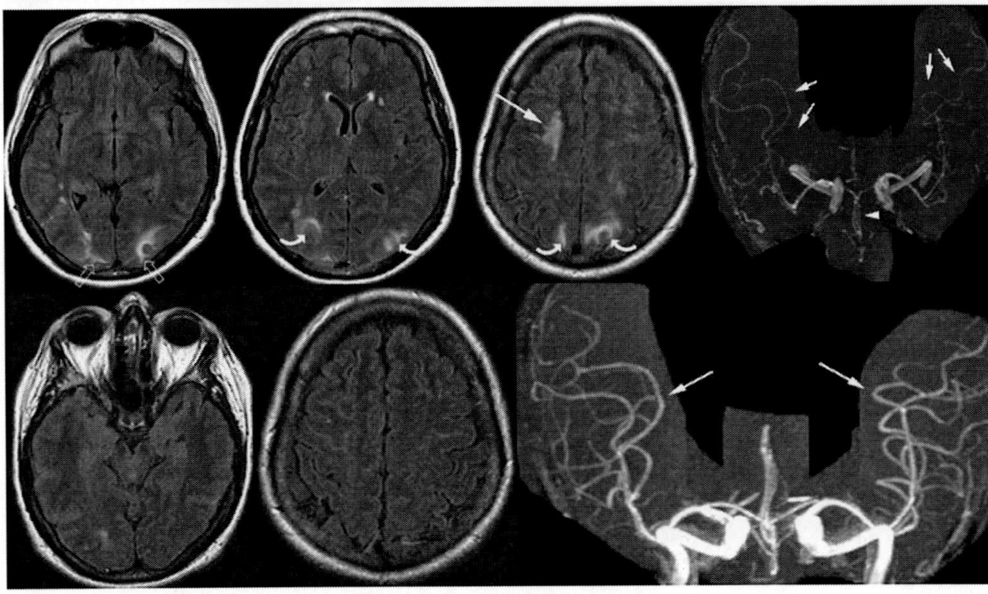

Figure 6.11 A 54-year-old female patient with bilateral multisegmental pneumonia as a cause of sepsis. An MRI performed 1 day after the onset of sepsis showed focal areas of vasogenic edema in the frontal, parietal, and occipital lobes on both sides (top row of FLAIR images). Signal abnormalities in the frontal lobe run linearly along the superior frontal sulcus and are unrelated to signal intensity in the parietal lobe, consistent with PRES, and classified as Grade 1. MRA (top row) shows extensive vasospasm of the first-, second-, and third-order branches in the anterior cerebral artery, middle cerebral artery, and posterior communicating artery on both sides. MRI images (bottom row of FLAIR) acquired at follow-up 11 days after the initial examination show regression of vasogenic edema in all regions. A repeat MRA shows that the extensive vasospasm has disappeared, and all vessels appear nearly normal (Bartynski et al., 2006).

Neuroradiological abnormalities showing ringlike enhancement

In some cases, in patients with sepsis and sterile CSF, the phenomenon of contrast accumulation is observed in the form of peripheral or linear patterns (Fig. 6.15). According to Hollinger et al. (2000), the neuroradiological abnormalities appear delayed in patients (3 or more weeks). At the same time, no convincing signs of diffusion restriction are detected (Hollinger et al., 2000).

In such cases, the presence of SAE cannot be inferred until other possible causes of encephalopathy have been ruled out, such as hypoxemia, liver failure, uremia, meningoencephalitis, endocarditis, drug intoxication, electrolyte imbalance, and cancer recurrence (Bolton et al., 1993). The pathophysiological basis of annular enhancement in SAE remains unclear. The possibility of vasogenic edema, subacute stage of ischemic edema, early cerebral stage cytotoxic edema, and late cerebral stage microabscess of the brain is discussed (Haimes et al., 1994; Schwartz et al., 1998; Warach et al., 1995). It should be noted that some authors classify microabscesses as SAE (Schwartz et al., 1998; Warach et al., 1995), and some researchers believe that this phenomenon is possibly a marker of disease progression in patients with a clinical diagnosis of SAE (Jackson et al., 1985).

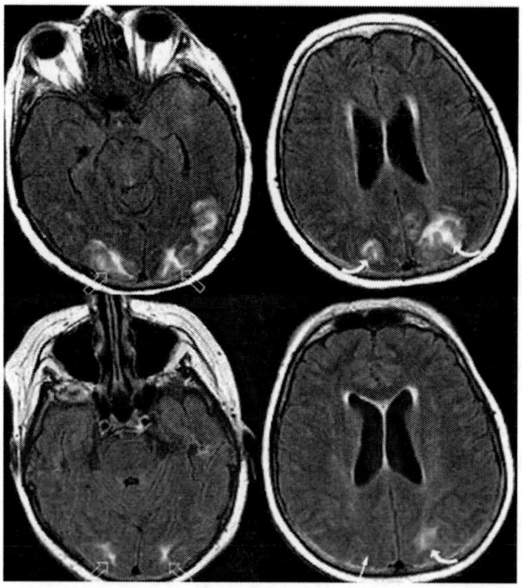

Figure 6.12 A 68-year-old female patient with a pancreatic abscess as a cause of sepsis. Axial FLAIR images show vasogenic edema in the occipital and parietal regions on both sides, typical of PRES with extension into the deep white matter but without extension to the ventricular surface, corresponding to a Grade 2 (top row of FLAIR images). MRI follow-up of the brain (bottom row of images from FLAIR), performed 1 month after the initial examination, showed almost complete resolution of edema in the occipital and left parietal regions and complete resolution in the right parietal region (Bartynski et al., 2006).

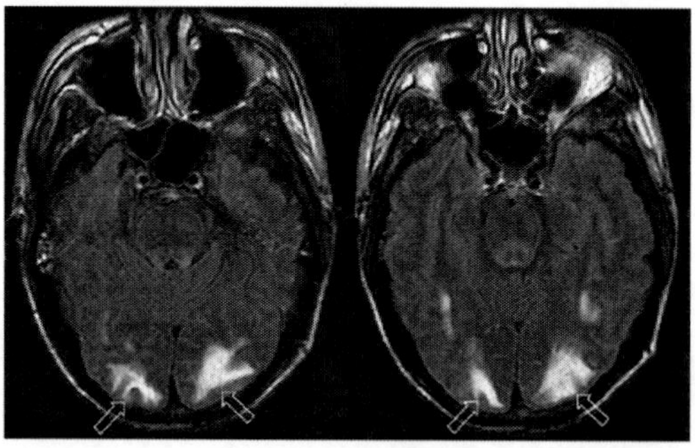

Figure 6.13 A 39-year-old male patient had severe pneumonia with bronchial obstruction as the cause of sepsis. Brain MR imaging (FLAIR sequence) showed a moderate signal intensity abnormality due to vasogenic edema in the occipital lobes, bilaterally typical of the PRES pattern with full extension to the ventricular surface and a moderate local cortical mass effect corresponding to Grade 3 (Bartynski et al., 2006).

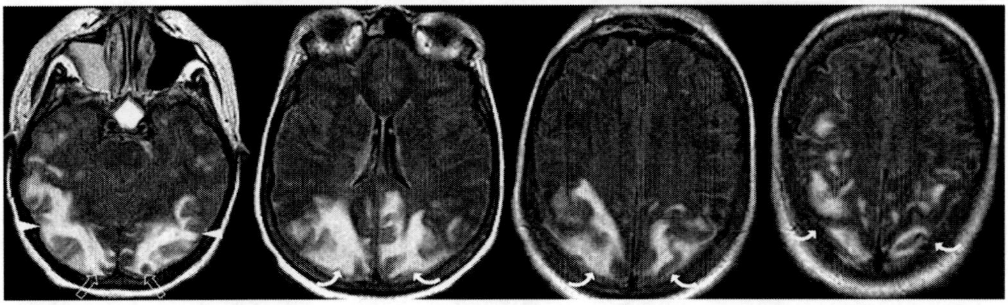

Figure 6.14 A 56-year-old female patient with a thigh abscess with culturally developed mixed flora. She developed MOD (coagulopathy, acute respiratory distress syndrome, acute renal failure, liver failure, and shock liver). Brain MR imaging (sequence FLAIR) performed 1 day after neurotoxicity showed severe and extensive vasogenic edema primarily involving the subcortical white matter of the parietal, occipital, and temporal regions bilaterally with ventricular distortions due to Grade 5 edema (Bartynski et al., 2006).

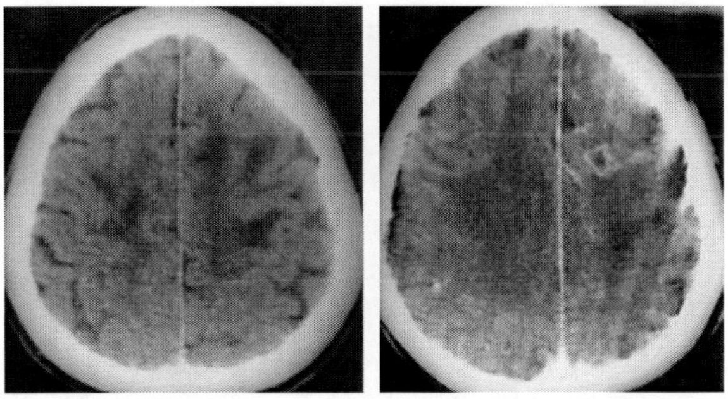

Figure 6.15 A 49-year-old male patient with fulminant pneumococcal septicemia 18 years after splenectomy for Hodgkin's disease, corresponding to the clinical syndrome of overwhelming post-splenectomy infection. Brain examination CT showed multiple non-enhancing hypodense areas in the white matter of both cerebral hemispheres 2 days after admission. Brain examination CT, performed 4 weeks after admission, showed regressive hypodense areas in the white matter and annular enhancement of lesions (Hollinger et al., 2000).

Brain hemorrhage

One of the unfavorable prognostic criteria for SAE is the development of intracranial hemorrhages. It should be noted that their spectrum and massiveness vary widely. They may be subarachnoid hemorrhages, focal intraparenchymal hemorrhages, or microhemorrhages, predominantly in cortical and subcortical areas.

Shindo et al. (2018) reported a 66-year-old man with persistent fever and diarrhea that had progressed to coma (GCS score was 11). MRI showed symmetrical areas of MRI signals (FLAIR) in the white matter of the cerebral hemispheres. SWI showed multiple microhemorrhages in the white matter (Fig. 6.16). Based on the history, clinical presentation, neuroimaging data, and instrumental examination, the diagnosis of SAE was made. An MRI scan at 60 days showed marked regression of the previously noted changes while maintaining the

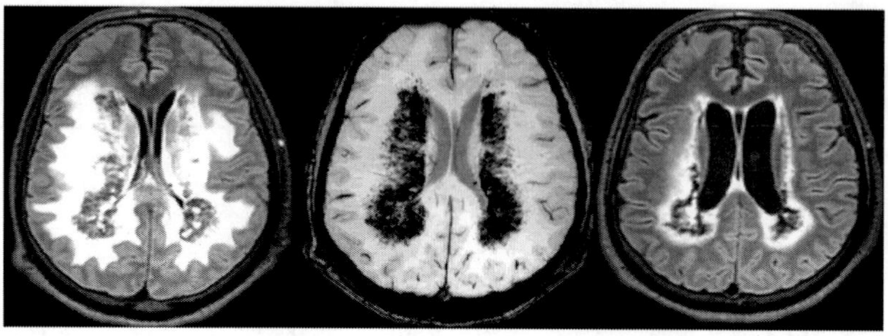

Figure 6.16 A 66-year-old male patient with sepsis-associated encephalopathy. The first two MRI scans of the brain (on Day 15) show areas of increased FLAIR signal in the white matter and multiple microhemorrhages in the same regions in the SWI. The third MRI scan shows decreased areas in white matter and cerebral atrophy at Day 60 (Shindo et al., 2018).

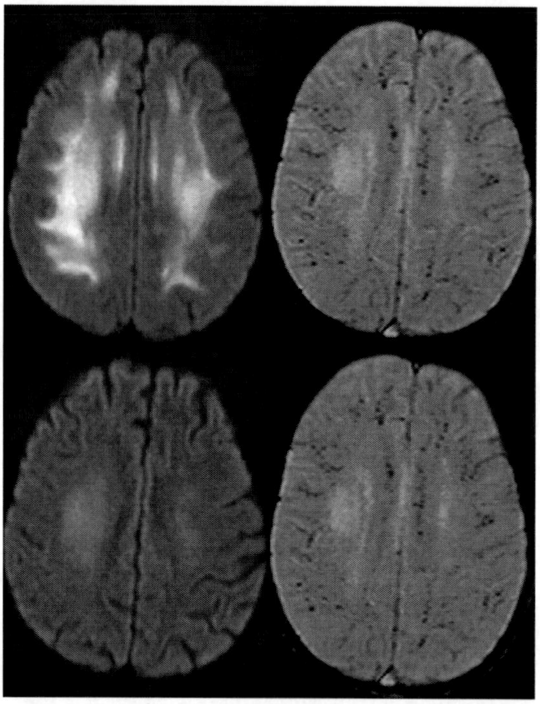

Figure 6.17 A 28-year-old woman underwent laparotomy for ruptured peritonitis. DWIs show extensive cytotoxic edema of the centrum semiovale and periventricular white matter on both sides. SWIs show extensive punctate efflorescent hypointensities suggestive of microhemorrhages in the subcortical white matter (top row). At follow-up (after 2 weeks), brain MRI images (DWI and SWI sequence) (bottom row) show a significant decrease in white matter cytotoxic edema and a decrease in petechial spots (Lekhra et al., 2015).

manifestations of the imaging patterns. Despite the positive dynamics of the MRI findings, the GCS score was 7 without significant recovery of the neurological deficit.

Lekhra et al. (2015) reported SAE in a 28-year-old woman with ruptured peritonitis. In the postoperative period, the patient developed sepsis and went into a coma. Analysis of cerebrospinal fluid (CSF) was normal. Because systemic septicemia was present, the possibility of SAE was considered. MRI abnormalities in the white matter in the centrum semiovale, periventricular area, which the authors felt were suggestive of cytotoxic edema. SWI imaging showed multiple petechial hemorrhages, which are rarely found at SAE. Repeat MRI scans of the brain showed that the prevalence of areas of cytotoxic edema on DWI decreased significantly, as did the resolution of petechial lesions on SWI. According to Lekhra et al. (2015), one possible explanation is that the infection triggers an autoimmune response that leads to perivascular demyelination and hemorrhage in the brain parenchyma.

The complete genesis of the hemorrhage remains unclear. Discussions include damage to the BBB in vasogenic edema, the late stages of cytotoxic edema, the role of disseminated intravascular coagulation (DIC), or the manifestations of fibrinoid necrosis of small vessels in sepsis. It is noteworthy that the severity of MRI changes does not always indicate a poor outcome in patients with SAE (Papadopoulos et al., 1999).

The cause of the hemorrhage may also be venous infarction after venous sinus thrombosis. The neuroradiologic picture is not different from the usual one.

In general, CT and MRI abnormalities in SAE are characterized by cortical swelling and loss of differentiation between gray and white matter. There are areas of increased MR signal in the basal ganglia, hippocampus (Fig. 6.18), subcortical and periventricular white matter on DWI, with a decrease in signal (restricted diffusion) on ADC maps, in areas with cytotoxic edema or without if the area is due to vasogenic edema.

During follow-up, the development of subarachnoid hemorrhage of varying severity is possible, as is the occurrence of the phenomenon of pseudo subarachnoid hemorrhage due to venous congestion (Fig. 6.19).

White matter necrosis

In addition, particularly in severe cases, areas of necrosis form in the white matter of the cerebral and cerebellar hemispheres and brainstem, showing a linear shape and typical MRI signal features. The following report presents a variant of severe SAE with diffuse edema, necrotic changes in the subcortical white matter, and signs of brain death.

Kondo et al. (2009) reported their experience with the diagnosis of SAE in pediatric practice. A 17-month-old boy was admitted to a hospital with generalized convulsions, and his level of consciousness was a Glasgow Coma Score (GCS) of 3. A brain CT performed one hour after the onset of convulsions, revealed diffuse cerebral edema. *Haemophilus influenzae* was detected in the blood culture. The brain edema progressively worsened despite the administration of mannitol. On day 56, CT showed persistent cerebral edema with evidence of massive subarachnoid hemorrhage. MRI performed on day 106 showed hyperdense, fissured lesions in the white matter of the hemispheres, cerebellum, and also in the brainstem, as well as an unclear corticomedullary junction. Thrombosis of the large intracranial venous sinus was also noted. On day 247, MR angiography showed a marked decrease in blood flow in the intracranial and extracranial arteries (Fig. 6.20). He was discharged one and a half years after the onset of the disease.

In the above case, the authors state that there is no clinical or laboratory evidence of a direct infectious process in the CNS and the clinical status and imaging data are explained

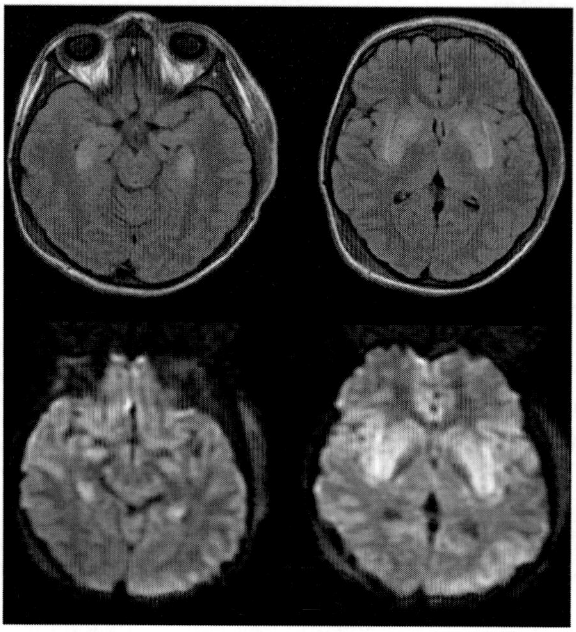

Figure 6.18 A X-year-old female patient with septic encephalopathy. FLAIR and DWI axial MRI sequences show diffuse abnormalities with increased intensity of MR signal in the basal nuclei, heads, and bodies of the hippocampus.

by disturbances of the BBB caused by bacterial toxins and cytokines. It is noteworthy that the angiography data are consistent with the concept of a sharp increase in intracranial pressure leading to the phenomenon of "stop contrast," which is one of the criteria for brain death (Kondo et al., 2009).

MRI findings varied widely between a single focal area (Fig. 6.21) with abnormally high signals in the white matter and massive confluent areas (Figs. 6.22, 6.23).

Sharshar et al. (2007) have attempted to systematize and order the MRI findings in patients with septic shock and establish a relationship between sepsis and leukoencephalopathy (Figs. 6.24–6.26).

In our opinion, the following can be added to the neuroradiological presentation of SAE: leukoencephalopathy, to necrotizing (Fig. 6.27), with the dynamic progression of white matter lesions; vasculopathy with minimal leptomeningeal enhancement (Fig. 6.28); hemorrhagic and ischemic lesions of varying severity associated with disseminated intravascular coagulation; diffuse cerebral edema due to a combination of vasogenic and cytotoxic edema; PRES; microabscesses.

It should be emphasized that the probability of the development of various types of hemorrhage is high, and one should always keep in mind the possibility of the development of the phenomenon of pseudo subarachnoid hemorrhage.

A particular topic of discussion is the development of small ischemic lesions and microabscesses as indicators of sepsis embolism (SEE) and metastatic sepsis encephalitis (SME).

Septic-embolic (SEE) and septic-metastatic encephalitis (SME)

The fairly common complications of sepsis include not only sepsis-associated encephalopathy (SAE) but also sepsis-embolic encephalitis (SEE) and sepsis-metastatic encephalitis (SME)

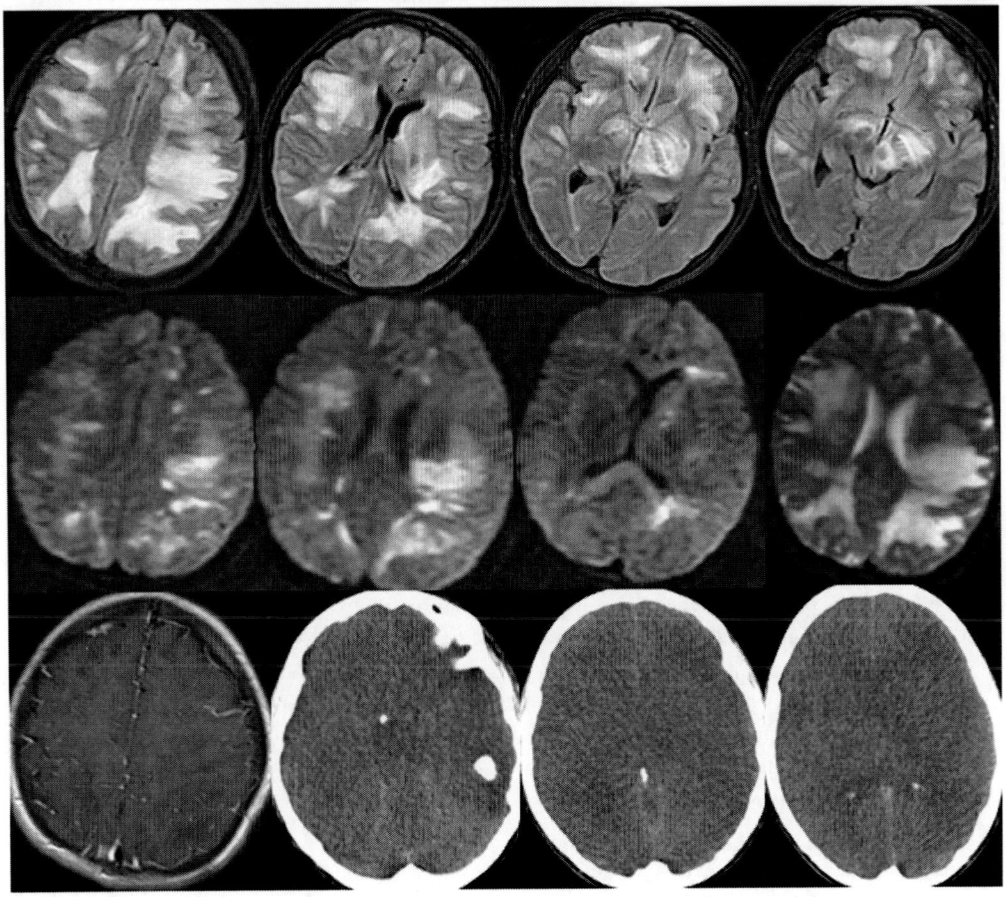

Figure 6.19 A 34-year-old female patient presented with puerperal sepsis, SAE, and coma (Glasgow score at 3). A detailed examination allowed the exclusion of autoimmune encephalitis, antiphospholipid syndrome, and systemic lupus erythematosus. MRI performed 4 days after emergence showed vasogenic edema with elements of cytotoxic edema and dislocation syndrome. Mild leptomeningeal enhancement was seen on postcontrast images. According to Sharshar et al. (2007), this presentation is a grade 3 leukoencephalopathy. CT on day 11 showed diffuse cerebral edema and the pseudo subarachnoid hemorrhage phenomenon.

(Tauber et al., 2020), which are part of the general pathophysiologic process observed in sepsis (Fig. 6.29).

Inflammation occurs in both SEE and SME, but ischemia and subsequent hemorrhage are predominant in SEE, whereas focal inflammation in the form of microabscesses or cerebris is more prominent in SME (Tauber et al., 2011). This gradation is reflected in the clinical presentation, since in septic encephalitis there is an increase in focal neurological deficits, while SAE is more characterized by delirium of varying severity. It should be noted that the division of SME and SEE is rather conditional.

Tauber et al. (2020) suggest that SEE most often develops as a complication of bacterial endocarditis with consecutive infected cerebral emboli leading to multiple strokes (Fig. 6.30).

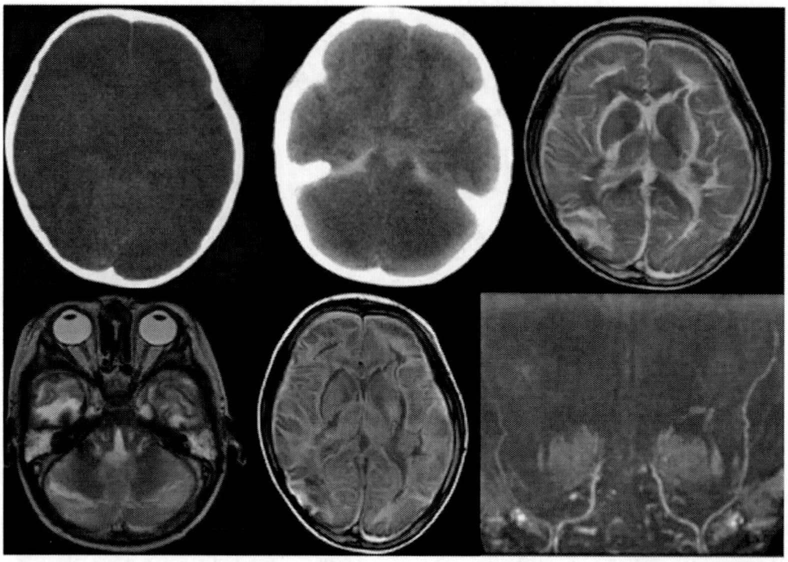

Figure 6.20 A 17-month-old male patient with sepsis. Brain CT performed on Day 1 shows a blurred corticomedullary junction and narrowed ventricles, suggestive of diffuse cerebral edema. Brain CT, performed on Day 56, shows persistent brain swelling and subarachnoid hemorrhage. A T2-W image (performed on Day 106) shows cracked lesions in the white matter, brainstem, and cerebellum. FLAIR imaging shows cracked lesions and extensive hyperintensity lesions in the white matter. MR angiography performed on day 247 shows a marked decrease in blood flow in the anterior, middle, and posterior cerebral arteries (Kondo et al., 2009).

The etiological causes of SME can be any bacterial or fungal focus and are characterized by microabscesses (Prange, 2006; Bitsch et al., 1996).

The propensity of SAE patients to develop intracerebral hemorrhage is explained by the special character of septic microemboli. Unlike other microemboli, they contain bacteria or fungi, and these pathogens penetrate the wall of the occluded microvessel and cause purulent arteriolitis with the destruction of the elastic fibers. Subsequently, spontaneous fragmentation of the embolus by autolysis contributes to focal intraparenchymal hemorrhage (Prange, 2006; Bitsch et al., 1996; Tauber et al., 2020). This mechanism is also observed in SAE, which determines the generality of these conditions. Like SAE, SME is characterized by diffuse axonal injury and demyelination in the subcortical white matter (Ehler et al., 2017; Tauber et al., 2020). Ehler et al. (2017) conducted a study that included a simulation of experimental sepsis in rats with fecal peritonitis, postmortem examinations of the brains of patients with sepsis, and a prospective cohort study of human sepsis in college laboratories and intensive care units. The authors identified two main types of changes: ischemic and diffuse neuroaxonal damage to the brain. Among these, diffuse axonal injury (DAI) was the predominant type in SAE.

Long-term outcome and neuroradiological findings

SAE can lead to diffuse brain atrophy (Fig. 6.31) and subsequent cognitive decline. Several cohort studies have reported a high prevalence of cognitive impairment in ICU survivors (Jackson et al., 2003; Hopkins et al., 2005; Devlin et al., 1999), but assessment is difficult because there

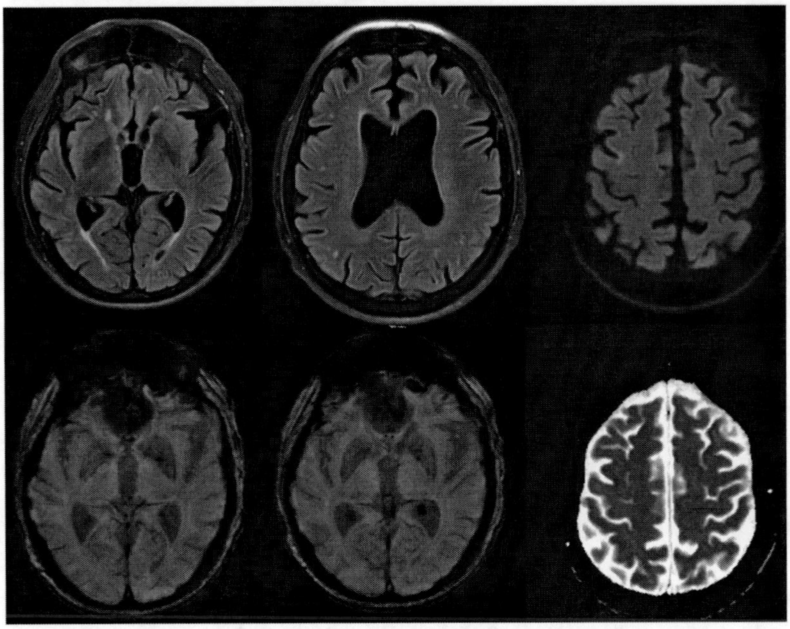

Figure 6.21 A 45-year-old male patient presented with septic encephalopathy after heart transplantation. After the clinical presentation, an MRI of the brain was performed. Axial FLAIR images showed multiple hypertensive lesions of varying sizes with clear contours in the subcortical regions of the frontal, parietal, and temporal lobes on both sides (a, b). DWI image showed a hypertensive lesion in the subcortical white matter of the right frontal lobe with abnormally low ADC values (abnormal diffusion restriction). SWI images showed punctate lesions as hypointense in the nucleus lentiformis and globus pallidus secondary to microhemorrhages.

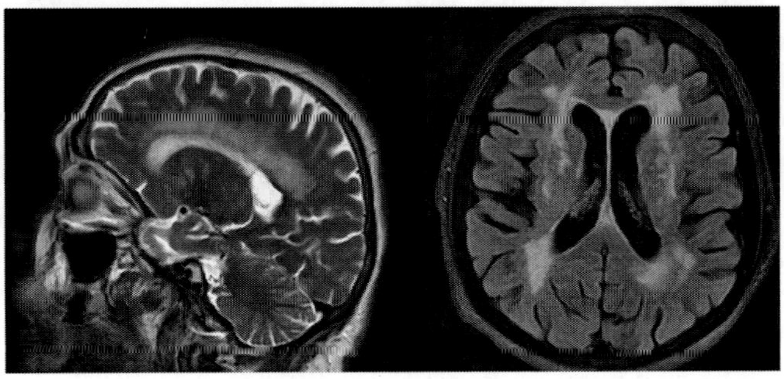

Figure 6.22 A 75-year-old woman with sepsis after coronary angioplasty and stent implantation. MRI performed 5 days after coronary intervention shows massive areas of abnormally high signal in the periventricular and centrum semiovale white matter on T2-weighted and FLAIR imaging. The difficulty in diagnosis, in this case, lies in the distinction between the manifestations of SAE and age-related changes.

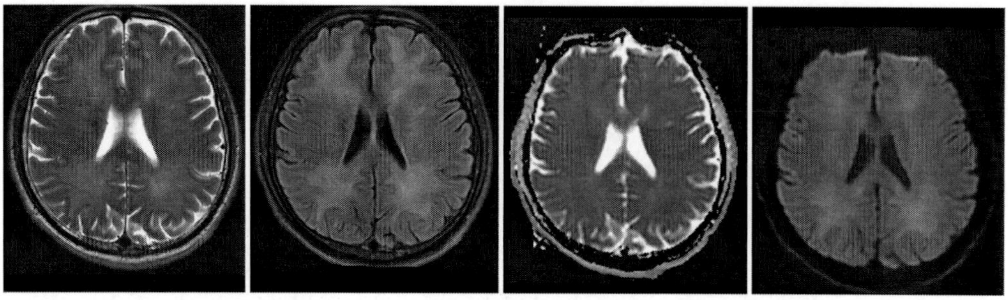

Figure 6.23 A 30-year-old man with ruptured peritonitis, sepsis, and delirium. T2-weighted and FLAIR images show massive confluent areas in the subcortical and deep white matter in the frontal and parietal regions on both sides. These areas are characterized by increased DWI signal without abnormally low ADC values (diffusion restriction).

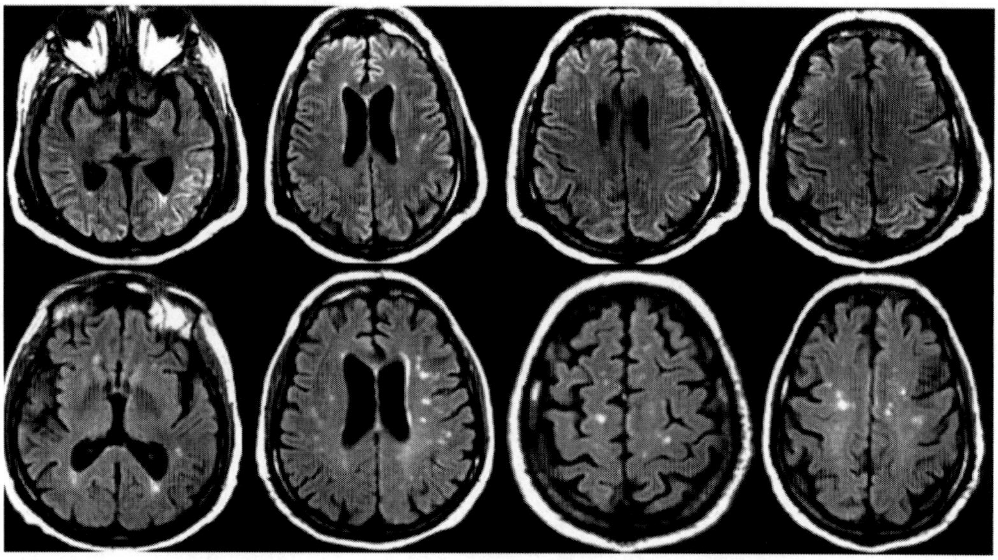

Figure 6.24 A 60-year-old man with cellulitis. Initial (top row) brain MRI respectively on Day 1 and after the onset of septic shock. Axial FLAIR images show few hyperintense lesions in the white matter of the frontal regions. Control MRI of the brain (bottom row) performed 24 days after the onset of septic shock shows many punctate hyperintense reductions, especially at the level of the centrum semiovale. They extend from the cortico-subcortical border into the deep white matter of the semioval centers with an orientation suggestive of the involvement of the Virchow-Robin spaces. This clinical presentation is termed Grade 1 leukoencephalopathy (Sharshar et al., 2007).

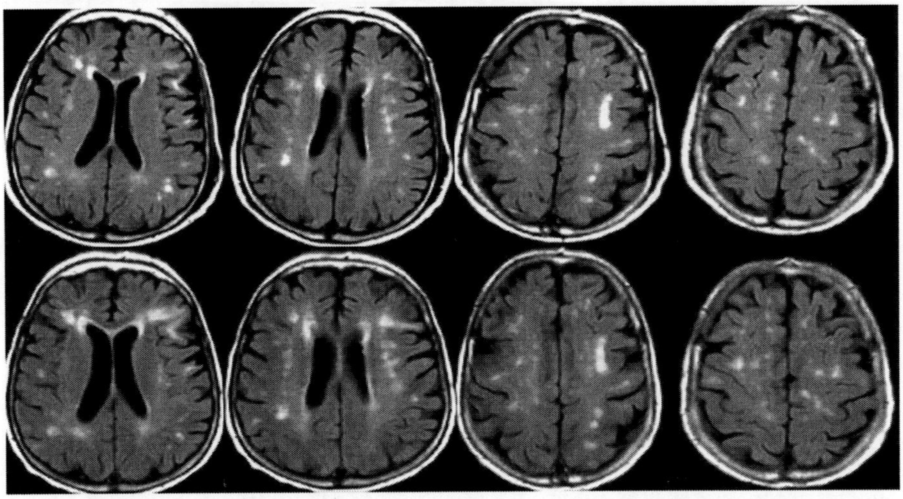

Figure 6.25 A 69-year-old woman with ARDS due to *Streptococcus pneumoniae*. Initial MRI of the brain (top row) respectively on day 3 after the onset of septic shock. Axial FLAIR images show multiple hyperintense lesions in the subcircular and centrum-semiovale white matter on both sides. Some lesions are punctate, while others are more extensive and confluent in some regions. This clinical presentation is termed Grade 2 leukoencephalopathy (Sharshar et al., 2007). Follow-up MRI shows some increase in the extent and conspicuity of the lesions (bottom row).

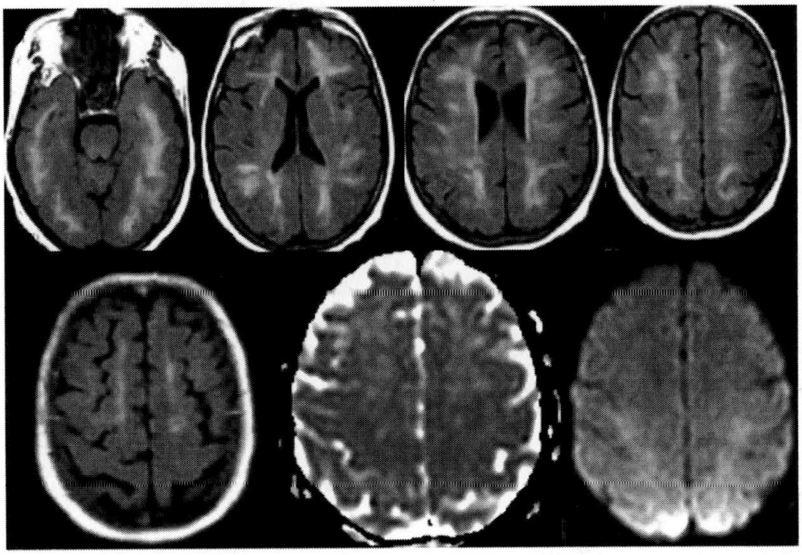

Figure 6.26 A 66-year-old woman with septicemia due to *Pseudomonas aeruginosa*. MRI was performed on Day 4 after the onset of septic shock. Axial FLAIR images showed hyperintense abnormalities in the subcortical, deep, and centrum semiovale white matter that were more extensive than those shown in Fig. 6.25, and the signal abnormalities were confluent. This presentation was termed Grade 3 leukoencephalopathy. The ADC map showed diffuse ADC enhancement in the white matter, indicating vasogenic edema in the areas of white matter with abnormal signals (Sharshar et al., 2007).

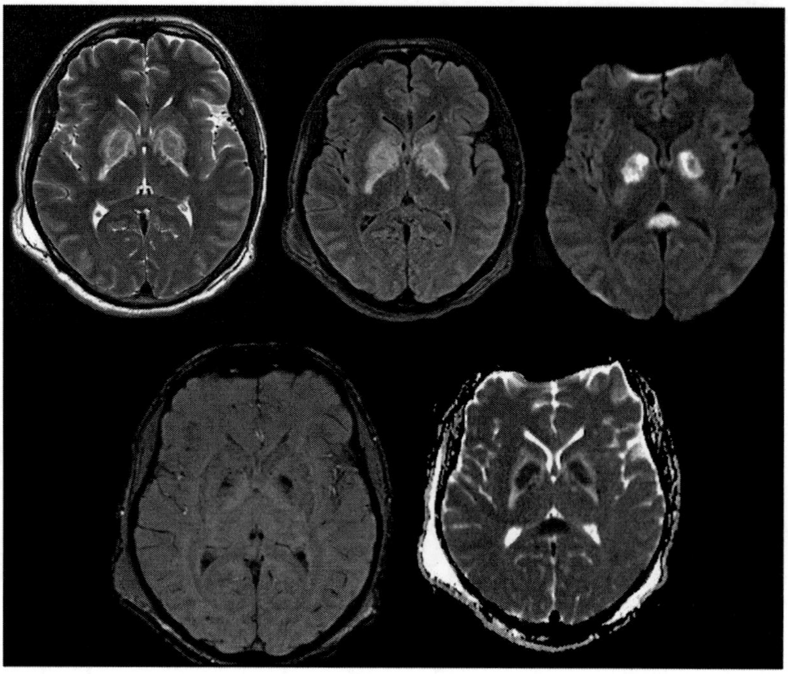

Figure 6.27 A 32-year-old woman with bilateral pyelonephritis, acute kidney failure, and sepsis. MRI performed on Day 3 shows symmetric necrosis of the basal nuclei due to severe hypoxia and toxemia. In addition, MRI shows a lenticular bifurcation sign suggestive of uremia.

is no data on premorbid cognitive status. There is evidence that executive dysfunction, like other forms of impairment, usually develops secondary to decreased blood flow to vulnerable subcortical structures, even in the absence of obvious ischemic injury (Alexander et al., 1986).

Conclusion

In this way, there are nonspecific but well-defined neuroradiologic patterns that should raise suspicion of SAE in a critically ill patient with sepsis and developing delirium.

An extremely serious problem is the difficulty in studying patients with sepsis, resulting in an extremely small and scattered number of cases and observations that rarely fit into an acceptable time scale of events. Therefore, neuroradiologic methods such as CT and MRI must be performed prospectively, with objective indicators to consider and monitor. MRI is the method of choice that allows early detection of a combination of areas of vasogenic and cytotoxic edema and/or hemorrhage due to hypotension, coagulopathy, and endotheliitis, signs of PRES, which are typical of SAE. CT is undoubtedly delayed and less specific. Further studies should be performed to gain a deeper understanding of the pathophysiological mechanisms underlying the neurological imaging patterns and to relate them to etiological factors, history, and possible iatrogens. The data obtained confirm the need for early diagnosis of SAE, taking into account its impact on the functional outcome of the disease.

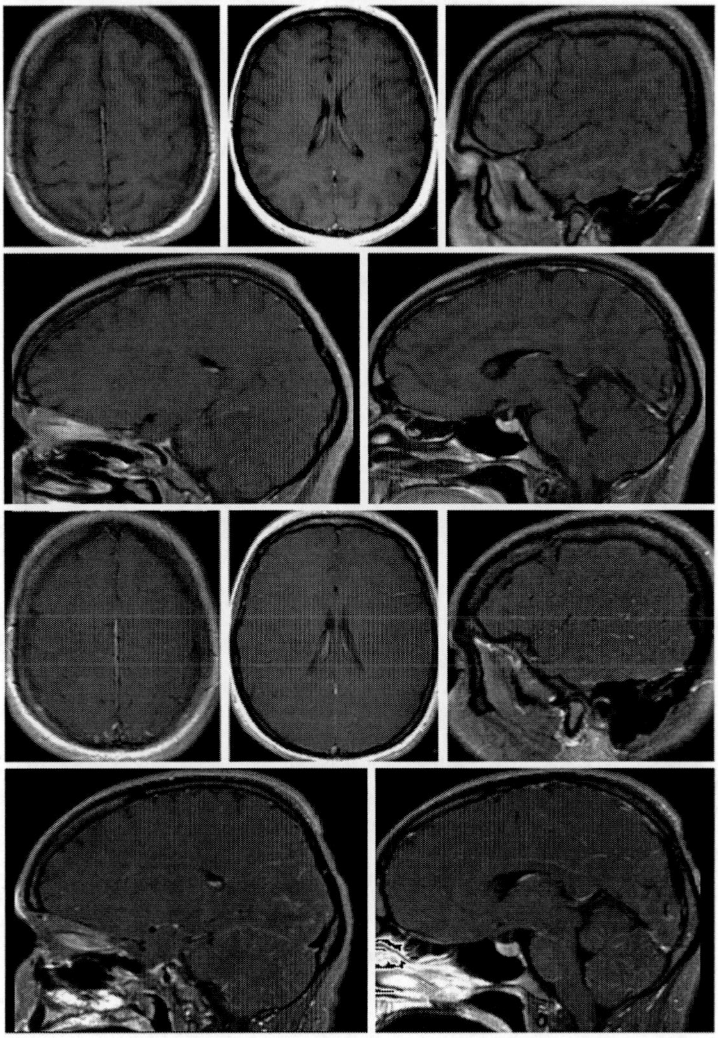

Figure 6.28 A 37-year-old female patient with pelvic peritonitis and septic encephalopathy. MRI performed on day 1 after the onset of septic was normal (top two rows of post-contrast T1W images). Follow-up MRI with an interval of a day shows gyriform enhancement of occipital and temporal lobes as well as the cerebellum on postcontrast T1-WI (bottom two rows of T1W post-contrast images).

Methods such as MR diffusion (DWI), diffusion tensor imaging (DTI, MR tractography), perfusion, magnetic resonance spectroscopy (MRS), and positron emission tomography (PET / CT, PET /MRI) will allow more detailed characterization of the temporal profile of key pathophysiological mechanisms in sepsis. For example, using arterial spin labeling (ASL) MR perfusion, Masse et al. (2018) found a loss of cerebral autoregulation with a corresponding increase in cerebral blood flow in the early stages of sepsis. This approach will allow us to determine the true significance of neuroradiological patterns in the diagnosis of sepsis, clarify prognostic criteria, and set the stage for building the evidence base needed to evaluate the efficacy of ongoing therapeutic trials and outcome measures.

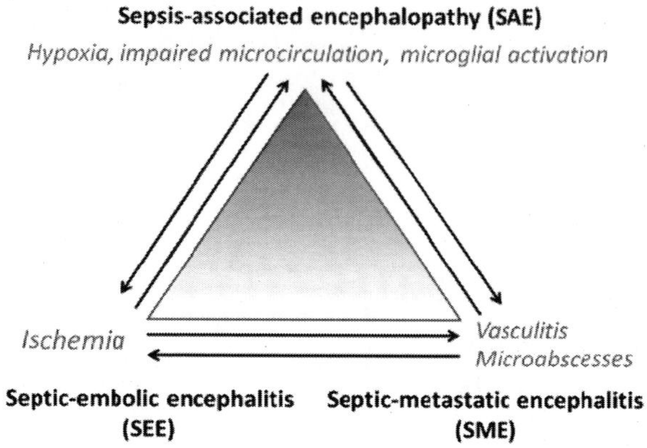

Figure 6.29 The continuum between septic-embolic (SEE) and septic-metastatic encephalitis (SME) and sepsis-associated encephalopathy (Tauber et al., 2020).

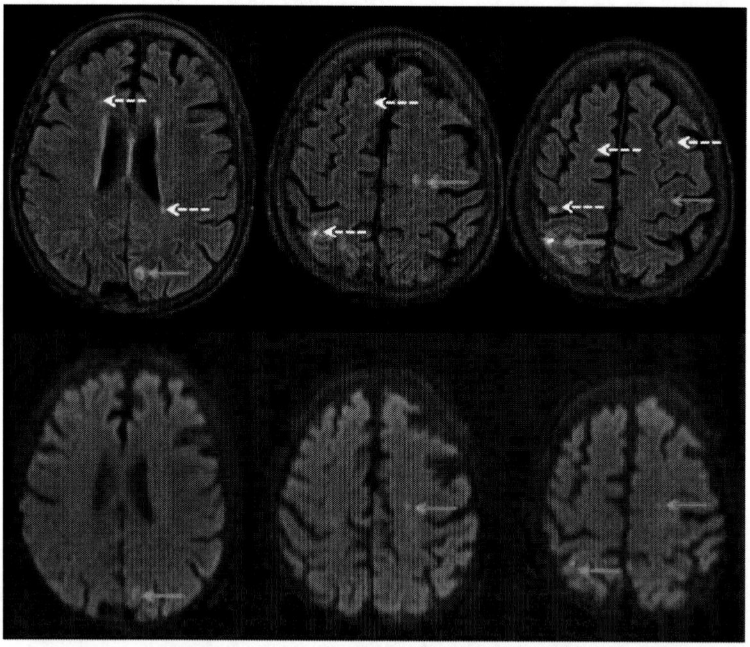

Figure 6.30 A 63-year-old female patient with thoracic spondylodiscitis, endocarditis of the mitral valve, and sepsis. MRI shows ischemic lesions visible on both FLAIR and DWI sequences in both cerebral hemispheres, whereas older ischemic lesions (≥ approximately 10 days) are visible only on FLAIR sequences. These abnormalities have been interpreted as septic-embolic encephalitis (an ischemic extreme variant of brain injury caused by sepsis) (Tauber et al., 2020).

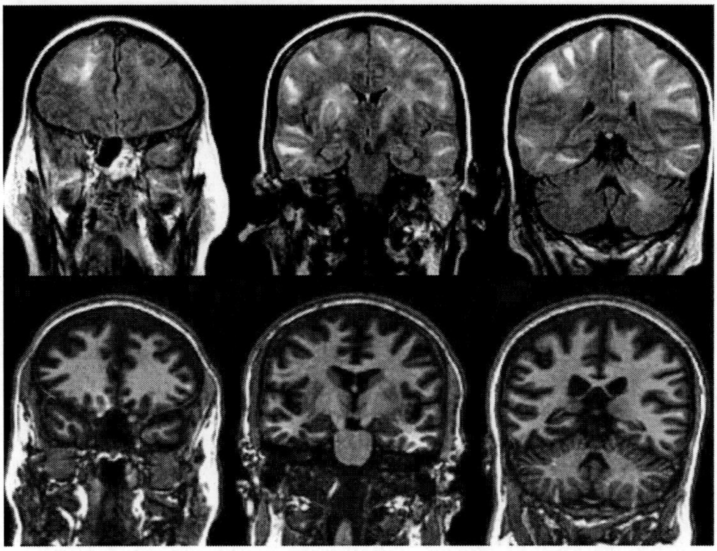

Figure 6.31 A 49-year-old woman was admitted to a local hospital with community-acquired pneumonia. Her condition progressed to severe sepsis with a diagnosis of ARDS. MRI 3 weeks after hospitalization showed diffuse hyperintense areas with abnormal subcortical and deep white matter of the brain and also in the left cerebellum (coronal FLAIR images – top row). There was no atrophy, intracranial hemorrhage, or ventricular enlargement. After discharge, the patient was unable to return to his previous social functioning despite an improved overall cognitive status. Control MRI (coronal T1-weighted brain imaging) at a 3.5-year follow-up (bottom row) showed marked atrophy of the cerebrum and cerebellum (also mild atrophy of the hippocampus) with sulcus widening and ventricular enlargement (Jackson et al., 2009).

Disclaimer

None

References

Abe, Shinpei, Akihisa Okumura, Tohru Fujii, Tomonosuke Someya, Rieko Tadokoro, Yasuhiro Arai, Tomoyuki Nakazawa, and Yuichiro Yamashiro. "Sepsis Associated Encephalopathy in an Infant with Biliary Atresia." *Brain and Development* 30, no. 8 (September 2008): 544–47. https://doi.org/10.1016/j.braindev.2007.12.015.

Ahmed, Munawwar, Jyoti Sureka, Vivek Mathew, RaviKanth Jakkani, and K. P. P. Abhilash. "Magnetic Resonance Imaging Findings in a Fatal Case of Salmonella Typhi-Associated Encephalopathy: A Case Report and Literature Review." *Neurology India* 59, no. 2 (2011): 270. https://doi.org/10.4103/0028-3886.79145.

Aird, William C. "The Role of the Endothelium in Severe Sepsis and Multiple Organ Dysfunction Syndrome." *Blood* 101, no. 10 (May 15, 2003): 3765–77. https://doi.org/10.1182/blood-2002-06-1887.

Alexander, G. E., M. R. DeLong, and P. L. Strick. "Parallel Organization of Functionally Segregated Circuits Linking Basal Ganglia and Cortex." *Annual Review of Neuroscience* 9, no. 1 (March 1986): 357–81. https://doi.org/10.1146/annurev.ne.09.030186.002041.

Barichello, Tatiana, Márcio R. Martins, Adalisa Reinke, Gustavo Feier, Cristiane Ritter, João Quevedo, and Felipe Dal-Pizzol. "Long-Term Cognitive Impairment in Sepsis Survivors:" *Critical Care Medicine* 33, no. 7 (July 2005): 1671. https://doi.org/10.1097/01.CCM.0000170192.54682.C1.

Bartynski, W. S., J. F. Boardman, Z. R. Zeigler, R. K. Shadduck, and J. Lister. "Posterior Reversible Encephalopathy Syndrome in Infection, Sepsis, and Shock." *AJNR: American Journal of Neuroradiology* 27, no. 10 (2006): 2179–90.

Bartynski, W. S., and J. F. Boardman. "Distinct Imaging Patterns and Lesion Distribution in Posterior Reversible Encephalopathy Syndrome." *American Journal of Neuroradiology* 28, no. 7 (August 1, 2007): 1320–27. https://doi.org/10.3174/ajnr.A0549.

Bitsch, A., R. Nau, R. A. Hilgers, R. Verheggen, G. Werner, and H. W. Prange. "Focal Neurologic Deficits in Infective Endocarditis and Other Septic Diseases." *Acta Neurologica Scandinavica* 94, no. 4 (October 1996): 279–86. https://doi.org/10.1111/j.1600-0404.1996.tb07066.x.

Bolton, Charles F., G. Young Bryan, and Douglas W. Zochodne. "The Neurological Complications of Sepsis." *Annals of Neurology* 33, no. 1 (January 1993): 94–100. https://doi.org/10.1002/ana.410330115.

Chacqueneau, A.-L., A. Desrumaux-Becquet, T. Debillon, M.-A. NGuyen, S. Bessaguet, C. Bost-Bru, P. Leroy, and I. Wroblewski. "Encéphalopathie associée au sepsis (EAS), un cas pédiatrique." *Archives de Pédiatrie* 20, no. 10 (October 2013): 1120–25. https://doi.org/10.1016/j.arcped.2013.06.027 [Chacqueneau, A.-L., A. Desrumaux-Becquet, T. Debillon, M.-A. NGuyen, S. Bessaguet, C. Bost-Bru, P. Leroy, and I. Wroblewski. "A Child with Sepsis-Associated Encephalopathy." *Arch Pediatr* 20, no. 10 (October 2013): 1120–25. https://doi.org/10.1016/j.arcped.2013.06.027]

Chaudhry, Neera, and Ashish Kumar Duggal. "Sepsis Associated Encephalopathy." *Advances in Medicine* 2014 (2014): 1–16. https://doi.org/10.1155/2014/762320.

Dekker, Gustaaf A., and Baha M. Sibai. "Etiology and Pathogenesis of Preeclampsia: Current Concepts." *American Journal of Obstetrics and Gynecology* 179, no. 5 (November 1998): 1359–75. https://doi.org/10.1016/S0002-9378(98)70160-7.

Devlin, John W., Gail Boleski, Mark Mlynarek, David R. Nerenz, Edward Peterson, Michelle Jankowski, H. Mathilda Horst, and Barbara J. Zarowitz. "Motor Activity Assessment Scale: A Valid and Reliable Sedation Scale for Use with Mechanically Ventilated Patients in an Adult Surgical Intensive Care Unit." *Critical Care Medicine* 27, no. 7 (July 1999): 1271–75. https://doi.org/10.1097/00003246-199907000-00008.

Eidelman, Leonid A. 'The Spectrum of Septic Encephalopathy: Definitions, Etiologies, and Mortalities'. *JAMA* 275, no. 6 (14 February 1996): 470. https://doi.org/10.1001/jama.1996.03530300054040.

Fugate, Jennifer E., Daniel O. Claassen, Harry J. Cloft, David F. Kallmes, Osman S. Kozak, and Alejandro A. Rabinstein. "Posterior Reversible Encephalopathy Syndrome: Associated Clinical and Radiologic Findings." *Mayo Clinic Proceedings* 85, no. 5 (May 2010): 427–32. https://doi.org/10.4065/mcp.2009.0590.

Haimes, Ab, Rd Zimmerman, S. Morgello, K. Weingarten, Rd Becker, R. Jennis, and Md Deck. "MR Imaging of Brain Abscesses." *American Journal of Roentgenology* 152, no. 5 (May 1, 1989): 1073–85. https://doi.org/10.2214/ajr.152.5.1073.

Hatta, S., H. Mochizuki, Y. Kuru, H. Miwa, T. Kondo, H. Mori, and Y. Mizuno. "Serial Neuroradiological Studies in Focal Cerebritis." *Neuroradiology* 36, no. 4 (May 1994): 285–88. https://doi.org/10.1007/BF00593261.

Heizmann, Claus W. "S100B Protein in Clinical Diagnostics: Assay Specificity." *Clinical Chemistry* 50, no. 1 (January 1, 2004): 249–51. https://doi.org/10.1373/clinchem.2003.027367.

Hinchey, Judy, Claudia Chaves, Barbara Appignani, Joan Breen, Linda Pao, Annabel Wang, Michael S. Pessin, Catherine Lamy, Jean-Louis Mas, and Louis R. Caplan. "A Reversible Posterior Leukoencephalopathy Syndrome." *New England Journal of Medicine* 334, no. 8 (February 22, 1996): 494–500. https://doi.org/10.1056/NEJM199602223340803.

Höllinger, P., R. Zürcher, G. Schroth, and H. P. Mattle. "Diffusion Magnetic Resonance Imaging Findings in Cerebritis and Brain Abscesses in a Patient with Septic Encephalopathy." *Journal of Neurology* 247, no. 3 (March 17, 2000): 232–34. https://doi.org/10.1007/s004150050573.

Hopkins, Ramona O., Lindell K. Weaver, Dave Collingridge, R. Bruce Parkinson, Karen J. Chan, and James F. Orme. "Two-Year Cognitive, Emotional, and Quality-of-Life Outcomes in Acute Respiratory Distress Syndrome." *American Journal of Respiratory and Critical Care Medicine* 171, no. 4 (February 15, 2005): 340–47. https://doi.org/10.1164/rccm.200406-763OC.

Hosokawa, Koji, Nicolas Gaspard, Fuhong Su, Mauro Oddo, Jean-Louis Vincent, and Fabio Silvio Taccone. "Clinical Neurophysiological Assessment of Sepsis-Associated Brain Dysfunction: A Systematic Review." *Critical Care (London, England)* 18, no. 6 (December 8, 2014): 674. https://doi.org/10.1186/s13054-014-0674-y.

Hotchkiss, R. S., R. C. Long, J. R. Hall, G. T. Shires, R. G. Brouillard, W. J. Millikan, and D. P. Jones. 'An in Vivo Examination of Rat Brain during Sepsis with 31P-NMR Spectroscopy'. *American Journal of Physiology-Cell Physiology* 257, no. 6 (1 December 1989): C1055–61. https://doi.org/10.1152/ajpcell.1989.257.6.C1055.

Iacobone, Emanuele, Juliette Bailly-Salin, Andrea Polito, Diane Friedman, Robert D. Stevens, and Tarek Sharshar. "Sepsis-Associated Encephalopathy and Its Differential Diagnosis:" *Critical Care Medicine* 37 (October 2009): S331–36. https://doi.org/10.1097/CCM.0b013e3181b6ed58.

Ito, T., T. Sakai, S. Inagawa, M. Utsu, and T. Bun. "MR Angiography of Cerebral Vasospasm in Preeclampsia." *AJNR: American Journal of Neuroradiology* 16, no. 6 (1995): 1344–46.

Iwashyna, Theodore J., E. Wesley Ely, Dylan M. Smith, and Kenneth M. Langa. "Long-Term Cognitive Impairment and Functional Disability Among Survivors of Severe Sepsis." *JAMA* 304, no. 16 (October 27, 2010): 1787. https://doi.org/10.1001/jama.2010.1553.

Jackson, Alan C., Joseph J. Gilbert, G. Bryan Young, and Charles F. Bolton. "The Encephalopathy of Sepsis." *Canadian Journal of Neurological Sciences/Journal Canadien Des Sciences Neurologiques* 12, no. 4 (November 1985): 303–7. https://doi.org/10.1017/S0317167100035381.

Jackson, James C., Robert P. Hart, Sharon M. Gordon, Ayumi Shintani, Brenda Truman, Lisa May, and E. Wesley Ely. "Six-Month Neuropsychological Outcome of Medical Intensive Care Unit Patients:" *Critical Care Medicine* 31, no. 4 (April 2003): 1226–34. https://doi.org/10.1097/01.CCM.0000059996.30263.94.

Jackson, James C., Ramona O. Hopkins, Russell R. Miller, Sharon M. Gordon, Arthur P. Wheeler, and E. Wesley Ely. "Acute Respiratory Distress Syndrome, Sepsis, and Cognitive Decline: A Review and Case Study:" *Southern Medical Journal* 102, no. 11 (November 2009): 1150–57. https://doi.org/10.1097/SMJ.0b013e3181b6a592.

Kondo, A., C. Sugiura, Y. Fujii, T. Inoue, Y. Maegaki, and K. Ohno. "Fulminant Sepsis-Associated Encephalopathy in Two Children: Serial Neuroimaging Findings and Clinical Course." *Neuropediatrics* 40, no. 04 (August 2009): 157–61. https://doi.org/10.1055/s-0029-1243626.

Larsson, Anders, Miklós Lipcsey, Jan Sjölin, Lars-Olof Hansson, and Mats B. Eriksson. "Slight Increase of Serum S-100B During Porcine Endotoxemic Shock May Indicate Blood-Brain Barrier Damage:" *Anesthesia & Analgesia* 101, no. 5 (November 2005): 1465–69. https://doi.org/10.1213/01.ANE.0000180193.29655.6A.

Lee, Vivien H., Eelco F. M. Wijdicks, Edward M. Manno, and Alejandro A. Rabinstein. "Clinical Spectrum of Reversible Posterior Leukoencephalopathy Syndrome." *Archives of Neurology* 65, no. 2 (February 1, 2008). https://doi.org/10.1001/archneurol.2007.46.

Lekhra, OmPrakash, and Pranav Chowdhary. "Sepsis Presenting as Acute Hemorrhagic Leukoencephalopathy: A Rare Case Report." *Journal of Dr. NTR University of Health Sciences* 4, no. 3 (2015): 196. https://doi.org/10.4103/2277-8632.165408.

Lin, Jen-Tsun, Shuu-Jiun Wang, Jong-Ling Fuh, Lian-Tsai Hsiao, Jiing-Feng Lirng, and Po-Min Chen. "Prolonged Reversible Vasospasm in Cyclosporin A-induced Encephalopathy." *AJNR: American Journal of Neuroradiology* 24, no. 1 (January 2003): 102–4.

Masse, Marie-Hélène, Marie Anne Richard, Frédérick D'Aragon, Charles St-Arnaud, Michael Mayette, Neill K. J. Adhikari, William Fraser, et al. "Early Evidence of Sepsis-Associated Hyperperfusion—A Study of Cerebral Blood Flow Measured with MRI Arterial Spin Labeling in Critically Ill Septic

Patients and Control Subjects*." *Critical Care Medicine* 46, no. 7 (July 2018): e663–69. https://doi.org/10.1097/CCM.0000000000003147.

Mo, Xiao, Xin Xiong, Yijie Wang, Heyi Gu, Yuhang Yang, and Jianfeng He. "Texture Feature-Based Machine Learning Classification on MRI Image for Sepsis-Associated Encephalopathy Detection: A Pilot Study." Edited by Luminita Moraru. *Computational and Mathematical Methods in Medicine* 2023 (February 2, 2023): 1–10. https://doi.org/10.1155/2023/6403556.

Mueller-Mang, Christina, Thomas Mang, Agnes Pirker, Katharina Klein, Christine Prchla, and Daniela Prayer. "Posterior Reversible Encephalopathy Syndrome: Do Predisposing Risk Factors Make a Difference in MRI Appearance?" *Neuroradiology* 51, no. 6 (June 2009): 373–83. https://doi.org/10.1007/s00234-009-0504-0.

Papadopoulos, M. C., F. J. Lamb, R. F. Moss, D. C. Davies, D. Tighe, and E. D. Bennett. "Faecal Peritonitis Causes Oedema and Neuronal Injury in Pig Cerebral Cortex." *Clinical Science (London, England: 1979)* 96, no. 5 (May 1999): 461–66.

Papadopoulos, Marios C., D. Ceri Davies, Ray F. Moss, Derek Tighe, and E. David Bennett. "Pathophysiology of Septic Encephalopathy: A Review:" *Critical Care Medicine* 28, no. 8 (August 2000): 3019–24. https://doi.org/10.1097/00003246-200008000-00057.

Piazza, O., E. Russo, S. Cotena, G. Esposito, and R. Tufano. "Elevated S100B Levels Do Not Correlate with the Severity of Encephalopathy During Sepsis." *British Journal of Anaesthesia* 99, no. 4 (October 2007): 518–21. https://doi.org/10.1093/bja/aem201.

Piazza, Ornella, Simona Cotena, Edoardo De Robertis, Ferdinando Caranci, and Rosalba Tufano. "Sepsis Associated Encephalopathy Studied by MRI and Cerebral Spinal Fluid S100B Measurement." *Neurochemical Research* 34, no. 7 (July 2009): 1289–92. https://doi.org/10.1007/s11064-008-9907-2.

Prange, H. W. "Die Septische Herdenzephalitis." *Intensivmedizin und Notfallmedizin* 43, no. 2 (March 2006): 85–93. https://doi.org/10.1007/s00390-006-0574-8 [Prange, H. W. "Septic focal encephalitis." Intensivmed 43, no. 2 (March 2006): 85–93. https://doi.org/10.1007/s00390-006-0574-8].

Primavera, A. "Reversible Posterior Leukoencephalopathy Syndrome in Systemic Lupus and Vasculitis." *Annals of the Rheumatic Diseases* 60, no. 5 (May 1, 2001): 534–37. https://doi.org/10.1136/ard.60.5.534.

Sasse, Kent C., Eric Nauenberg, Alan Long, Bette Anton, Harvey J. Tucker, and Teh-wei Hu. "Long-Term Survival after Intensive Care Unit Admission with Sepsis:" *Critical Care Medicine* 23, no. 6 (June 1995): 1040–47. https://doi.org/10.1097/00003246-199506000-00008.

Schwartz, R. B., K. M. Jones, P. Kalina, R. L. Bajakian, M. T. Mantello, B. Garada, and B. L. Holman. "Hypertensive Encephalopathy: Findings on CT, MR Imaging, and SPECT Imaging in 14 Cases." *American Journal of Roentgenology* 159, no. 2 (August 1992): 379–83. https://doi.org/10.2214/ajr.159.2.1632361.

Schwartz, R. B., R. V. Mulkern, H. Gudbjartsson, and F. Jolesz. "Diffusion-Weighted MR Imaging in Hypertensive Encephalopathy: Clues to Pathogenesis." *AJNR: American Journal of Neuroradiology* 19, no. 5 (May 1998): 859–62.

Sharshar, Tarek, Nicholas S Hopkinson, David Orlikowski, and Djillali Annane. "Science Review: The Brain in Sepsis – Culprit and Victim." *Critical Care* 9, no. 1 (2004): 37. https://doi.org/10.1186/cc2951.

Sharshar, Tarek, Robert Carlier, Francis Bernard, Céline Guidoux, Jean-Philippe Brouland, Olivier Nardi, Geoffroy Lorin De La Grandmaison, et al. "Brain Lesions in Septic Shock: A Magnetic Resonance Imaging Study." *Intensive Care Medicine* 33, no. 5 (May 2007): 798–806. https://doi.org/10.1007/s00134-007-0598-y.

Shindo, Akihiro, Kei Suzuki, Yoshiaki Iwashita, and Hidekazu Tomimoto. "Sepsis-Associated Encephalopathy with Multiple Microbleeds in Cerebral White Matter." *The American Journal of Medicine* 131, no. 7 (July 2018): e297–98. https://doi.org/10.1016/j.amjmed.2018.02.012.

Sprung, Charles L., Peter N. Peduzzi, Clayton H. Shatney, Roland M. H. Schein, Michael F. Wilson, John N. Sheagren, and Lerner B. Hinshaw. "Impact of Encephalopathy on Mortality in the Sepsis Syndrome:" *Critical Care Medicine* 18, no. 8 (August 1990): 801–6. https://doi.org/10.1097/00003246-199008000-00001.

Stubbs, Daniel J., Adam K. Yamamoto, and David K. Menon. "Imaging in Sepsis-Associated Encephalopathy—Insights and Opportunities." *Nature Reviews Neurology* 9, no. 10 (October 2013): 551–61. https://doi.org/10.1038/nrneurol.2013.177.

Tauber, S. C., S. Bunkowski, W. Brück, and R. Nau. "Septic Metastatic Encephalitis: Coexistence of Brain Damage and Repair: Brain Damage and Repair in Septic Metastatic Encephalitis." *Neuropathology and Applied Neurobiology* 37, no. 7 (December 2011): 768–76. https://doi.org/10.1111/j.1365-2990.2011.01196.x.

Tauber, Simone C., Marija Djukic, Johannes Gossner, Helmut Eiffert, Wolfgang Brück, and Roland Nau. "Sepsis-Associated Encephalopathy and Septic Encephalitis: An Update." *Expert Review of Anti-Infective Therapy* 19, no. 2 (February 1, 2021): 215–31. https://doi.org/10.1080/14787210.2020.1812384.

Trommer, B. L., D. Homer, and M. A. Mikhael. "Cerebral Vasospasm and Eclampsia." *Stroke* 19, no. 3 (March 1988): 326–29. https://doi.org/10.1161/01.STR.19.3.326.

Warach, Steven, Jochen Gaa, Bettina Siewert, Piotr Wielopolski, and Robert R. Edelman. "Acute Human Stroke Studied by Whole Brain Echo Planar Diffusion-Weighted Magnetic Resonance Imaging." *Annals of Neurology* 37, no. 2 (February 1995): 231–41. https://doi.org/10.1002/ana.410370214.

Wu, Huiying, Yikai Xu, and Wenbiao Xu. "Imaging Manifestations of Sepsis-Associated Encephalopathy." *International Journal of Imaging Systems and Technology* 28, no. 3 (September 2018): 196–206. https://doi.org/10.1002/ima.22270.

Young, G. B., C. F. Bolton, T. W. Austin, Y. M. Archibald, J. Gonder, and G. A. Wells. "The Encephalopathy Associated with Septic Illness." *Clinical and Investigative Medicine. Medecine Clinique Et Experimentale* 13, no. 6 (December 1990): 297–304.

Young, G. Bryan. "Encephalopathy of Infection and Systemic Inflammation." *Journal of Clinical Neurophysiology: Official Publication of the American Electroencephalographic Society* 30, no. 5 (October 2013): 454–61. https://doi.org/10.1097/WNP.0b013e3182a73d83.

Young, G. Bryan, Charles F. Bolton, Yvonne M. Archibald, Thomas W. Austin, and George A. Wells. "The Electroencephalogram in Sepsis-Associated Encephalopathy:" *Journal of Clinical Neurophysiology* 9, no. 1 (January 1992): 145–52. https://doi.org/10.1097/00004691-199201000-00016.

Zauner, Christian, Alexandra Gendo, Ludwig Kramer, Georg C. Funk, Edith Bauer, Peter Schenk, Klaus Ratheiser, and Christian Madl. "Impaired Subcortical and Cortical Sensory Evoked Potential Pathways in Septic Patients*." *Critical Care Medicine* 30, no. 5 (May 2002): 1136–39. https://doi.org/10.1097/00003246-200205000-00030.

Chapter 7

Positron emission tomography in sepsis-associated encephalopathy

Daria V. Ryzhkova[1]*, MD., Ph.D., Kristina M. Bykova[2], MD

[1]Department of Nuclear Medicine and Radiation Technologies with a Clinic, Research Institute of Nuclear Medicine and Theranostics, Almazov National Medical Research Centre of Ministry of Health Care of Russian Federation, Saint Petersburg, Russian Federation,

[2] Department of Anesthesiology and Intensive Care, Almazov National Medical Research Centre of Ministry of Health Care of Russian Federation, Saint Petersburg, Russian Federation

Abstract

Despite significant advances in the treatment of sepsis, sepsis-associated encephalopathy is still associated with high mortality and the development of severe cognitive impairment.

The research results demonstrate promising directions in the field of studying brain metabolism and specific aspects of the functioning of the blood-brain barrier.

In our study, patients with sepsis-associated encephalopathy revealed a pattern of hypometabolism in various parts of the cerebral cortex.

Keywords: positron emission tomography, 18F-fluorodeoxyglucose, sepsis-associated encephalopathy, cerebral metabolism

Abbreviations

[18F]-FDG – [18F]-fluorodeoxyglucose
[99mTc]-HMPAO – technetium 99m-hexamethylpropyleneamine oxime
CAM-ICU – Confusion Assessment Method for the ICU
CT – computed tomography
ICU – intensive care unite

* Corresponding author: Daria V. Ryzhkova, Professor, MD., Ph.D.
e-mail address: d_ryjkova@mail.ru

Editor: Irina A. Savvina, Natalia V. Beloborodova and Tatyana N. Trofimova
In: Sepsis-Associated Encephalopathy
ISBN: 979-8-89113-178-1

PET – positron emission tomography
RASS – Richmond Agitation-Sedation Scale
SAPS II – Simplified Acute Physiology Score
SOFA – Sequential Organ Failure Assessment
TSPO – Translocator protein

Introduction

The possibility of early diagnosis of brain dysfunction is very significant due to high mortality and poor prognosis for the septic patient if brain damage progresses. Along with clinical and laboratory diagnosis of acute cerebral insufficiency, neuroimaging and the study of brain metabolism, neurotransmitter function, and cerebral perfusion are of particular importance. In this regard, the X-ray and positron emission tomography (PET) technologies complement the data on sepsis-associated encephalopathy.

The chapter discusses the results of experimental and clinical studies of cerebral metabolism, perfusion, and neurotransmission in sepsis-associated encephalopathy using PET. The results of PET studies of Almazov National Medical Research Centre of patients with sepsis are also described.

Currently, the experience of diagnosing sepsis-associated encephalopathy with PET is rather limited and is based on the results of PET with 18F-fluorodeoxyglucose (18F-FDG).

PET and brain glucose metabolism, cerebral perfusion and neuronal damage in experimental models of sepsis-associated encephalopathy

Early diagnosis of sepsis-associated encephalopathy (SAE) is essential for the treatment and prognosis of septic patients. Positron emission tomography combined with computed tomography (PET/CT) of the brain has demonstrated promising results for the early diagnosis of septic encephalopathy in vivo experiments on a rodent model.

A study by Semmler et al. (2008) demonstrated the effect of sepsis on the induction of neuroinflammation, which led to a concomitant decrease in brain metabolism [1]. The study investigated the relationship between electrophysiological, metabolic, and morphological changes in the brain caused by sepsis-associated encephalopathy in experimental animals exposed to bacterial lipopolysaccharide (LPS). 18F-FDG PET was used to assess brain glucose metabolism by a small animal PET scanner with an effective resolution of 0.7 mm. The authors found that brain glucose uptake was reduced in all areas of the neocortex, but persisted in the caudate nucleus, hippocampus, and thalamus, indicating differences in regional vulnerability of different brain areas in the experimental model used.

Szöllősi D et al. (2018) investigated the ability to assess the early effects of systemic inflammation on the brain in a mouse model of sepsis-associated encephalopathy using nuclear medicine technologies [2]. Scintigraphy and PET of the brain of each animal were performed 4 hours after intravenous administration of bacterial LPS using the following radiopharmaceuticals: [99mTc]HMPAO and [125I]iomazenil to measure brain perfusion and neuronal damage, respectively; [18F]-FDG has been used to study glucose metabolism in the brain. The microglial activity was assessed using the radiopharmaceutical [125I]CLINME. The authors demonstrated a marked decrease in perfusion and a significantly increased uptake of [18F]-FDG and [125I] CLINME. Increased [125I]iomazenil uptake has been noted in the hippocampus and cerebellum after perfusion normalization. The authors demonstrated a negative correlation between [18F]-FDG and [125I]iomazenil uptake and brain perfusion. Based on the results of the study, the authors concluded that [125I]CLINME and [99mTc]HMPAO SPECT can be used to detect microglial activation and assess brain perfusion, respectively, at an early stage of systemic inflammation. The authors also suggested that increased uptake of [18F]-FDG and [125I] iomazenil in sepsis-associated encephalopathy has not necessarily reflected neuronal hypermetabolism and the absence of neuronal damage. The most likely cause of that are processes occurring during neuroinflammation, such as microglial activation and brain matter infiltration by immune cells.

Weberpals et al. (2009) studied the long-term effects of septic encephalopathy on cerebral metabolism, cognition, learning, and memory using a mouse model of bacterial LPS injection-induced sepsis [3]. The authors noted that behavioral disturbances were independent of [18F]-FDG uptake in the brain 2 months after LPS injection. Moreover, immunohistochemical analysis showed that LPS did not lead to neuronal death, but caused sustained activation of microglia in wild-type mice.

It is well known that microglial activation is one of the earliest changes seen in sepsis-associated encephalopathy, and prolonged microglial activation can adversely affect other brain cells. One of the markers reflected microglial activation is overexpression of TSPO. TSPO is mainly expressed in the outer mitochondrial membrane of steroid-synthesizing cells in the central nervous system such as microglia, astrocytes, and endothelial cell. It is involved in many physiological processes including transporting cholesterol into mitochondria, steroid hormone synthesis, and bioenergetics [4, 5].

Currently, a large number of labeled ligands for TSPO have been developed. [11C]PK-11195 is the first generation TSPO tracer, which has been widely used in preclinical and clinical studies. However, this radiopharmaceutical has some disadvantages such as low blood-brain barrier permeability and high non-specific plasma binding resulting in low signal-to-noise ratio in the PET images [6]. The second-generation TSPO tracers, including [11C]DAA1106, [1(F] FEDAA1106, [125I]CLINDE [11C]PBR06, [11C]PBR28, [18F] PBR111, [18F]DPA-713, [18F] DPA- 714, [18F]F-DPA, [11C]AC5216, [18F]FEMPA, and [18F]FEPPA, were developed for overcoming the limitations of [11C]PK11195 [7–14].

Several studies have compared the binding properties of second- and third-generation TSPO indicators. Nevertheless, the binding affinity of second-generation TSPO tracers in the human brain was influenced by the rs6971 gene polymorphism, resulting in high inter-subject variability. In addition, [11C]PBR28 binding appears to be dependent on chromosome 1 variant rs2997325 on microglial activation [15].

A comparative PET study by Zanotti-Fregonara et al. (2018) showed higher permeability of [11C]PBR28 across the blood-brain barrier compared to [18F]GE-180 in humans [16].

Third-generation TSPO tracers such as [18F]GE-180, (S)-[18F]GE-387, and [11C]ER176 solve the problem of ligand-dependent affinity attenuation [17–19] because these radiopharmaceuticals are insensitive to TSPO rs6971 polymorphisms in an in vitro experiment [20].

Chaney et al. (2019) showed that [11C]DPA-713 PET is superior to [18F]GE-180 PET in detecting microglial activation in a mouse model of stroke [21]. James et al. (2017) demonstrated higher sensitivity of [18F]GE180 compared to [18F]PBR06 in detecting microglial activation [22]. It should be noted that radiopharmaceuticals have found their application for the diagnosis of multiple sclerosis, Alzheimer's disease, amyloidosis, and brain pathologies, associated with the deposition of tau-protein.

There are a few articles devoted to the possibilities of PET for assessing microglial activation in case of systemic bacterial infection. Experimental studies of Hannestad et al. (2012) in nonhuman primates using PET with [11C]-PBR28, which is the ligands that bind to a translocator protein (TSPO), have shown the ability to diagnose very early microglial activation in the brain [23]. Six female baboons were scanned before and 1 hour and/or 4 hours and/or 22 hours after intravenous administration of 0.1 mg/kg *E. coli* LPS causing systemic inflammation. In the group of experimental animals there was revealed an increase in [11C]PBR28 binding to TSPO by 29±16% and 62±34% in 1 hour and 4 hours (and=3) respectively after the administration of LPS. A positive correlation was observed between serum levels of IL-1β and IL-6 and uptake of [11C]PBR28 in the animal's brain. The authors concluded that in the brain of nonhuman primates, LPS-induced systemic inflammation causes a strong increase in TSPO levels in microglia, which is easily detected by [11C]PBR28 PET. However, the authors noted that one disadvantage of [11C]PBR28 in humans is that approximately 3.4% of the population will not bind this radiotracer and approximately 30% will have low binding due to a substitution polymorphism in the TSPO gene, citing to a study by Owen et al. (2011) [24]. The authors suggest that labeled TSPO ligands can be used to characterize the effects of systemic inflammation on the human brain to develop new neuroprotective and anti-inflammatory drugs and monitor their efficacy.

PET can also detect changes in neurotransmitter function in sepsis, with the possibility of developing specific treatment targets [25].

PET and clinical investigations of the human brain in sepsis: 18F-FDG PET/CT in the diagnosis of sepsis-associated encephalopathy

A study by Sandiego et al. (2015) was performed on eight volunteers who underwent PET with [11C]PBR28 twice: at baseline and 3 hours after LPS injection (1 ng/kg, iv bolus). The authors demonstrated an increase in the accumulation of [11C]PBR28 in the human brain by an average of 46 ± 8% after LPS injection, which reflected the activation of microglia as a response to systemic inflammation [26].

In our study, [18F]-FDG PET/CT was performed on 10 critically ill patients diagnosed with sepsis and septic shock according to the Third International Consensus Definitions for Sepsis and Septic Shock (Sepsis-3, 2016).

When analyzing PET images using the 3D-SSP method (regional [18F]-FDG uptake is normalized to the level of radiopharmaceutical accumulation in the brainstem), [18F]-FDG hypoaccumulation was noted in the lateral, parasagittal regions of the prefrontal cortex of both hemispheres of the brain; in the sensorimotor cortex of both hemispheres of the brain; in the anterior and posterior parts of both cingulate gyri; in the cortex of the upper and lower sections of both parietal lobes of the brain; in the lateral cortex of the occipital lobes of both hemispheres of the brain; in the lateral and medial cortex of the temporal lobes of both cerebral hemispheres. The pattern of hypometabolism in various parts of the cerebral cortex was recorded regardless of the use of sedatives in the structure of intensive care for sepsis and the degree of deprivation of the level of consciousness, from minimal cognitive and behavioral disorders to delirium and coma.

PET FDG Test Results

Patient : A
Patient Id :
Ordering Provider : Not Available
Reading Physician : Not Available
Inj.Dose : 158.87 MBq/ml FDG

Age : 65
Test Date : 11 Oct 2022
Birth Date :
Exam : 18F-FDG Brain
Scanner : GE MEDICAL SYSTEMS Discovery 710

Region	Uptake Ratio	Z-Score
Prefrontal Lateral R	1.21	-2.61
Prefrontal Lateral L	1.18	-2.67
Prefrontal Medial R	1.17	-2.03
Prefrontal Medial L	1.20	-1.85
Sensorimotor R	1.25	-1.67
Sensorimotor L	1.20	-2.00
Anterior Cingulate R	1.14	-1.24
Anterior Cingulate L	1.13	-1.30
Posterior Cingulate R	1.28	-2.11
Posterior Cingulate L	1.32	-1.78
Precuneus R	1.29	-2.16
Precuneus L	1.25	-2.17
Parietal Superior R	1.06	-2.35
Parietal Superior L	1.08	-2.12
Parietal Inferior R	1.10	-2.82
Parietal Inferior L	1.00	-3.31
Occipital Lateral R	1.25	-2.12
Occipital Lateral L	1.24	-2.03
Primary Visual R	1.49	-1.31
Primary Visual L	1.55	-0.95
Temporal Lateral R	1.08	-2.61
Temporal Lateral L	1.03	-2.80
Temporal Mesial R	1.02	-0.55
Temporal Mesial L	0.99	-0.95
Cerebellum Whole	1.21	-0.59
Pons	1.00	0.00
Reference Region: Pons		

Z-Score Images

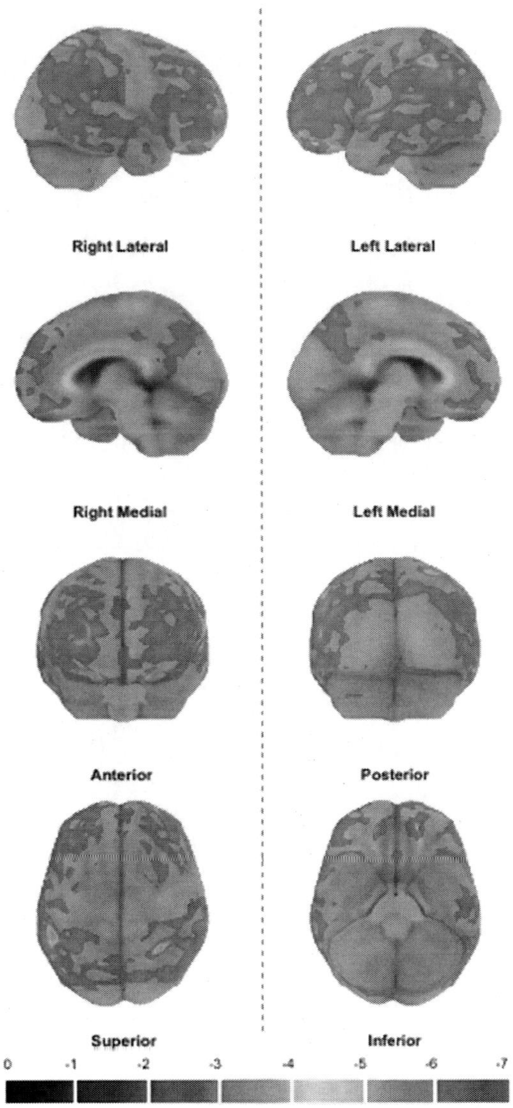

Images shown have a 2 SD threshold applied

Figure 7.1 PET signs of glucose hypometabolism in the cortex of both frontal lobes, in the sensorimotor cortex of the left hemisphere, in both precuneus, in the posterior part of the right cingulate gyrus, in the cortex of both parietal and occipital lobes, in the lateral cortex of both temporal lobes. Metabolism of glucose in other parts of the brain within age limits.

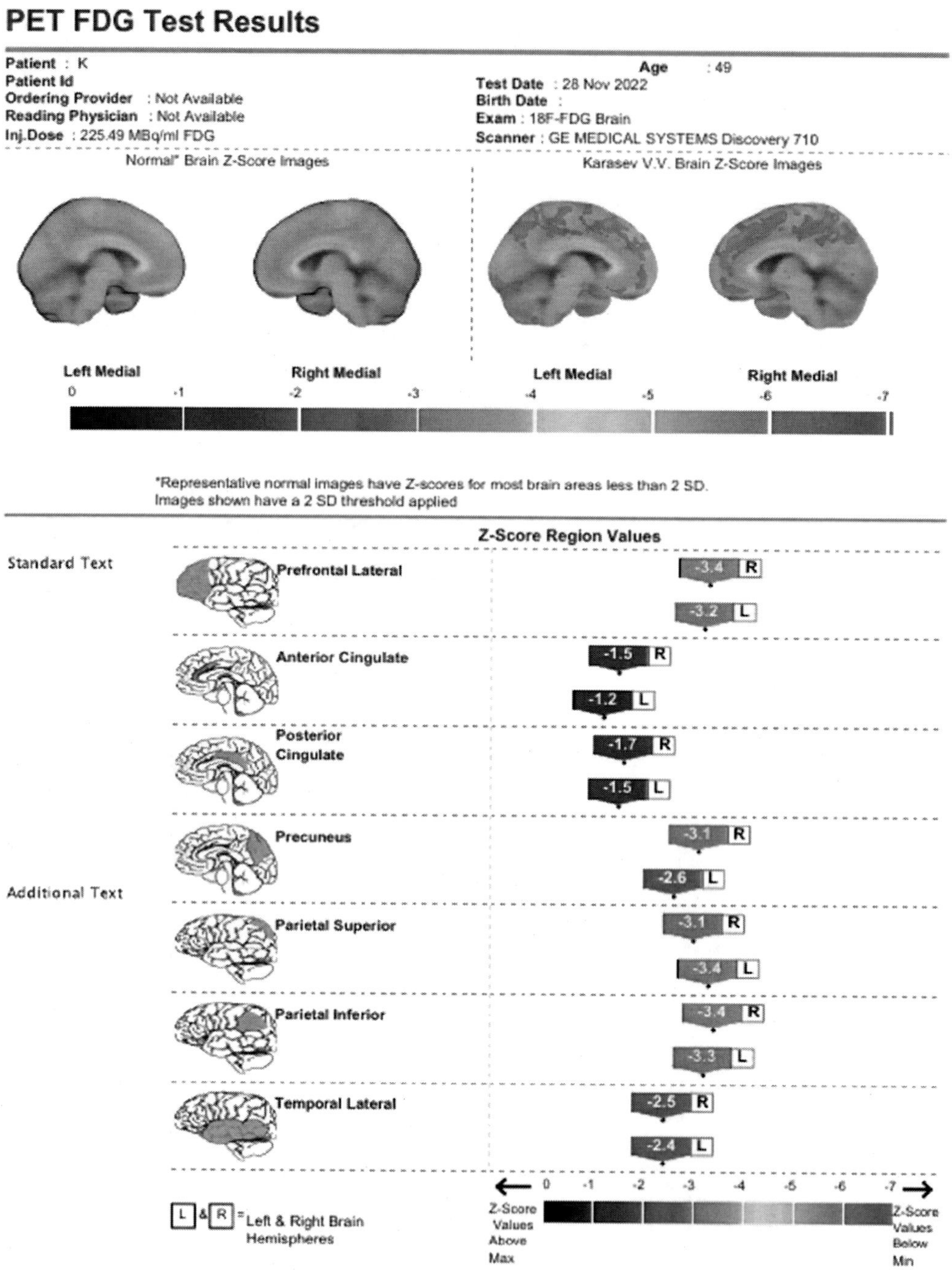

Figure 7.2 PET signs of glucose hypometabolism in the associative cortex of both frontal lobes, in the sensorimotor cortex of both hemispheres of the brain, in both precuneus, in the cortex of both parietal lobes, in the lateral cortex of both temporal lobes and in the lateral cortex of the left occipital lobe. Metabolism of glucose in other parts of the brain within age limits.

PET FDG Test Results

Patient : S
Patient Id :
Ordering Provider : Not Available
Reading Physician : Not Available
Inj.Dose : 168.77 MBq/ml FDG

Age : 47
Test Date : 15 Nov 2022
Birth Date :
Exam : 18F-FDG Brain
Scanner : GE MEDICAL SYSTEMS Discovery 710

Region	Uptake Ratio	Z-Score
Prefrontal Lateral R	1.31	-3.67
Prefrontal Lateral L	1.32	-3.61
Prefrontal Medial R	1.21	-3.53
Prefrontal Medial L	1.21	-3.60
Sensorimotor R	1.18	-4.37
Sensorimotor L	1.17	-4.26
Anterior Cingulate R	1.17	-2.42
Anterior Cingulate L	1.20	-2.24
Posterior Cingulate R	1.34	-3.72
Posterior Cingulate L	1.32	-3.74
Precuneus R	1.31	-3.99
Precuneus L	1.29	-4.25
Parietal Superior R	0.93	-6.00
Parietal Superior L	1.02	-5.07
Parietal Inferior R	1.25	-3.92
Parietal Inferior L	1.23	-4.07
Occipital Lateral R	1.32	-3.50
Occipital Lateral L	1.32	-3.42
Primary Visual R	1.48	-2.70
Primary Visual L	1.53	-2.30
Temporal Lateral R	1.19	-3.14
Temporal Lateral L	1.19	-3.07
Temporal Mesial R	0.99	-2.10
Temporal Mesial L	0.98	-2.48
Cerebellum Whole	1.17	-1.82
Pons	1.00	0.00
Reference Region: Pons		

Z-Score Images

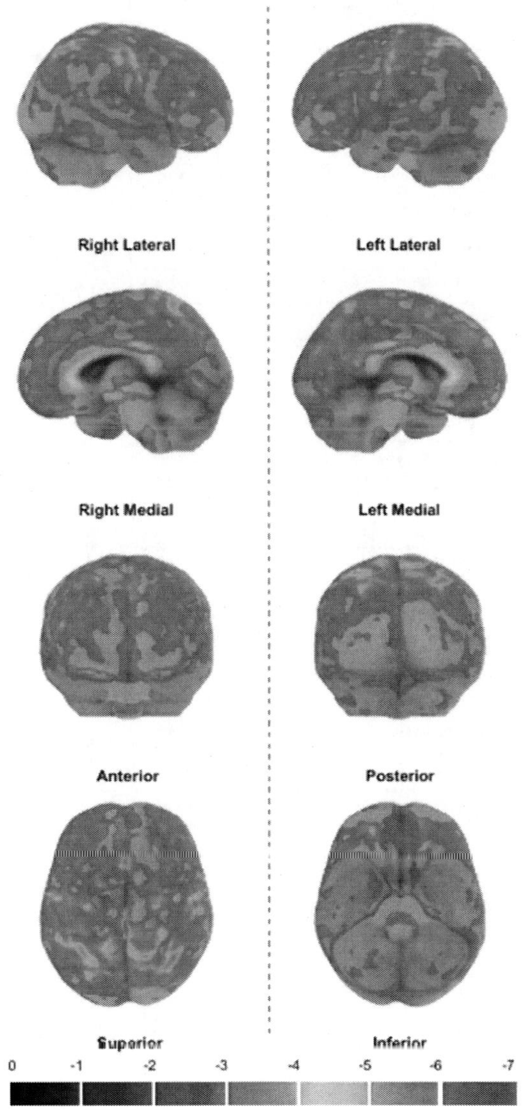

Figure 7.3 PET signs of total glucose hypometabolism in the cerebral cortex.

PET FDG Test Results

Patient : H
Patient Id :
Ordering Provider : Not Available
Reading Physician : Not Available
Inj.Dose : 168.87 MBq/ml FDG

Age : 71
Test Date : 18 Nov 2022
Birth Date :
Exam : 18F-FDG Brain
Scanner : GE MEDICAL SYSTEMS Discovery 710

Region	Uptake Ratio	Z-Score
Prefrontal Lateral R	1.30	-1.84
Prefrontal Lateral L	1.29	-1.89
Prefrontal Medial R	1.19	-1.92
Prefrontal Medial L	1.21	-1.78
Sensorimotor R	1.36	-0.99
Sensorimotor L	1.36	-0.92
Anterior Cingulate R	1.22	-0.26
Anterior Cingulate L	1.19	-0.52
Posterior Cingulate R	1.53	-0.78
Posterior Cingulate L	1.53	-0.71
Precuneus R	1.32	-2.10
Precuneus L	1.33	-2.01
Parietal Superior R	1.23	-1.41
Parietal Superior L	1.30	-0.79
Parietal Inferior R	1.26	-1.72
Parietal Inferior L	1.23	-1.84
Occipital Lateral R	1.29	-1.96
Occipital Lateral L	1.30	-1.80
Primary Visual R	1.32	-2.27
Primary Visual L	1.38	-1.89
Temporal Lateral R	1.16	-1.81
Temporal Lateral L	1.15	-1.71
Temporal Mesial R	1.04	-0.04
Temporal Mesial L	1.06	0.33
Cerebellum Whole	1.19	-0.66
Pons	1.00	0.00
Reference Region: Pons		

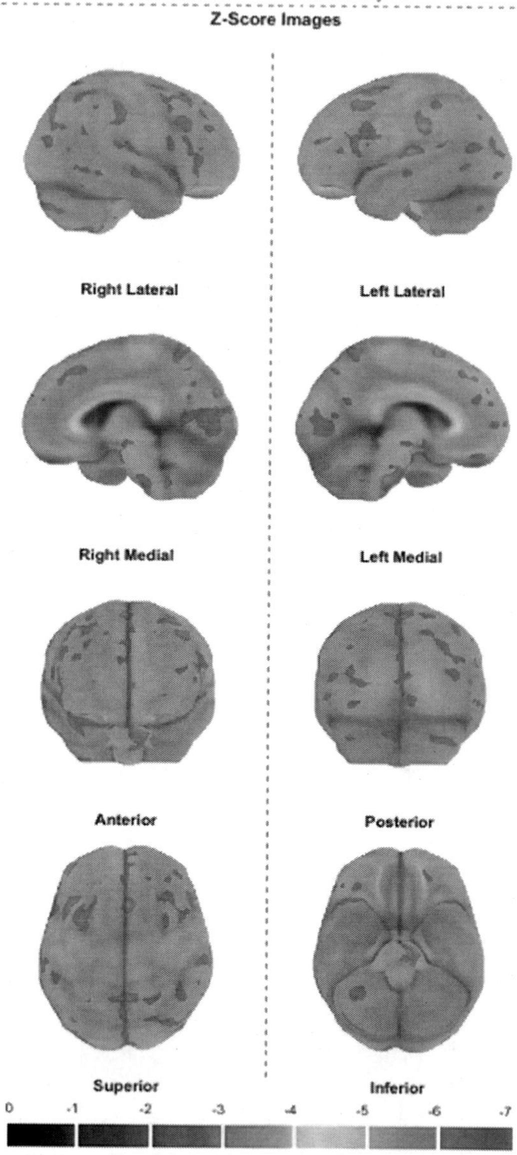

Figure 7.4 PET signs of glucose hypometabolism in the precuneus of both hemispheres and in the visual cortex of the right hemisphere of the brain. Hypermetabolism of glucose in the basal ganglia. Metabolism of glucose in other parts of the brain within age limits.

As a result of the study, according to PET/CT with [18F]-FDG, multiple areas of glucose hypometabolism were identified in all patients with sepsis (in 100% of cases).

It should be noted that in patients with SAE, hypometabolism was detected mainly in the precuneus (in 100% of cases), in the cortex of the right and left parietal lobes (83% and 66%, respectively), in the occipital lateral cortex (on the left 83%, on the right 66%), in temporal lateral cortex (left 83%, right 66%).

Following the results obtained, the severity of the condition and multiple organ failure in patients with SAE (the SOFA scale was used) correlates directly with the presence of zones of hypometabolism of the cerebral cortex (in particular, more pronounced hypometabolism is observed in the cortex of the lower parts of both parietal lobes ($p<0.045$), occipital lateral cortex ($p<0.031$), precuneus ($p<0.031$), and posterior cingulate gyrus ($p<0.013$).

The higher the value of the total score in patients with SAE on the scale of multiple organ failure SAPS II, the more pronounced hypometabolism of glucose was observed in the occipital lateral cortex ($p<0.045$).

Below we present various clinical examples of patients examined by us.

Patient A., 65 years old, was diagnosed with sepsis. The primary focus of the infectious process is nosocomial bilateral polysegmental pneumonia. The study was performed on the 9th day from the onset of sepsis. According to the SOFA scale 10 points, SAPS II 35 points, RASS - 1 point. The study was performed without the use of sedatives. The period of general hospitalization is 35 days. Discharged with clinical improvement.

Patient K., 49 years old, was diagnosed with sepsis on the background of infective endocarditis. The study was performed on the 4th day from the onset of sepsis. According to the SOFA scale 7 points, SAPS II 28 points, RASS 0 points, CAM-ICU no delirium. The study was performed without the use of sedatives. The period of general hospitalization was 59 days. Discharged with clinical improvement.

Patient Sh., aged 47, was diagnosed with sepsis against the background of duodenal ulcer perforation with diffuse fibrinous peritonitis. The study was performed on the 11th day from the onset of sepsis. According to the SOFA scale 7 points, SAPS II 36 points, RASS 0 points, CAM-ICU no delirium. The study was performed without the use of sedatives. The period of general hospitalization was 18 days. Discharged with clinical improvement.

Patient H., aged 72, was diagnosed with sepsis due to perforation of the duodenal stump with diffuse peritonitis. The study was performed on the 21st day from the onset of sepsis. According to the SOFA scale 8 points, and SAPS II 40 points. On the first day of the diagnosis of sepsis according to the RASS scale +2 points, CAM-ICU delirium is present. At the time of the study RASS 0 points, and CAM-ICU had no delirium. The study was performed without the use of sedatives. The period of general hospitalization was 46 days. Discharged with clinical improvement.

Conclusion

As a result of our study, it was established that one of the links in the pathogenesis of the development of acute cerebral insufficiency in SAE is metabolic disorders of the cerebral cortex. The pattern of hypometabolism in various parts of the cerebral cortex was recorded regardless of the use of sedatives.

The identified pattern of reduced glucose metabolism associated with cognitive impairment can be further used to monitor the effectiveness of neurometabolic therapy. [18F]-FDG PET/CT performed in patients with sepsis confirms metabolic abnormalities in the cerebral cortex requiring early proactive neurometabolic therapy to improve both cognitive and overall disease outcomes.

Undoubtedly, the future in clinical medicine, including critical care medicine and sepsis, belongs to high-tech methods of hardware diagnostics. We will use a subtle tool for diagnosing cerebral dysfunction and complement the clinicians' understanding of the state of the patient's brain in the different stages of sepsis.

Conflict of interest: The authors declare that there is no conflict of interest.

References

[1] Semmler A, Hermann S, Mormann F, et al. Sepsis causes neuroinflammation and a concomitant decrease in cerebral metabolism. *J Neuroinflammation* 2008; 5: 38. doi:10.1186/1742-2094-5-38

[2] Szöllősi D, Hegedűs N, Veres D, et al. Evaluation of brain nuclear medicine imaging tracers in a murine model of sepsis-associated encephalopathy. *Mol Imaging Biol* 2018; 20. doi:10.1007/s11307-018-1201-3

[3] Weberpals M, Hermes M, Hermann S, et al. NOS2 gene deficiency protects from sepsis-induced long-term cognitive deficits. *J Neurosci Off J Soc Neurosci* 2009; 29: 14177–14184. doi:10.1523/JNEUROSCI.3238-09.2009

[4] Notter T, Schalbetter SM, Clifton NE, et al. Neuronal activity increases translocator protein (TSPO) levels. *Mol Psychiatry* 2021; 26: 2025–2037. doi:10.1038/s41380-020-0745-1

[5] Gui Y, Marks JD, Das S, et al. Characterization of the 18 kDa translocator protein (TSPO) expression in post-mortem normal and Alzheimer's disease brains. *Brain Pathol Zurich Switz* 2020; 30: 151–164. doi:10.1111/bpa.12763

[6] Vivash L, O'Brien TJ. Imaging microglial activation with TSPO PET: Lighting up neurologic diseases? *J Nucl Med Off Publ Soc Nucl Med* 2016; 57: 165–168. doi:10.2967/jnumed.114.141713

[7] Hamelin L, Lagarde J, Dorothée G, et al. Distinct dynamic profiles of microglial activation are associated with the progression of Alzheimer's disease. *Brain J Neurol* 2018; 141: 1855–1870. doi:10.1093/brain/awy079

[8] Ni R, Röjdner J, Voytenko L, et al. In vitro characterization of the regional binding distribution of amyloid PET tracer Florbetaben and the glia tracers Deprenyl and PK11195 in autopsy Alzheimer's brain tissue. *J Alzheimers Dis JAD* 2021; 80: 1723–1737. doi:10.3233/JAD-201344

[9] Hagens MHJ, Golla SV, Wijburg MT, et al. In vivo assessment of neuroinflammation in progressive multiple sclerosis: A proof of concept study with [18F]DPA714 PET. *J Neuroinflammation* 2018; 15: 314. doi:10.1186/s12974-018-1352-9

[10] Varrone A, Oikonen V, Forsberg A, et al. Positron emission tomography imaging of the 18-kDa translocator protein (TSPO) with [18F]FEMPA in Alzheimer's disease patients and control subjects. *Eur J Nucl Med Mol Imaging* 2015; 42: 438–446. doi:10.1007/s00259-014-2955-8

[11] Miyoshi M, Ito H, Arakawa R, et al. Quantitative analysis of peripheral benzodiazepine receptor in the human brain using PET with (11)C-AC-5216. *J Nucl Med Off Publ Soc Nucl Med* 2009; 50: 1095–1101. doi:10.2967/jnumed.109.062554

[12] Giridharan VV, Collodel A, Generoso JS, et al. Neuroinflammation trajectories precede cognitive impairment after experimental meningitis—Evidence from an in vivo PET study. *J Neuroinflammation* 2020; 17: 5. doi:10.1186/s12974-019-1692-0

[13] Dani M, Wood M, Mizoguchi R, et al. Microglial activation correlates in vivo with both tau and amyloid in Alzheimer's disease. *Brain J Neurol* 2018; 141: 2740–2754. doi:10.1093/brain/awy188

[14] Toppala S, Ekblad LL, Tuisku J, et al. Association of early β-amyloid accumulation and neuroinflammation measured with [11C]PBR28 in elderly individuals without dementia. *Neurology* 2021; 96: e1608–e1619. doi:10.1212/WNL.0000000000011612

[15] Felsky D, Roostaei T, Nho K, et al. Neuropathological correlates and genetic architecture of microglial activation in elderly human brain. *Nat Commun* 2019; 10: 409. doi:10.1038/s41467-018-08279-3

[16] Zanotti-Fregonara P, Pascual B, Rizzo G, et al. Head-to-head comparison of 11C-PBR28 and 18F-GE180 for quantification of the translocator protein in the human brain. *J Nucl Med Off Publ Soc Nucl Med* 2018; 59: 1260–1266. doi:10.2967/jnumed.117.203109

[17] López-Picón FR, Snellman A, Eskola O, et al. Neuroinflammation appears early on PET imaging and then plateaus in a mouse model of Alzheimer disease. *J Nucl Med Off Publ Soc Nucl Med* 2018; 59: 509–515. doi:10.2967/jnumed.117.197608

[18] Kleinberger G, Brendel M, Mracsko E, et al. The FTD-like syndrome causing TREM2 T66M mutation impairs microglia function, brain perfusion, and glucose metabolism. *EMBO J* 2017; 36: 1837–1853. doi:10.15252/embj.201796516

[19] Fan Z, Calsolaro V, Atkinson RA, et al. Flutriciclamide (18F-GE180) PET: First-in-human PET study of novel third-generation in vivo marker of human translocator protein. *J Nucl Med Off Publ Soc Nucl Med* 2016; 57: 1753–1759. doi:10.2967/jnumed.115.169078

[20] Qiao L, Fisher E, McMurray L, et al. Radiosynthesis of (R, S)-[18 F]GE387: A potential PET radiotracer for imaging translocator protein 18 kDa (TSPO) with low binding sensitivity to the human gene polymorphism rs6971. *ChemMedChem* 2019; 14: 982–993. doi:10.1002/cmdc.201900023

[21] Chaney A, Cropper HC, Johnson EM, et al. 11C-DPA-713 versus 18F-GE-180: A preclinical comparison of translocator protein 18 kDa PET tracers to visualize acute and chronic neuroinflammation in a mouse model of ischemic stroke. *J Nucl Med Off Publ Soc Nucl Med* 2019; 60: 122–128. doi:10.2967/jnumed.118.209155

[22] James ML, Belichenko NP, Shuhendler AJ, et al. [18F]GE-180 PET detects reduced microglia activation after LM11A-31 therapy in a mouse model of Alzheimer's disease. *Theranostics* 2017; 7: 1422–1436. doi:10.7150/thno.17666

[23] Hannestad J, Gallezot J-D, Schafbauer T, et al. Endotoxin-induced systemic inflammation activates microglia: [^{11}C]PBR28 positron emission tomography in nonhuman primates. *NeuroImage* 2012; 63: 232–239. doi:10.1016/j.neuroimage.2012.06.055

[24] Papadopoulos V, Fan J, Zirkin B. Translocator protein (18 kDa): An update on its function in steroidogenesis. *J Neuroendocrinol* 2018; 30. doi:10.1111/jne.12500

[25] Stubbs DJ, Yamamoto AK, Menon DK. Imaging in sepsis-associated encephalopathy–insights and opportunities. *Nat Rev Neurol* 2013; 9: 551–561. doi:10.1038/nrneurol.2013.177

[26] Sandiego CM, Gallezot J-D, Pittman B, et al. Imaging robust microglial activation after lipopolysaccharide administration in humans with PET. *Proc Natl Acad Sci U S A* 2015; 112: 12468–12473. doi:10.1073/pnas.1511003112

Chapter 8

Sepsis-associated encephalopathy as a component of multiple organ failure in ICU patients

Ivan A. Ryzhkov*, MD., Ph.D.,
Artem N. Kuzovlev, MD., Ph.D.
Federal Research and Clinical Center of Intensive Care Medicine and Rehabilitology, Moscow, Russia

Abstract

Multiple organ dysfunction (MOD) is more common in sepsis than single-system dysfunction. Sepsis-associated encephalopathy (SAE) is a component of a dynamic pattern of organ dysfunction in a particular patient. Clinical manifestations of SAE vary widely from subtle behavioral disturbances, hypo- or hyperactive delirium, to coma. All these manifestations, however, are nonspecific for SAE. It is often difficult to isolate one specific cause in a given case of acute encephalopathy because most ICU patients have been exposed to a variety of both predisposing (advanced age, dementia, severe comorbidity, depression, alcohol abuse, and poor nutrition) and precipitating risk factors (surgery, decompensation of chronic disease, pain, immobility, metabolic abnormalities, infection, sedation, ICU environment, etc.). Each of these factors can exacerbate the severity of SAE. Thus, the occurrence and severity of encephalopathy in a patient with sepsis largely depend on the severity of dysfunction in other organs, and on the other hand, delirium (or other manifestations of SAE) can significantly change the clinical presentation, treatment strategy, and prognosis in this cohort of patients. Timely control of infection, correction of hypoxia, and circulatory and metabolic disorders, along with control of reversible risk factors for delirium, are the basis for successful treatment of SAE and improvement of long-term outcomes.

Keywords: sepsis, multiple organ dysfunction, multiple organ failure, sepsis-associated encephalopathy, delirium, ICU, pathophysiology

* Corresponding author: Ivan A. Ryzhkov, MD., Ph.D.
e-mail address: iryzhkov@fnkcrr.ru

Editor: Irina A. Savvina, Natalia V. Beloborodova and Tatyana N. Trofimova
In: Sepsis-Associated Encephalopathy
ISBN: 979-8-89113-178-1

Abbreviations

AKI – acute kidney injury
ARDS – acute respiratory distress syndrome
CT – computed tomography
DAMPs – damage-associated molecular patterns
DIC – disseminated intravascular coagulation
DSM-5 – Diagnostic and Statistical Manual of the American Psychiatric Association
FOUR – Full Outline of UnResponsiveness score
GCS – Glasgow Coma Scale
ICU – intensive care unit
IL – interleukin
LODS – Logistic Organ Dysfunction Score
MOD – multiple organ dysfunction
MODS – Multiple Organ Dysfunction Score
MOF – multiple organ failure
MRI – magnetic resonance imaging
PAMPs – pathogen-associated molecular patterns
qSOFA – quick SOFA
RASS – Richmond Agitation-Sedation Scale
SAE – sepsis-associated encephalopathy
SIRS – systemic inflammatory response syndrome
SOFA – Sequential Organ Failure Assessment
SpO_2 – arterial oxygen saturation
TNF – tumor necrosis factor

Introduction

According to current concepts, the presence of organ dysfunction is the key feature that distinguishes sepsis from uncomplicated infection [1]. Within this definition, damage to tissues and organs in sepsis is due not so much to the virulence of the causative pathogen as to a dysregulated/maladaptive host response to infection. An imbalance between pro- and anti-inflammatory pathways creates a background for the development of other types of homeostasis disorders and can be considered a manifestation of immune system dysfunction [2]. Infection and inadequate immune response in combination with some other pathogenetic factors (hypoxia, oxygen free radicals, acidosis, etc.) lead to microvascular and cellular disorders in various tissues and organs (up to necrosis and apoptosis), which is clinically expressed as a disorder of their function [3]. The severity of organ dysfunction in sepsis varies widely from asymptomatic laboratory abnormalities (moderate hypoxemia or thrombocytopenia) to septic shock with severe multiple organ dysfunction (MOD) or failure (MOF). Among the most common disorders in sepsis, it is worth noting the circulatory, renal, pulmonary, gastrointestinal and hepatic, hematologic, and central nervous systems failures. MOD is more common than single-system dysfunction [4, 5].

From this perspective, sepsis-associated encephalopathy (SAE) should always be considered only as a component of a complex and dynamic pattern of organ dysfunction in a particular patient. In a narrow sense, SAE has been defined as a general cerebral dysfunction that accompanies sepsis in the absence of direct central nervous system infection, structural abnormality, or other types of encephalopathy [6]. This definition emphasizes the importance of excluding primary infectious and non-infectious brain pathology (encephalitis, meningitis, septic emboli, stroke, etc.) before making a diagnosis of SAE in a patient with a suspected or proven infection. Clinical manifestations of brain dysfunction in SAE vary widely from subtle behavioral disturbances, hypo- or hyperactive delirium, to sopor and coma. All these manifestations, however, are nonspecific and often occur in ICU patients due to other disease processes and detrimental factors, such as hypoxia, hepatic encephalopathy, pancreatitis, adverse effects of drugs (antibiotics, sedatives), and many others. It is often difficult to isolate one specific cause in a given case of delirium because most patients have been exposed to a variety of both predisposing and precipitating risk factors [7]. Thus, the occurrence and severity of encephalopathy in a patient with sepsis largely depend on the severity of dysfunction in other organs, and on the other hand, delirium (or other manifestations of SAE) can significantly change the clinical presentation, treatment strategy, and prognosis in this cohort of patients.

The purpose of this chapter is to highlight the role of organ dysfunction/failure in the development of SAE in critically ill patients with sepsis, as well as the impact of SAE on the severity and pattern of MOF. The focus is on the clinical pathophysiology of MOF in sepsis and modern strategies for their diagnosis and therapy.

The pathophysiology of organ dysfunction in sepsis

The cause of any infection is a pathogenic or opportunistic microorganism. The pathogen causes primary alteration of host tissues and provokes inflammation, which is clinically manifested in the form of local and systemic (fever, weakness, leukocytosis) signs and symptoms of infection. However, in critically ill patients, pathogen virulence is not always the main factor determining disease severity and prognosis. The dynamic interplay between three variable factors (infection, host response, and intensive care measures) creates a unique clinical presentation of organ dysfunction in a particular septic patient [5].

The importance of the infection itself in the pathogenesis of sepsis is emphasized by the fact that the early administration of empiric antimicrobial therapy improves the outcome of patients with sepsis and septic shock [8]. Pathogen species, the degree of bacterial contamination, and the site of infection may give specificity to the clinical presentation of sepsis and guide patient management. In particular, rapid surgical control of the infection often prevents the development of severe consequences.

The first phase of the host response involves the detection of pathogen-associated molecular patterns (PAMPs) by innate immune cells, followed by the activation of numerous intracellular signaling pathways. Damage-associated molecular patterns (DAMPs) are released from damaged tissues (e.g., heat shock proteins, mitochondrial DNA) and may activate the same sequence of events as PAMPs, amplifying the initial host response to infection [9, 10]. Immune dysregulation in sepsis can manifest itself either as an exaggerated pro-inflammatory response with hyperproduction of the corresponding mediators (TNF, IL-1, IL-6, etc.) or, conversely, as immunosuppression, especially after the patient has passed the acute phase of the critical illness. Exaggerated systemic inflammation provokes secondary tissue alteration, leading through several general pathological processes to the development of organ dysfunction in various organs.

Microcirculatory alterations in sepsis are manifested by a decrease in the proportion of perfused vessels, an increase in the proportion of vessels with intermittent flow, a decrease in total vessel density, and an increase in the heterogeneity of blood flow distribution [11]. Endothelial dysfunction plays an important role in the development of these abnormalities and, in turn, can be induced by hypoxia, PAMPs, DAMPs, oxidative stress, altered nitric oxide (NO) production, and some other factors (e.g., activation of leukocytes and platelets) [12]. Destruction of the glycocalyx, an increase in endothelial permeability, and impaired autoregulation of microvascular tone lead to the development of interstitial edema, vasoplegia, and impaired peripheral perfusion. Hypovolemia, myocardial dysfunction, and other systemic hemodynamic disorders may also play a major role in the development of peripheral hypoperfusion (especially in septic shock). Notably, microcirculatory alterations and hypoperfusion of many organs may persist even after restoration of systemic hemodynamic parameters such as blood pressure and cardiac output [11].

Infection, immune dysregulation, and circulatory disorders induce a complex of metabolic disorders, among which hyperlactatemia and associated metabolic acidosis are the most important from a clinical point of view. Hyperlactatemia in sepsis develops not only as a consequence of hypoxia and anaerobic glycolysis but also as a result of the metabolic reprogramming of cells from oxidative phosphorylation to aerobic glycolysis [13]. Aerobic glycolysis (Warburg effect) is the oxidation of glucose through glycolysis despite the availability of oxygen. A metabolic shift toward aerobic glycolysis in immune cells and some other tissues has some advantages, allowing the host to develop an adequate inflammatory response in the early stages of sepsis. On the other side, failure to restore oxidative phosphorylation at later stages of sepsis has been shown to perpetuate a pro-inflammatory state that limits organ function and survival [12]. Assessment of serum lactate levels is included in current guidelines for the diagnosis and treatment of sepsis and septic shock. This parameter helps to recognize patients with sepsis promptly, assess the severity of their condition, as well as evaluate the effectiveness of therapeutic measures and prognosis [1, 8].

Many other cellular and molecular mechanisms (oxidative stress, mitochondrial dysfunction, cell death by necrosis or apoptosis, etc.) can be involved in the development of organ damage and dysfunction in sepsis and are discussed in detail in several review papers [3, 10, 12].

Thus, the pathogenesis of organ dysfunction in sepsis is largely universal, although the relative role of individual pathogenetic factors may vary in different organ systems. MOF is defined as the failure of two or more organ systems. It is worth noting that MOF is not a disease or even a syndrome, but rather a clinical concept that clinicians and researchers use to refer to the complex and heterogeneous set of complications that occur in a critically ill patient [14]. MOF is associated with extremely high mortality in ICU patients, and the pathogenesis of this serious condition involves not only the universal mechanisms described above (e.g., hypoxia) but also such a biological phenomenon as organ crosstalk [12, 15]. It implies that the failure of one organ can affect (deteriorate) the function of another remote organ through neuroendocrine, immune, and other regulatory mechanisms. For example, the vagal nerve influences the immune response in sepsis in the so-called cholinergic anti-inflammatory pathway [16, 17]. In this process, stimulation of the afferent part of the vagus nerve by inflammatory mediators leads to efferent signaling to the spleen and other organs via the efferent part, resulting in the release of acetylcholine. In turn, acetylcholine activates cholinergic receptors on macrophages, inhibiting the excessive release of pro-inflammatory cytokines [10]. In animal models of sepsis, blockade of this reflex pathway by vagotomy increased systemic inflammation, while vagal nerve stimulation improved survival [18].

Primary acute brain injury can lead to a deterioration in the function of distant organs and contribute to the development of severe complications. For example, traumatic brain injury triggers the activation of sympathetic pathways, which leads to an increase in capillary permeability and pulmonary vasoconstriction. One of the major complications is neurogenic pulmonary edema which requires urgent diagnosis and treatment [15]. Other examples of organ crosstalk in sepsis are given in the relevant sections below.

Assessment of the severity of organ dysfunction in the ICU

Since the 1980s, several scoring systems have been proposed to assess the severity of multiple organ dysfunction in critically ill patients, quantifying the dysfunction of a particular organ system based on clinical findings, laboratory data, or therapeutic interventions [14]. The Multiple Organ Dysfunction Score (MODS), the Logistic Organ Dysfunction Score (LODS), and the Sequential Organ Failure Assessment (SOFA) have gained the most popularity for assessing the severity of organ dysfunction in sepsis [19, 20].

The SOFA score is the predominant tool in current use for this purpose. It quantitatively (from 0 to 4 points) evaluates the degree of dysfunction of each of the six organ systems (the respiratory, cardiovascular, hematological, liver, renal, and neurological systems), followed by the calculation of the total score [21]. An acute change in total SOFA score ≥2 points consequent to the infection is a diagnostic criterion for sepsis [1]. The important advantages of this scoring system are its ease of use (the assessed variables are routinely used in the ICU) and the ability to assess the patient's condition over time. Although the SOFA score was developed as a measure of the severity of organ dysfunction, it also has prognostic value and has been used in many clinical studies [10]. This, in turn, makes it possible to standardize the assessment of organ dysfunction in the ICU and improve the comparability of results from different studies. The evolution of clinical practice and the emergence of some new diagnostic tools and therapeutic interventions dictate the need to develop and validate modified versions of SOFA that would take these changes into account [20].

The epidemiology of MOD/MOF in sepsis varies depending on the patient population studied and approaches to assessing the patient's condition and the function of individual organ systems. Sakr et al. reported that cardiovascular (24%) and respiratory (22%) systems failures were most commonly present on the day of admission to the ICU, whereas respiratory (43%) and renal (36%) organ failures were the most prevalent during the ICU stay [22]. In the same study, hospital mortality increased according to the severity of organ dysfunction and the number of failing organs. In an earlier study, almost 80% of ICU patients with sepsis had MOF, which was also dominated by respiratory and cardiovascular failure [4]. Hospital mortality in these cases exceeded 50%.

The epidemiology and clinical presentation of MOF in neonates and children may differ from those in adults, with asphyxia and sepsis being two major causes and a mortality rate as high as 13–50%. Central nervous system damage is the major MOF-associated adverse outcome in newborns, with gestational age and the timing of treatment initiation being key factors affecting the risk of MOF development [23].

Special scoring systems have been developed to assess the severity of injury and dysfunction of individual organ systems. The Glasgow Coma scale (GCS) has been used for many years to assess the severity of cerebral dysfunction in traumatic brain injury and other brain injuries. It has also been used as a neurological component of most scoring systems for assessing organ dysfunction in the ICU, including the SOFA score [19]. Richmond's agitation-sedation scale (RASS) and confusion assessment method for the ICU (CAM-ICU) were developed later and are used to diagnose delirium and assess the depth of sedation in the ICU. Their inclusion in scoring systems (as a neurological component) will improve the performance of the systems [20].

The difference between "dysfunction" and "failure" of an organ is rather arbitrary. In general, failure of an organ system implies a severe degree of its dysfunction, in which temporary replacement of the function is vital (e.g., mechanical ventilation for respiratory failure or dialysis for acute renal failure). However, about heart or cerebral failure, this is not always applicable in clinical practice.

The treatment of MOD/MOF in sepsis is currently mainly based on supportive intensive care, rather than the use of specific pharmacological agents to purposefully adjust the molecular or cellular pathways of the disease. An exception is rational antimicrobial therapy aimed at eliminating the inciting pathogen. This circumstance indicates that there is no "magic bullet" that will dramatically improve the outcomes of treatment of organ dysfunction in sepsis. The most justified strategy for the management of ICU patients is the application of the principles of clinical pathophysiology and personalized medicine for the timely recognition of pathological processes in a particular patient and their controlled correction, considering the functional reserves of the patient and the dynamics of his condition [24].

SAE or critical illness-associated acute encephalopathy?

Clinically, cerebral dysfunction in ICU patients can manifest itself as delirium or decreased level of consciousness of varying severity (from obtundation to coma). To standardize approaches to diagnosing cerebral dysfunction in clinical practice and trials, an interdisciplinary group issued a consensus statement on nomenclature in 2020 [25]. The statement proposes to use only three terms: acute encephalopathy, delirium, and coma, which are defined in Table 8.1. Acute encephalopathy thus refers to the brain disorder underlying delirium or coma.

Dozens of predisposing and precipitating risk factors for delirium have been identified [7]. Predisposing factors include advanced age, dementia, severe comorbidity, frailty, depression, alcohol abuse, and poor nutrition. Precipitating factors can be both relating to presenting illness (acute infections, major and/or emergency surgery, decompensation of chronic disease) and a variety of abnormalities, environmental factors, and therapeutic interventions that affect the patient during hospitalization (pain, immobility, metabolic abnormalities, nosocomial infection, sedation, ICU environment, etc.). Delirium is common in hospitalized older adults, with an overall prevalence of 23%. Delirium prevalence is high in the ICU, with a systematic review of studies reporting a pooled prevalence of 31% [26].

Because of the above, SAE is only one of many possible scenarios for acute encephalopathy that can occur in ICU patients. Patients with infection and sepsis are exposed to the same predisposing and precipitating risk factors of brain dysfunction as any other critically ill patient. In particular, non-infectious systemic inflammation (such as in severe trauma or pancreatitis) may be an independent major risk factor for organ dysfunction and outcome in critically ill patients. Dulhunty et al. reported that central nervous system failure occurred more frequently in ICU patients with non-infectious systemic inflammatory response syndrome (SIRS) (33 vs. 22%, $P < 0.001$) and resulted in death more commonly than in patients with confirmed sepsis [27].

Table 8.1 Recommended definitions for acute encephalopathy, delirium, and coma. Modified from [25].

Term	Definition	Comments
Acute encephalopathy	A rapidly developing (over less than 4 weeks, but usually within hours to a few days) pathobiological process in the brain.	This can lead to a clinical presentation of subsyndromal delirium, delirium, or in case of a severely decreased level of consciousness, or coma; all representing a change from baseline cognitive status.
Delirium	A clinical state is characterized by a combination of features defined by diagnostic systems such as the DSM-5.	The DSM-5 criteria for delirium include A. Disturbance in attention and awareness. B. The disturbance develops over a short period (usually hours to a few days), represents a change from baseline attention and awareness, and tends to fluctuate in severity during the day. C. An additional disturbance in cognition (e.g., memory deficit, disorientation, language, visuospatial ability, or perception). D. The disturbances in criteria A and C are not explained by another preexisting, established, or evolving neurocognitive disorder, and do not occur in the context of a severely reduced level of arousal, such as coma. E. There is evidence from the history, physical examination, or laboratory findings that the disturbance is a direct consequence of another medical condition, substance intoxication or withdrawal, exposure to a toxin, or is because of multiple etiologies.
Coma	A clinical state of severely depressed responsiveness is defined by diagnostic systems such as the GCS or FOUR scores.	

Note. DSM-5 – Diagnostic and Statistical Manual of the American Psychiatric Association. GCS – Glasgow Coma Score; FOUR – Full Outline of UnResponsiveness score.

Perhaps due to the difficulties of differential diagnosis of acute encephalopathies, data on the epidemiology of the SAE vary among different authors. On the one hand, signs of acute encephalopathy in septic ICU patients were detected in 30–50% of the cases and were strongly associated with confirmed bacteremia [6, 28]. Since altered mentation (Glasgow Coma Scale score <15) is often one of the earliest manifestations of sepsis, this variable, along with blood pressure and respiratory rate, is included in the qSOFA score for identifying adult patients with suspected sepsis outside the ICU [1]. On the other hand, two large multicenter studies reported a prevalence of cerebral dysfunction of 12–26% among ICU patients with sepsis [4, 22]. Nevertheless, there is strong evidence that SAE is associated with severe consequences for patients with prolonged cognitive, physical, and social impairments, carrying a substantial mortality risk, as high as 70–80% for patients with MOF [6, 22, 29].

Critical illness polyneuropathy and myopathy is a type of neurological dysfunction in sepsis that is likely underappreciated clinically. Sepsis, hyperglycemia, use of neuromuscular blocking agents, and systemic steroids are risk factors for polyneuropathy, so this complication develops in the majority of critically ill patients with MOD/MOF [30]. A big clinical problem is weaning from the ventilator and rehabilitation of patients with critical-illness polyneuropathy and myopathy.

In the pathogenesis of SAE, brain bioenergetics disorders, increased permeability of the blood-brain barrier, neurotransmitter imbalance, neuroinflammation, and microglial activation play an important role. The pathophysiological mechanisms of SAE largely overlap with those of acute encephalopathy of other etiologies, losing specificity as the disease progresses [6, 7]. A detailed discussion of the cellular and molecular mechanisms of SAE is beyond the scope of this chapter.

There is a correlation between the severity of the clinical presentation of SAE and the affected brain structures [29, 31]. Mild forms of SAE are manifested by "sickness behavior," which is induced by the action of pro-inflammatory cytokines (IL-1α, IL-1β, TNF-α, and IL-6) on the subcortical structures of the brain (hippocampus, limbic system), followed by the activation of the neuroendocrine system. Disorders in the connectivity of brain regions and alterations in the frontal cortex underlie the various manifestations of delirium. Coma is the most severe form of neurological impairment during sepsis. Irreversible pathological changes in the hippocampus and brainstem can develop, which in turn is associated with persistent severe neurological deficits and a high risk of death. Sickness behavior is induced by the action of pro-inflammatory cytokines in the brain. In chronically critically ill patients with previous severe brain injury, exacerbation of encephalopathy occurs against the background of already existing severe cerebral dysfunction and depleted functional reserves of the body [32].

In the following sections of this chapter, dysfunction of major organ systems and some methods of intensive care are considered extracerebral pathogenetic factors of SAE in critically ill ICU patients (Figure 8.1).

Respiratory failure

In clinical studies focusing on MOF in critically ill patients, the lungs and respiratory system were most commonly affected in sepsis, with a prevalence of up to 43–75% [4, 22]. Respiratory failure in sepsis can be the result of primary pulmonary infection (pneumonia, purulent tracheobronchitis), exacerbation of chronic pulmonary disease (COPD), as well as hypoventilation and pulmonary atelectasis due to immobilization, pain, general weakness, etc. However, the most common cause of respiratory failure in patients with sepsis is acute respiratory distress syndrome (ARDS), which develops against the background of a systemic inflammatory response to the infection of a distant organ [8]. It is characterized by radiographic evidence of bilateral pulmonary infiltrates not attributable to cardiac failure, and progressive hypoxemia, often resulting in mechanical ventilation [33]. Sepsis is the most common cause of ARDS. In the pathogenesis of infectious ARDS, activation of the microvascular endothelium, platelets, and coagulation play an important role in disease progression and poor outcomes [34]. Hypoxia and in severe cases hypercapnia may contribute to dysfunction in other organ systems, resulting in the high mortality rate of ARDS [5].

The brain is one of the vulnerable organs in ARDS, regardless of the presence of sepsis [35, 36]. The mechanisms involved in the development of ARDS-associated brain injury, in addition to hypoxemia, include exacerbation of inflammation, hypotension, and adverse events of lung mechanical ventilation. Hypoxemia is a contributing cause of the emergence of acute brain injury and long-term cognitive impairment in critically ill patients [37]. Morphologically, hypoxic brain injury against the background of systemic infection (in particular, COVID-19) is manifested by non-specific damage to neurons and microglia with severe disorders of the cerebral circulation and a high risk of both stroke and intracranial hemorrhage [35]. Hypoxemia

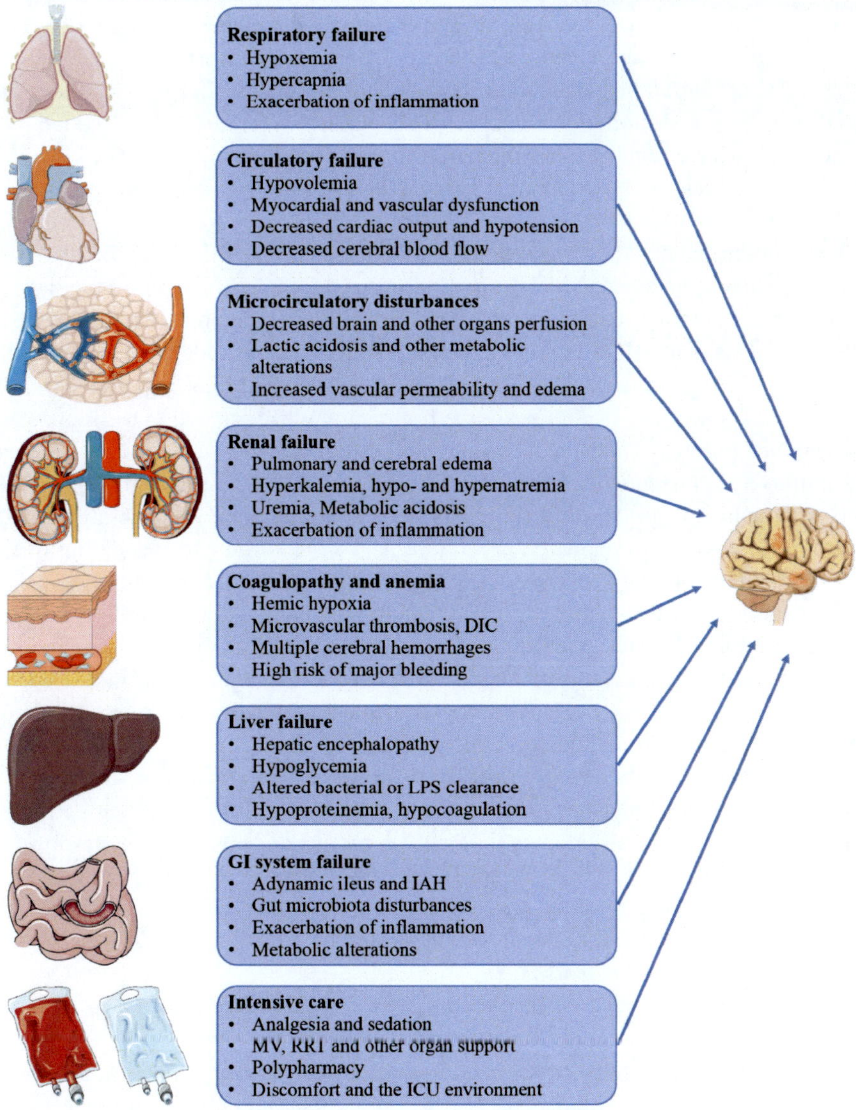

Figure 8.1 Dysfunction/failure of distant organs and methods of intensive care as extracerebral pathogenetic factors of sepsis-associated encephalopathy.

Note. DIC – disseminated intravascular coagulation, GI – gastrointestinal, IAH – intra-abdominal hypertension, ICU – intensive care unit, LPS – lipopolysaccharide, MV – mechanical ventilation, RRT – renal replacement therapy. Parts of the figure were drawn using pictures from Servier Medical Art. Servier Medical Art by Servier is licensed under a Creative Commons Attribution 3.0 Unported License (https://creativecommons.org/licenses/by/3.0/).

in most patients can be corrected with oxygen therapy and mechanical ventilation, but there is insufficient evidence to make a recommendation on the use of conservative (PaO_2 55–70 mmHg; SpO_2 88–92%) or liberal oxygen strategies in adults with sepsis-induced respiratory failure [8]. Potentiation of inflammation in sepsis and ARDS is due to the release of activated neutrophils from the pulmonary circulation and increased production of pro-inflammatory cytokines into the systemic circulation, in particular, IL-1β and TNF-α [36]. Pro-inflammatory cytokines can enhance neuroinflammation by acting on brain structures via a circumventricular area that lacks the blood-brain barrier. In an experimental model of ARDS, the levels of laboratory markers of brain damage and cell death in the hippocampus were higher in animals with ARDS compared with hypoxemic animals without ARDS (inhalation of hypoxic oxygen concentrations) [38]. This suggests that ARDS leads to neuropathologic changes independent of hypoxemia. In another experimental study in pigs, the combination of intracranial hypertension and ARDS caused mutual aggravation of damage in the brain and lungs (damage in the hippocampus and cerebral edema, pulmonary edema, and increased dystelectatic/atelectatic lung regions) [39].

Treatment of hypoxemia in patients with sepsis and ARDS begins with oxygen therapy (in patients without hypercapnia), while noninvasive ventilation (NIV) or high-flow oxygen in some cases provides additional opportunities to improve oxygenation and ventilation of the lungs. However, most patients with severe ARDS require tracheal intubation and invasive mechanical ventilation. Mechanical ventilation despite being lifesaving can exacerbate pulmonary and systemic inflammation, leading to lung and distant organ injury [36]. Additional brain damage in ventilated patients with SAE may occur through the mechanisms of increased release of pro-inflammatory cytokines, excessive alveolar stretch, and over-distension with activation of maladaptive vagal reflexes and other neurohumoral responses.

A protective ventilation strategy is used to minimize the side effects of mechanical ventilation in patients with sepsis and ARDS. The main elements of this strategy are mechanical ventilation using lower tidal volumes (4–8 ml/kg predicted body weight) and lower inspiratory pressures (plateau pressure < 30 cm H_2O), prone positioning for more than 12 h a day, and higher positive end-expiratory pressure [8, 33]. Currently, there is no consistent data on the effectiveness of specific pharmacological therapy for ARDS in sepsis, which would target underlying pathologic mechanisms [5, 8].

Although there are guidelines for the treatment of ARDS and acute brain injury independently, guidance on concomitant management is limited [40]. Treatment strategies aimed at managing severe ARDS may at times conflict with the management of acute brain injury. For example, in some patients with severe ARDS, protective ventilation can cause hypercapnia, which in turn can exacerbate intracranial hypertension. Therefore, the treatment strategy for such patients should be personalized with an assessment of the risks and benefits of the interventions, in particular, mechanical ventilation and fluid therapy.

Circulatory failure, microvascular disturbances, and septic shock

Cardiovascular abnormalities in sepsis may develop due to hypovolemia, vascular dysfunction, and myocardial dysfunction. A significant cause of hypovolemia in sepsis, in addition to obvious external and perspiration losses, is leakage of fluid into the interstitium due to increased capillary permeability with the development of edema. Sepsis-induced vascular dysfunction is manifested by systemic vasodilation and impaired autoregulation of organ blood flow [10].

The main clinical manifestations of hemodynamic instability in sepsis are arterial hypotension, tachycardia, and signs of peripheral hypoperfusion in the form of mottled clammy skin, oliguria, and altered mental state [41]. Septic shock is defined as a subset of sepsis in which circulatory, cellular, and metabolic abnormalities are associated with a greater risk of mortality than sepsis alone. The need for vasopressor therapy to maintain a mean arterial pressure of 65 mm Hg or greater and having a serum lactate level greater than 2 mmol/L despite fluid resuscitation are clinical criteria for the diagnosis of septic shock [1]. Thus, septic shock is characterized by fluid-resistant hypotension with severe impairment of tissue perfusion and metabolism.

Since microcirculatory disturbances and decreased organ perfusion are important pathogenic factors for MOF in sepsis, clinical assessment of these variables has received increasing attention. Microvascular alterations are characterized by a decrease in vascular density and the presence of non-perfused capillaries close to well-perfused vessels [42]. These alterations can be detected using modern point-of-care technologies of non-invasive intravital microscopy, such as side stream dark-field imaging. The persistence of microcirculatory and metabolic (increased serum lactate) disturbances after the restoration of blood pressure and cardiac output is a predictive marker of poor outcomes in sepsis [42].

Decreased systemic vascular resistance determines the hemodynamic profile of distributive shock with preserved or even increased cardiac output in the early stages of sepsis [5]. However, the development of technologies for the clinical assessment of hemodynamics and, in particular, the echocardiography has revealed a major role of myocardial dysfunction and impaired hemodynamic coherence in the pathogenesis of septic shock. In addition to the traditional variables of preload and myocardial contractility (such as end-diastolic volume, stroke volume, and left ventricular ejection fraction), indices such as ventricular and arterial elastance are currently used for a more differentiated assessment of cardiac performance and afterload [43].

Hemodynamic management in sepsis includes careful monitoring of circulatory variables and serum lactate levels; fluid resuscitation with a bolus of crystalloid solutions (30 ml/kg) at the initial stage, followed by personalized fluid administration regimen using dynamic measures with a passive leg raise or a fluid bolus; the administration of vasopressors (norepinephrine is a first-line drug) to maintain perfusion of vital organs when fluid resuscitation is ineffective; and the administration of inotropes (dobutamine) if there are signs of heart failure [8].

Cerebral circulation disorders within the framework of SAE can occur not only due to such obvious causes as severe arterial hypotension. Disturbances in autoregulation of cerebral blood flow and microvascular alterations can cause brain hypoperfusion even against the background of relatively stable systemic hemodynamics [7, 44]. The combination of macro- and microcirculatory alterations, endothelial dysfunction, and neurovascular uncoupling contribute to brain ischemic lesions in septic shock. These ischemic lesions were found not only in brain areas sensitive to ischemia (the hippocampus, the basal ganglia, frontal cortex) but also in the nuclei of the autonomic nervous system (i.e., amygdala, anterior and posterior hypothalamus, locus coeruleus) [31]. Decreased heart rate variability, reflecting the dysfunction of the autonomic nervous system, is also associated with a worse outcome in sepsis [31]. Both impaired cerebral autoregulation during sepsis and increased cerebrovascular resistance were associated with delirium during sepsis [45]. Comorbid patients with preexisting cerebrovascular atherosclerosis and neurodegenerative diseases are particularly prone to delirium and have a high risk of progressive cognitive impairment after sepsis resolves [7].

Thus, disorders of systemic and cerebral hemodynamics undoubtedly contribute to the development of acute encephalopathy in patients with sepsis and MOF. Timely correction of hypovolemia and hypotension followed by personalized fluid therapy, adequate oxygenation, and ventilation in combination with other reasonable intensive care measures contribute to the speedy normalization of brain perfusion and reduce the risk of severe complications and death. It is especially worth noting the importance of maintaining fluid balance in patients with sepsis. There is an association between a more positive fluid balance and mortality risk in sepsis [46]. On the other hand, an overly restrictive fluid management strategy may worsen neurological outcomes in patients with sepsis and ARDS in the long term [47]. Therefore, the random allocation of patients into groups of liberal and restrictive fluid management strategies is not always justified in clinical trials.

Renal failure, fluid, electrolyte, and acid-base disorders

Sepsis is the most common cause of acute kidney injury (AKI), which, in turn, is one of the most common organ failures in ICU patients with a prevalence of up to 36% [22]. AKI is associated with an overall mortality rate of 50% when found as a component of MOD in sepsis [48]. It has long been believed that arterial hypotension and a decrease in renal blood flow, leading to ischemia and acute tubular necrosis, play a key role in the pathogenesis of renal failure in sepsis and other critical illnesses. However, some animal and human studies indicate that total renal blood flow is not universally impaired during sepsis, and AKI can develop in the presence of normal or even increased renal blood flow [49]. Inflammation, microvascular alterations, and maladaptive responses of tubular epithelial cells to injurious signals are more specific pathogenetic factors for sepsis-associated AKI [48].

The main clinical manifestations of renal dysfunction in critically ill patients are oliguria (urine output less than 0.5 ml/kg/h) and a rapid increase (1.5–3.0 times baseline) in serum creatinine levels. Anuria, pulmonary and cerebral edema, hyperkalemia, and metabolic acidosis are characteristic of severe cases of renal failure. All these disturbances of homeostasis are additional factors of brain damage in critically ill patients with acute encephalopathy, and in particular, in SAE [7]. Thus, in a prospective cohort study of ICU patients with respiratory failure and/or shock AKI was shown to be associated with delirium and coma during critical illness [50]. Sodium is the main cation of the extracellular fluid, which determines the osmotic balance. Therefore, the damaged brain is very vulnerable to abrupt changes in serum sodium concentration, which occur, for example, with the rapid correction of hypernatremia with hypoosmotic fluids or as a result of an inadequate regimen of renal replacement therapy. Due to the widespread use of renal replacement therapy in the ICU, uremic coma is currently rarely the direct cause of acute encephalopathy and death.

More specific mechanisms of kidney-brain crosstalk were observed in animal models of AKI. Exacerbation of inflammation and neurotransmitter imbalance are of the greatest pathophysiological significance [12]. Local renal inflammation led to increased levels of the pro-inflammatory chemokines in the cerebral cortex and hippocampus, increased expression of glial fibrillary acidic protein in astrocytes, and the disruption of the blood-brain barrier in mice with AKI [51]. Renal failure can also reduce the elimination of drugs (antibiotics, analgesics, and sedatives), and elevated levels of these drugs can result in neurotoxicity [10].

On the other hand, brain injury may deteriorate renal function leading to hyponatremia or AKI induced by an overly activated sympathetic nervous system. Excessive release of epinephrine and norepinephrine from renal sympathetic nerves activates the renin-angiotensin-aldosterone system and leads to the contraction of afferent arterioles and renal ischemia [15].

Treatment of renal failure in sepsis is currently non-specific and includes elimination of causes (antibiotics), fluid management to correct hypovolemia and electrolyte imbalance, judicious use of diuretics, and various options for renal replacement therapy (hemodialysis, hemofiltration, or their combined use). In adults with sepsis or septic shock and AKI, with no definitive indications for renal replacement therapy (i.e., anuria, uremic complications, refractory acidosis, refractory fluid overload or hyperkalemia), Surviving Sepsis Campaign guidelines suggest against using renal replacement therapy [8].

Coagulopathy and anemia

The interplay between hemostasis and inflammation is implicated in the pathogenesis of MOD/MOF in sepsis due to the mutually aggravating effect of the disorder of one component on another [52]. The coagulopathy in sepsis is manifested in a hypercoagulation with the consumption of platelets and clotting factors (in severe cases), commonly referred to as disseminated intravascular coagulation (DIC) [5]. Laboratory signs of coagulopathy may include thrombocytopenia, prolonged global coagulation assays (prothrombin time or the activated partial thromboplastin time), high fibrin degradation products, and low levels of physiological anticoagulants, such as antithrombin and protein C. DIC is manifested by widespread microvascular thrombosis in small and mid-size vessels and simultaneous profuse hemorrhage from various sites [52]. Since the severity of sepsis correlates strongly with thrombocytopenia, this parameter is included as a hematological component in the SOFA and many other scoring systems. Hematological failure along with liver failure and total LODS score were the main factors associated with early death in ICU patients with sepsis [4].

Severe coagulopathy along with endothelial dysfunction and disorders of the cerebral microcirculation may contribute to the exacerbation of SAE. Post-mortem morphological examination of the brain of patients who died from sepsis and MOF revealed multiple microthrombi with ischemic lesions and multiple hemorrhages [31].

Timely administration of antibiotics and control of the source is the basis for the successful treatment of coagulopathy in sepsis. The need for the use of donor plasma, platelets, and clotting factors arises when these hemostatic factors are depleted in patients with bleeding or the need for invasive interventions [52].

Anemia in critically ill patients develops as a result of impaired hematopoiesis, for example, with sepsis and renal dysfunction, as well as due to accelerated destruction of red blood cells (hemolysis) and blood loss (including due to frequent blood sampling). Anemia can contribute to the aggravation of hypoxic damage to the brain and other organs, especially in combination with hypoxemia and circulatory disorders. A restrictive transfusion strategy recommended for sepsis typically includes a hemoglobin concentration transfusion trigger of 70g/L. However, for some patients with acute myocardial ischemia, severe hypoxemia, or acute hemorrhage, the target hemoglobin values will be higher [8].

Liver and gastrointestinal system failure

Hepatic dysfunction in most scoring systems is assessed by the degree of increase in serum concentrations of bilirubin and transaminases. However, given the many functions of the liver, some other clinical and laboratory variables can be used as markers of hepatic dysfunction: ascites, pathological changes in the liver according to CT or MRI, hepatic encephalopathy, elevated serum gamma-GT, alkaline phosphatase and ammonia, decreased serum albumin, prothrombin index, and other clotting factors [20].

Sepsis-induced liver injury has a substantial effect on the outcome of sepsis, owing mostly to altered bacterial or lipopolysaccharide clearance, and the imbalance of pro- and anti-inflammatory cytokines [10]. In large clinical trials, the combination of hepatic and cerebral failures (as assessed by the SOFA scoring system) in patients with sepsis was associated with the highest mortality [4, 22]. Liver failure increases the risk of severe hypoglycemia in patients with sepsis, which is a recognized precipitating factor for delirium and hypoglycemic coma [7]. Hepatic encephalopathy is a distinct type of acute encephalopathy in patients with the end-stage of liver disease (e.g., cirrhosis). In this regard, the differential diagnosis of hepatic encephalopathy and SAE is difficult in this patient population.

The main manifestations of gastrointestinal system dysfunction/failure in critically ill patients are impaired gastrointestinal motility (gastro stasis, adynamic ileus), stress ulcers with gastrointestinal bleeding, as well as pancreatitis and acalculous cholecystitis [5]. Intra-abdominal hypertension and compartment syndrome are pathogenic factors in the development of MOF in patients with abdominal sepsis and polytrauma. The severity of gastrointestinal system dysfunction is not considered a component of MOF when assessed using the original SOFA score. However, both specialized scoring systems (GastroIntestinal Dysfunction Score [GIDS]) and specific laboratory markers of gastrointestinal dysfunction (citrulline, intestinal fatty acid binding protein [I-FABP]) have been proposed for use in clinical and research practice [20]. A separate problem in the management of patients with sepsis is *Clostridioides difficile* colitis. It occurs due to a disturbance of the normal bacterial flora of the colon on the background of antimicrobial therapy and is characterized by mucosal inflammation, diarrhea, and a pronounced systemic inflammatory response. Early enteral nutrition (in the absence of contraindications) and the reasonable use of proton pump inhibitors are the main therapeutic measures to preserve the integrity of the intestinal wall and decrease the incidence of stress ulcers and nosocomial infections in patients with sepsis [8].

Increased permeability of the intestinal wall is one of the primary pathogenetic factors of MOD/MOF in sepsis. Some experimental data point to the role of the mesenteric lymph as a carrier of gut-derived DAMPs to the lung and systemic circulation. The gut becomes a pro-inflammatory organ, driving the systemic inflammatory response, without the need for systemic bacterial translocation [53]. The study of the role of gut microbiota disturbances in the pathogenesis of distant organ dysfunction in sepsis has become one of the mainstreams of research in this area [54]. Quantitative and qualitative changes in the taxonomic composition of the microbiome may result in dysregulation of gut-brain cross-talk, enhancing neuroinflammation, abnormal blood-brain barrier permeability, neurotransmitter imbalance, and metabolic alterations in the brain [55]. Microbial phenolic metabolites can target brain function in critically ill patients with severe brain injury by the direct and indirect modulation of inflammation and metabolism [56].

Intensive care and the ICU environment

Intensive care, on the one hand, saves the patient's life, gaining time and allowing the patient to recover while organ support is being carried out. On the other hand, aggressive measures of organ support, such as mechanical ventilation or dialysis, themselves become additional pathogenetic factors that modify the host response and the clinical picture of MOD [5]. For example, mechanical ventilation itself is a major risk factor for delirium in ICU patients [36, 57].

Many ICU patients require analgesics (e.g., in the postoperative period) and sedative agents to promote sleep, relieve discomfort from invasive procedures (mechanical ventilation, monitoring), and combat anxiety and agitation. At the same time, many studies have shown that analgesics, sedatives, medication changes, and withdrawal are associated with delirium [37, 58]. In the study of Girard et al. [37] sedative-associated delirium was most common, and a longer duration of sedative-associated delirium predicted a worse outcome in terms of the patient's cognitive abilities 12 months later. Benzodiazepines, L-type calcium channel blockers, antihistamines, opioids, and steroids may convey the highest risk of delirium, especially in elderly patients [7]. A meta-analysis of randomized trials showed that the use of a dexmedetomidine or propofol sedation regimen rather than a benzodiazepine sedation regimen in critically ill adults might reduce ICU length of stay and duration of mechanical ventilation [59]. Apart from the above, the common use of sedative agents in the ICU can make it difficult to recognize SAE.

Other specific ICU-related factors, such as hypo- and hyperglycemia, polypharmacy, sleep deprivation, and lack of communication with family are risk factors for hospital-acquired delirium [7]. Light rather than deep sedation and brief cessation of sedation for daily wake-up tests are recommended for reducing the risk of acute encephalopathy and length of stay in the ICU [36].

Conclusion

SAE is a special case of organ dysfunction in patients with sepsis. Most of these patients present with MOD and homeostasis disorders, which require urgent admission to the ICU and complex intensive care. This population of critically ill patients has many predisposing and precipitating risk factors for acute encephalopathy, the clinical manifestations of which range from subclinical delirium to deep coma. Each of these factors can exacerbate the severity of SAE and should therefore be considered when planning a diagnosis and treatment strategy. Timely control of infection, correction of hypoxia, and circulatory and metabolic disorders, along with control of reversible risk factors for delirium, are the basis for successful treatment of SAE and improvement of long-term outcomes.

References

1. Singer M, Deutschman CS, Seymour CW, Shankar-Hari M, Annane D, Bauer M, et al. The third international consensus definitions for sepsis and septic shock (sepsis-3). *JAMA*. 2016 Feb 23;315(8):801. doi: 10.1001/jama.2016.0287
2. Hotchkiss RS, Monneret G, Payen D. Sepsis-induced immunosuppression: From cellular dysfunctions to immunotherapy. *Nat Rev Immunol*. 2013 Dec;13(12):862–74. doi: 10.1038/nri3552
3. Abraham E, Singer M. *Mechanisms of Sepsis-Induced Organ Dysfunction and Recovery*. Berlin, Heidelberg: Springer-Verlag Berlin Heidelberg; 2007. (Update in Intensive Care and Emergency Medicine).
4. Blanco J, Muriel-Bombín A, Sagredo V, Taboada F, Gandía F, Tamayo L, et al. Incidence, organ dysfunction and mortality in severe sepsis: A Spanish multicentre study. *Crit Care Lond Engl*. 2008;12(6):R158. doi: 10.1186/cc7157

5. Ziesmann MT, Marshall JC. Multiple organ dysfunction: The defining syndrome of sepsis. *Surg Infect.* 2018;19(2):184–90. doi: 10.1089/sur.2017.298
6. Gofton TE, Young GB. Sepsis-associated encephalopathy. *Nat Rev Neurol.* 2012 Oct;8(10):557–66. doi: 10.1038/nrneurol.2012.183
7. Wilson JE, Mart MF, Cunningham C, Shehabi Y, Girard TD, MacLullich AMJ, et al. Delirium. *Nat Rev Dis Primer.* 2020 Nov 12;6(1):90. doi: 10.1038/s41572-020-00223-4
8. Evans L, Rhodes A, Alhazzani W, Antonelli M, Coopersmith CM, French C, et al. Surviving sepsis campaign: International guidelines for the management of sepsis and septic shock 2021. *Intensive Care Med.* 2021 Nov;47(11):1181–247. doi: 10.1007/s00134-021-06506-y
9. Timmermans K, Kox M, Scheffer GJ, Pickkers P. Danger in the intensive care unit: Damps in critically ill patients. *Shock Augusta Ga.* 2016 Feb;45(2):108–16. doi: 10.1097/SHK.0000000000000506
10. Lelubre C, Vincent JL. Mechanisms and treatment of organ failure in sepsis. *Nat Rev Nephrol.* 2018 Jul;14(7):417–27. doi: 10.1038/s41581-018-0005-7
11. De Backer D, Orbegozo Cortes D, Donadello K, Vincent JL. Pathophysiology of microcirculatory dysfunction and the pathogenesis of septic shock. *Virulence.* 2014 Jan 1;5(1):73–9. doi: 10.4161/viru.26482
12. Pool R, Gomez H, Kellum JA. Mechanisms of organ dysfunction in sepsis. *Crit Care Clin.* 2018 Jan;34(1):63–80. doi: 10.1016/j.ccc.2017.08.003
13. Levy B. Lactate and shock state: The metabolic view. *Curr Opin Crit Care.* 2006 Aug;12(4):315–21. doi: 10.1097/01.ccx.0000235208.77450.15
14. Baue AE. History of MOF and definitions of organ failure. In: Baue AE, Faist E, Fry DE, editors. *Multiple Organ Failure.* New York: Springer New York; 2000, pp. 3–13.
15. Kotfis K, Siwicka-Gieroba D, Dąbrowski W. Brain–multiorgan cross-talk in critically ill patients with acute brain injury. In: Vincent JL, editor. *Annual Update in Intensive Care and Emergency Medicine 2022.* Cham: Springer International Publishing; 2022, pp. 317–31. (Annual Update in Intensive Care and Emergency Medicine). doi:10.1007/978-3-030-93433-0_25
16. Borovikova LV, Ivanova S, Zhang M, Yang H, Botchkina GI, Watkins LR, et al. Vagus nerve stimulation attenuates the systemic inflammatory response to endotoxin. *Nature.* 2000;405(6785):458–62. doi: 10.1038/35013070
17. Wang DW, Yin YM, Yao YM. Vagal modulation of the inflammatory response in sepsis. *Int Rev Immunol.* 2016 Sep 2;35(5):415–33. doi: 10.3109/08830185.2015.1127369
18. Huston JM, Gallowitsch-Puerta M, Ochani M, Ochani K, Yuan R, Rosas-Ballina M, et al. Transcutaneous vagus nerve stimulation reduces serum high mobility group box 1 level and improves survival in murine sepsis. *Crit Care Med.* 2007 Dec;35(12):2762–8. doi: 10.1097/01.CCM.0000288102.15975.BA
19. Pellathy TP, Pinsky MR, Hravnak M. Intensive care unit scoring systems. *Crit Care Nurse.* 2021;41(4):54–64. doi: 10.4037/ccn2021613
20. Reintam Blaser A, Bachmann KF, Arabi YM. Organ dysfunction scores in the adult ICU. In: Vincent JL, editor. *Annual update in intensive care and emergency medicine 2023.* Cham: Springer Nature Switzerland; 2023, pp. 93–108. (Annual Update in Intensive Care and Emergency Medicine). doi: 10.1007/978-3-031-23005-9_8
21. Vincent JL, Moreno R, Takala J, Willatts S, De Mendonça A, Bruining H, et al. The SOFA (sepsis-related organ failure assessment) score to describe organ dysfunction/failure: On behalf of the working group on sepsis-related problems of the European society of intensive care medicine. *Intensive Care Med.* 1996 Jul;22(7):707–10.
22. Sakr Y, Lobo SM, Moreno RP, Gerlach H, Ranieri VM, Michalopoulos A, et al. Patterns and early evolution of organ failure in the intensive care unit and their relation to outcome. *Crit Care Lond Engl.* 2012 Nov 16;16(6):R222. doi: 10.1186/cc11868
23. Golomidov AV, Grigoriev EV, Moses VG, Moses KB. Pathogenesis, prognosis, and outcomes of multiple organ failure in newborns (review). *Gen Reanimatol.* 2022 Dec 20;18(6):37–49. doi: 10.15360/1813-9779-2022-6-37-49
24. Zilber AP. *Etudes of Critical Medicine.* Moscow: MEDpress-inform; 2006, 568 p.

25. Slooter AJC, Otte WM, Devlin JW, Arora RC, Bleck TP, Claassen J, et al. Updated nomenclature of delirium and acute encephalopathy: Statement of ten Societies. *Intensive Care Med.* 2020 May;46(5):1020–2. doi: 10.1007/s00134-019-05907-4
26. Krewulak KD, Stelfox HT, Leigh JP, Ely EW, Fiest KM. Incidence and prevalence of delirium subtypes in an adult ICU: A systematic review and meta-analysis. *Crit Care Med.* 2018 Dec;46(12):2029–35. doi: 10.1097/CCM.0000000000003402
27. Dulhunty JM, Lipman J, Finfer S; Sepsis Study Investigators for the ANZICS Clinical Trials Group. Does severe non-infectious SIRS differ from severe sepsis? Results from a multi-center Australian and New Zealand intensive care unit study. *Intensive Care Med.* 2008 Sep;34(9):1654–61. doi: 10.1007/s00134-008-1160-2
28. Eidelman LA, Putterman D, Putterman C, Sprung CL. The spectrum of septic encephalopathy: Definitions, etiologies, and mortalities. *JAMA.* 1996 Feb 14;275(6):470–3.
29. Annane D, Sharshar T. Cognitive decline after sepsis. *Lancet Respir Med.* 2015 Jan;3(1):61–9. doi: 10.1016/S2213-2600(14)70246-2
30. Sweis R, Ortiz J, Biller J. Neurology of sepsis. *Curr Neurol Neurosci Rep.* 2016 Mar;16(3):21. doi: 10.1007/s11910-016-0623-z
31. Heming N, Mazeraud A, Verdonk F, Bozza FA, Chrétien F, Sharshar T. Neuroanatomy of sepsis-associated encephalopathy. *Crit Care.* 2017 Dec;21(1):65. doi: 10.1186/s13054-017-1643-z
32. Parfenov AL, Petrova MV, Pichugina IM, Luginina EV. Comorbidity development in patients with severe brain injury resulting in chronic critical condition (review). *Gen Reanimatol.* 2020 Aug 29;16(4):72–89. doi: 10.15360/1813-9779-2020-4-72-89
33. Fan E, Del Sorbo L, Goligher EC, Hodgson CL, Munshi L, Walkey AJ, et al. An official American thoracic society/European society of intensive care medicine/society of critical care medicine clinical practice guideline: Mechanical ventilation in adult patients with acute respiratory distress syndrome. *Am J Respir Crit Care Med.* 2017 May 1;195(9):1253–63. doi: 10.1164/rccm.201703-0548ST
34. Babkina AS, Ostrova IV, Yadgarov MY, Kuzovlev AN, Grechko AV, Volkov AV, et al. The role of Von Willebrand factor in the pathogenesis of pulmonary vascular thrombosis in COVID-19. *Viruses.* 2022 Jan 21;14(2):211.
35. Babkina AS, Golubev AM, Ostrova IV, Volkov AV, Kuzovlev AN. Brain morphological changes in COVID-19. *Gen Reanimatol.* 2021 Jul 3;17(3):4–15. doi: 10.3390/v14020211
36. Ziaka M, Exadaktylos A. ARDS associated acute brain injury: From the lung to the brain. *Eur J Med Res.* 2022 Aug 13;27(1):150. doi: 10.1186/s40001-022-00780-2
37. Girard TD, Thompson JL, Pandharipande PP, Brummel NE, Jackson JC, Patel MB, et al. Clinical phenotypes of delirium during critical illness and severity of subsequent long-term cognitive impairment: A prospective cohort study. *Lancet Respir Med.* 2018 Mar;6(3):213–22. doi: 10.1016/S2213-2600(18)30062-6
38. Fries M, Bickenbach J, Henzler D, Beckers S, Dembinski R, Sellhaus B, et al. S-100 protein and neurohistopathologic changes in a porcine model of acute lung injury. *Anesthesiology.* 2005 Apr;102(4):761–7. doi: 10.1097/00000542-200504000-00011
39. Heuer JF, Pelosi P, Hermann P, Perske C, Crozier TA, Brück W, et al. Acute effects of intracranial hypertension and ARDS on pulmonary and neuronal damage: A randomized experimental study in pigs. *Intensive Care Med.* 2011 Jul;37(7):1182–91. doi: 10.1007/s00134-011-2232-2
40. Kim JA, Wahlster S, LaBuzetta JN, Nobleza COS, Johnson NJ, Rubinos C, et al. Focused management of patients with severe acute brain injury and ARDS. *Chest.* 2022 Jan;161(1):140–51. doi: 10.1016/j.chest.2021.08.066
41. Vincent JL, De Backer D. Circulatory shock. *N Engl J Med.* 2013 Oct 31;369(18):1726–34. doi: 10.1056/NEJMra1208943
42. De Backer D. Novelties in the evaluation of microcirculation in septic shock. *J Intensive Med.* 2023 Apr 30;3(2):124–30. doi: 10.1016/j.jointm.2022.09.002
43. Guarracino F, Baldassarri R, Pinsky MR. Pathophysiological determinants of cardiovascular dysfunction in septic shock. In: Vincent JL, editor. *Annual Update in Intensive Care and Emergency*

Medicine 2016. Cham: Springer International Publishing; 2016, pp. 177–84. (Annual Update in Intensive Care and Emergency Medicine). doi: 10.1007/978-3-319-27349-5
44. Taccone FS, Su F, De Deyne C, Abdellhai A, Pierrakos C, He X, et al. Sepsis is associated with altered cerebral microcirculation and tissue hypoxia in experimental peritonitis. *Crit Care Med.* 2014 Feb;42(2):e114–122. doi: 10.1097/CCM.0b013e3182a641b8
45. Wood MD, Boyd JG, Wood N, Frank J, Girard TD, Ross-White A, et al. The use of near-infrared spectroscopy and/or transcranial doppler as non-invasive markers of cerebral perfusion in adult sepsis patients with delirium: A systematic review. *J Intensive Care Med.* 2022 Mar;37(3):408–22. doi: 10.1177/0885066621997090
46. Sakr Y, Rubatto Birri PN, Kotfis K, Nanchal R, Shah B, Kluge S, et al. Higher fluid balance increases the risk of death from sepsis: Results from a large international audit. *Crit Care Med.* 2017 Mar;45(3):386–94. doi: 10.1097/CCM.0000000000002189
47. Mikkelsen ME, Christie JD, Lanken PN, Biester RC, Thompson BT, Bellamy SL, et al. The adult respiratory distress syndrome cognitive outcomes study: Long-term neuropsychological function in survivors of acute lung injury. *Am J Respir Crit Care Med.* 2012 Jun 15;185(12):1307–15. doi: 10.1164/rccm.201111-2025OC
48. Zarbock A, Gomez H, Kellum JA. Sepsis-induced acute kidney injury revisited: Pathophysiology, prevention and future therapies. *Curr Opin Crit Care.* 2014 Dec;20(6):588–95. doi: 10.1097/MCC.0000000000000153
49. Gomez H, Ince C, De Backer D, Pickkers P, Payen D, Hotchkiss J, et al. A unified theory of sepsis-induced acute kidney injury: Inflammation, microcirculatory dysfunction, bioenergetics, and the tubular cell adaptation to injury. *Shock Augusta Ga.* 2014 Jan;41(1):3–11. doi: 10.1097/SHK.0000000000000052
50. Siew ED, Fissell WH, Tripp CM, Blume JD, Wilson MD, Clark AJ, et al. Acute kidney injury as a risk factor for delirium and coma during critical illness. *Am J Respir Crit Care Med.* 2017 Jun 15;195(12):1597–607. doi: 10.1164/rccm.201603-0476OC
51. Liu M, Liang Y, Chigurupati S, Lathia JD, Pletnikov M, Sun Z, et al. Acute kidney injury leads to inflammation and functional changes in the brain. *J Am Soc Nephrol JASN.* 2008 Jul;19(7):1360–70. doi: 10.1681/ASN.2007080901
52. Levi M, van der Poll T. Coagulation and sepsis. *Thromb Res.* 2017 Jan;149:38–44. doi: 10.1016/j.thromres.2016.11.007
53. Assimakopoulos SF, Triantos C, Thomopoulos K, Fligou F, Maroulis I, Marangos M, et al. Gut-origin sepsis in the critically ill patient: Pathophysiology and treatment. *Infection.* 2018 Dec;46(6):751–60. doi: 10.1007/s15010-018-1178-5
54. Chernevskaya EA, Beloborodova NV. Gut microbiome in critical illness (review). *Gen Reanimatol.* 2018 Oct 28;14(5):96–119. doi: 10.15360/1813-9779-2018-5-96-119
55. Braniste V, Al-Asmakh M, Kowal C, Anuar F, Abbaspour A, Tóth M, et al. The gut microbiota influences blood-brain barrier permeability in mice. *Sci Transl Med.* 2014 Nov 19;6(263):263ra158. doi: 10.1126/scitranslmed.3009759
56. Chernevskaya E, Klimenko N, Pautova A, Buyakova I, Tyakht A, Beloborodova N. Host-microbiome interactions mediated by phenolic metabolites in chronically critically ill patients. *Metabolites.* 2021 Feb 20;11(2):122. doi: 10.3390/metabo11020122
57. Almeida ICT, Soares M, Bozza FA, Shinotsuka CR, Bujokas R, Souza-Dantas VC, et al. The impact of acute brain dysfunction in the outcomes of mechanically ventilated cancer patients. Lim M, editor. *PLoS ONE.* 2014 Jan 22;9(1):e85332. doi: 10.1371/journal.pone.0085332
58. Sampson EL, West E, Fischer T. Pain, and delirium: Mechanisms, assessment, and management. *Eur Geriatr Med.* 2020 Feb;11(1):45–52. doi: 10.1007/s41999-019-00281-2
59. Fraser GL, Devlin JW, Worby CP, Alhazzani W, Barr J, Dasta JF, et al. Benzodiazepine versus nonbenzodiazepine-based sedation for mechanically ventilated, critically ill adults: A systematic review and meta-analysis of randomized trials. *Crit Care Med.* 2013 Sep;41(9 Suppl 1): S30–38. doi: 10.1097/CCM.0b013e3182a16898

Chapter 9

Features of sepsis-associated encephalopathy in children

Irina A. Savvina[1,2,3]*, MD., Ph.D.,
Victoria I. Gurskaya[1], MD., Ph.D.,
William A. Khachatryan[4], MD., Ph.D.,
Eleonora T. Nazaralieva[4], MD., Ph.D.

[1] Department of Anesthesiology and Intensive Care, Almazov National Medical Research Centre of Ministry of Health Care of Russian Federation, Saint Petersburg, Russian Federation

[2] Department of Pathomorphology of Nervous System, Russian Polenov Scientific Research Neurosurgical Institute – the branch of Almazov National Medical Research Centre of Ministry of Health Care of Russian Federation, Saint Petersburg, Russian Federation

[3] Department of Anesthesiology and Intensive Care named after V.L. Vanevskiy of the North-Western State Medical University named after Ilya I. Mechnikov of the Ministry of Health of Russian Federation, St. Petersburg, Russian Federation

[4]Department of Pediatric Neurosurgery, Almazov National Medical Research Centre of Ministry of Health Care of Russian Federation, Saint Petersburg, Russian Federation

Abstract

Pediatric sepsis is accompanied by a high mortality rate. Among the most significant causes of adverse outcomes, sepsis-associated encephalopathy (SAE) is an acute cerebral dysfunction in the form of delirium and coma. The immaturity of the central nervous system (CNS) in young children in morphofunctional terms explains the tendency to generalize responses to infection, the focus of which is located outside the CNS, and the systemic inflammatory response in the form of a convulsive syndrome, turning off consciousness; damage to the blood-brain barrier (BBB) due to endotoxemia leads to the development of intrathecal inflammation and cerebral edema, accompanied by the aggravation of neurotransmitter imbalance, hypoperfusion and fixation of cognitive deficit, and activation of neuronal apoptosis, which normally occurs up to 2 years of a child's life. In this chapter, the authors describe the clinical picture of SAE in children, taking into account age characteristics, the methods of functional diagnostics used in pediatrics to verify cerebral dysfunction, bedside neuromonitoring methods, and laboratory diagnostic panels to confirm the diagnosis of SAE.

---

* Corresponding author: Irina A. Savvina, Professor, MD., Ph.D.
e-mail address: irinasavvina@mail.ru

Editor: Irina A. Savvina, Natalia V. Beloborodova and Tatyana N. Trofimova
In: Sepsis-Associated Encephalopathy
ISBN: 979-8-89113-178-1

Keywords: sepsis-associated encephalopathy, pediatric patients, infant brain development, septic cognitive impairment, neurological assessment, laboratory markers of cerebral damage.

Introduction

The number of publications on sepsis-associated encephalopathy (SAE) is growing rapidly, but the vast majority of them concern the adult population. However, the problem of sepsis and complications after a septic condition in children is no less relevant for clinicians. The data of foreign colleagues indicate the development of SAE among the adult population in every third patient with sepsis, and the development of acute cerebral insufficiency is accompanied by long-term disorders of consciousness and an increase in mortality [1]. We did not find similar statistics for children.

The heterogeneity of the age population of pediatric patients and the inherent uneven development of the physiological systems of the body, including the central and autonomic parts of the nervous system in the main age groups of children, make it extremely important to conduct neuromonitoring and interpret its results for diagnosing dysfunction of the central and autonomic nervous system in sepsis in the pediatric population.

Definition of sepsis-associated encephalopathy: epidemiology in pediatrics

Septic encephalopathy is a multifocal or diffuse brain lesion in patients with an infectious status, which is accompanied by the development and course of sepsis, but without clinical and/or laboratory verification of the focus of infection in the brain [2]. As for the epidemiology of septic encephalopathy among pediatric patients, the data found in the literature are ambiguous and sometimes can vary, reaching, according to some survey analyses, up to 30% among children in the ICU with sepsis [3]. It should be borne in mind that the study of the development and incidence of septic encephalopathy among the pediatric population is of significant socio-economic importance. The consequences of sepsis-associated encephalopathy in children may include cognitive and behavioral disorders, a decrease in the physiological parameters of various functional systems, the rate of physical development and stress resistance, and impaired memory and verbal and adaptive skills for a long period after discharge from a medical institution [4, 5]. Moreover, due to the peculiarities of the rate of metabolic processes and their disturbances in the ICU, this group of children poses a high risk for the development of concomitant diseases, such as arterial hypertension, renal failure, and endocrine polyglandular insufficiency, which, in turn, leads to an increase in disability [6, 7].

Acute cerebral injury in sepsis in children cannot be considered without taking into account the characteristics of the maturation and development of the child's brain. Since the pathophysiological processes underlying SAE are realized at the level of intrathecal and systemic inflammation in sepsis, neurotransmitter imbalance, impaired permeability of the blood-brain barrier, neuronal death, the processes of neuronal differentiation and myelination of the nerve tracts, synaptogenesis, and the rate of apoptosis, neuroregulatory mechanisms of activity will be vulnerable. We consider it necessary to reflect in this chapter on some aspects of brain ontogenesis, taking into account the above mechanisms for the development of acute cerebral insufficiency in sepsis in children.

Some physiological aspects of brain development

Perinatal development of the brain begins with the formation of the neural tube, one of the most important stages in the development of the embryo. The final formation of the neural tube stops by the 26th day after conception [8]. Later, the hemispheres of the brain are formed and the structuring of the subcortical regions occurs.

The generation of neurons occurs between the 10th and 20th weeks of pregnancy [9]. Thus, by the end of brain maturation, about 86 billion neurons are formed, which usually do not change during the life of the organism, except for the hippocampus region [10]. Critical moments of maturation of the central nervous system occur in the last trimester of intrauterine development and the first two years of a child's life [11]. The process of neuron generation is also considered critical in the stages of fetal development (Figure 9.1).

After birth, until the end of the first year of life, the child has an active migration of immature neurons to the frontal cortex, where they further differentiate and mature [12]. Thus, identifying the formation of cognitive abilities with the development of the frontal lobes of the brain, the role of late migration to the frontal cortex is of decisive importance in the formation of intellectual abilities or the occurrence of cognitive deficits of varying severity [13]. The processes of neuron migration are very complexly organized and require certain energy consumption of the cell. Thus, migrating neurons and glial filaments themselves contain glycogen, which provides them with energy for movement [14]. Glial tissue is an excellent source of energy for neurons. It contains glycogen, which under anaerobic conditions can supply neurons with energy through glycolysis processes [13]. Also, glial tissue can absorb an excessive amount of secreted transmitters, which can adversely affect the further maturation of the brain [13]. It is believed that neuroglial cells are capable of growing up to 2 years after birth [12]. Glial cells are divided into

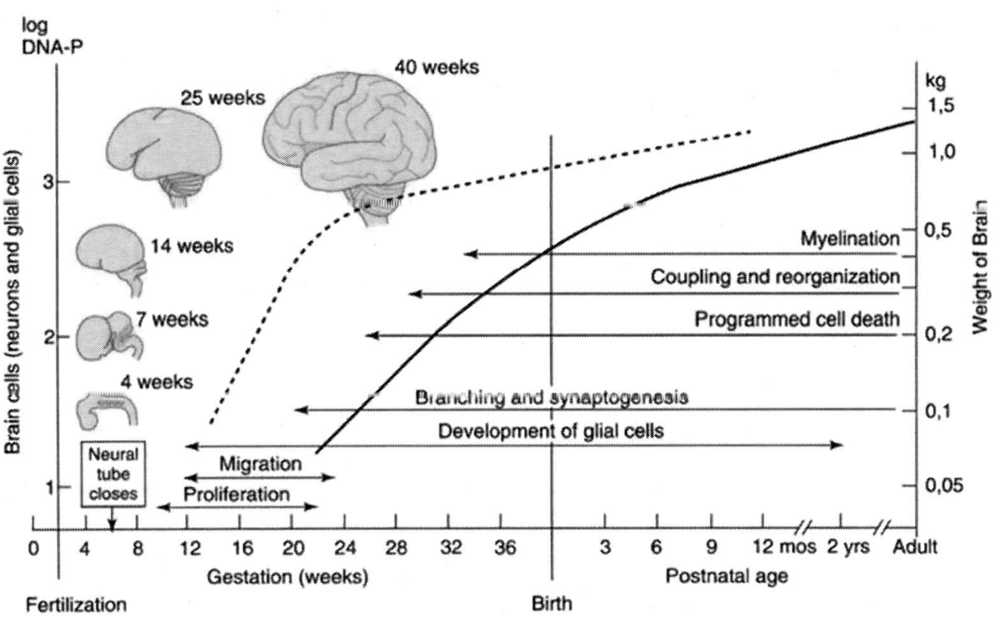

Figure 9.1 Stages of brain development (H. Lagercrantz, 2016).

two groups: microglia and macroglia, which include oligodendrocytes, astrocytes, and ependymal cells [12]. In young children, under the influence of various negative external factors or disruption of the processes of maturation of the nervous tissue, the development of glial tumors of the brain is possible in utero [15].

By the time of birth, the most functionally mature is the brain stem [16]. The process of myelination of nerve fibers begins approximately from the 23rd week of pregnancy and continues until puberty. Each neuron is embedded in a thin sheet of myelin, which consists mainly of phospholipids. Functionally, the neonate has the least developed cerebral cortex [17]. This neurophysiological phenomenon is based on a unique mechanism of synaptogenesis. This term was proposed by the British physiologist Charles Sherrington [18]. The process of synaptogenesis is very complex and consists of several stages. The first synapses appear at about 6–8 weeks of gestation (first phase of synaptogenesis); then, at 12–17 weeks of gestation, the second phase occurs, which is similar to the process of neuronal migration; at 20–24 weeks of gestation, the third phase begins, which ends approximately between 8 and 12 months of life after birth, when increased synapse formation occurs. Then comes the fourth phase, which continues throughout life. In the course of mastering a new skill or action, the impulse wanders through more fibers and gradually takes the shortest and most efficient route; thus, the skill is consolidated [18].

The transmission of a nerve impulse during synaptogenesis depends on the environment that determines this synapse [9]. In the developing synapse, brain-derived neurotrophic factor (BDNF) regulates a wide range of functions, including increased neurotransmitter release and cholesterol biosynthesis [19]. Cholesterol is a structural component of the neuronal cell membrane and is involved in various signal interactions [8, 14]. Also, matrix metalloproteinases, which regulate many signaling processes, take part in the process of synaptogenesis [20].

Neurotransmitter systems during brain development

The nervous system is responsible for the perception of information from the environment and the internal environment, the analysis of this information, and the initiation of the response (including motor) of the body to the incoming signal [17]. Neurons can generate and conduct electrical signals that are transmitted to the innervated cell in the area of specialized intercellular contacts (synapses). The vast majority of these contacts are the so-called chemical synapses, in which an electrical signal leads to the release of a chemical messenger (neurotransmitter) from the end of the neuron, which, diffusing through the synaptic cleft, interacts with specific receptor proteins on the postsynaptic membrane of the innervated cell [11]. Depending on the nature of the receptor, an electrical signal is generated on the postsynaptic membrane, and/or a signaling cascade of reactions is triggered, leading to a change in metabolism in the innervated cell [21]. Thus, interneuronal communication in the nervous system is based on the alternation of electrical and chemical processes that provide synaptic transmission of information. An action potential is generated in a neuron and sent along the axon, which is then transmitted to the synapse through the release of neurotransmitters, leading to a change in metabolism in the innervated cell and causing a response in another neuron or effector cell (e.g., muscle cells, most exocrine and endocrine cells) [21]. The released neurotransmitters bind to receptors on another neuron. Neurons that release neurotransmitters are called presynaptic; neurons that receive neurotransmitter signals are called postsynaptic. Depending on the type of neurotransmitter and receptor, the signal can either activate or inhibit the receiving cell [21].

The best-known neurotransmitters include the following:

Acetylcholine (ACh) is one of the major neurotransmitters in the brain, playing an important role in cortical activation, attention, learning, and pain perception (Figure 9.2). Cholinergic innervation of the cortex begins to manifest itself from the 20th week of gestation, somewhat later than aminergic. Brainstem neurons fire during wakefulness and are released during REM sleep. Cholinergic receptors – muscarinic and nicotinic – undergo important changes during development. Nicotinic receptors play an important role during the development and formation of brain neuroplasticity mechanisms.

Catecholamines and serotonin

Norepinephrine regulates the development of Cajal-Retzius cells, which are important for neuronal migration. Noradrenergic neurons are mainly located in the locus coeruleus, from which they branch into the cortex and brainstem.

Dopamine also appears early in development and is found at 6–8 weeks of gestation in the human embryo. The bodies of dopaminergic neurons are localized in the substantia nigra and ventral tegmentum and penetrate the basal ganglia, hippocampus, cortex, and many other structures (Figure 9.3). Dopamine plays an important role in motor and cognitive processes [22].

Serotonin is involved in early morphogenesis and affects neuronal proliferation. Neurons are located in the midbrain, hypothalamus, and raphe nuclei that coordinate complex sensory and motor patterns during various behavioral states (Figure 9.3) [23].

GABA (γ-aminobutyric acid) is considered the major inhibitory neurotransmitter in adult mammals. However, at an early age, the opposite happens: since the concentration of intracellular chlorides is high, GABA opens chloride channels and depolarization occurs, i.e., excitation. During maturation, the chloride concentration decreases, resulting in the opposite effect of GABA. GABA-induced depolarization is required for the proper formation of excitatory synapses and the development of dendrites in cortical neurons [21].

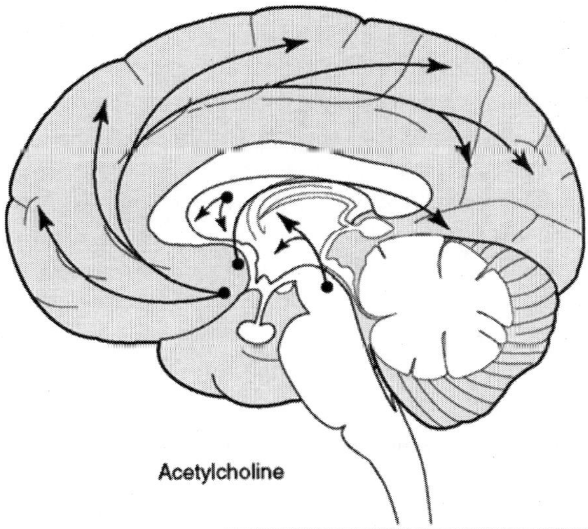

Figure 9.2 Distribution of cholinergic nerves in the brain. Nerves in the brain stem are projected toward the cortex. There are also local circuits in the basal ganglia (H. Lagercrantz, 2016).

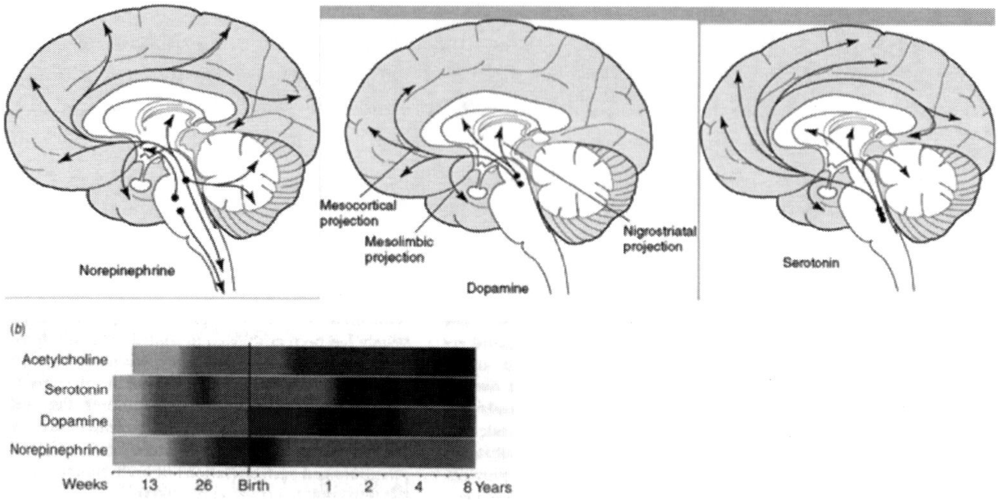

Figure 9.3 Distribution of norepinephrine (noradrenaline), dopamine, and serotonin nerves in the brain. Below neurotransmitter concentrations versus gestational age in the human brain (H. Lagercrantz, 2016).

Exciting amino acids

Glutamate and aspartate are the dominant excitatory amino acids and primary neurotransmitters in approximately half of all mammalian forebrain synapses. The highest level of excitatory amino acids is observed at the age of 1–2 years in the human brain, which is probably due to the high generation of synapses during this period [17].

Congenital opioids

There are various types of innate opioids, some of them are endorphins, predominantly localized in the pituitary gland, and enkephalins and their receptors, localized in the periaqueductal gray matter. Their main role is in pain modulation and perception, but they may also be involved in cardiorespiratory control. The endogenous opioid system matures later than others, and this may explain why the pain threshold is lower in the early stages of child development [24].

Many neuroactive molecules change their functional role in the central nervous system (CNS) during development and make a significant contribution to the process of neuron growth and differentiation in the immature CNS. Catecholamines are known to appear in mammalian embryos before neuronal differentiation [17]. Norepinephrine and acetylcholine are considered classic neurotransmitters and predominate in the peripheral nervous system. They appear at an early stage both in phylogeny and ontogenesis. The rapid release of noradrenaline at birth is believed to play an important role in initiating infant attachment to the mother by increasing the ability to smell [21]. The complex structure of the human brain requires more neurotransmitters with fast and accurate signal transmission, acting directly on ion channels. Therefore, excitatory and inhibitory amino acids predominate in the mature CNS, where monoamines and neuropeptides may act more as neuromodulators [24]. It is known that some of the neurotransmitters described and studied to date can change their function during brain development or depending on the innervated neurons in a particular area of the brain. The effect of the neurotransmitter on the postsynaptic neuron also changes accordingly. It is also known that neurotransmitters can be expressed in large quantities in the early stages of development, as described above, but by the time of full maturation of the brain, only some of them remain in synapses [24].

Modern scientific evidence has refuted the previously known Dale principle, which was based on the fact that one neuron produces and stores one neurotransmitter [21]. Already by the beginning of the 1990s, the analysis of the results of experimental studies led to the formation of a modern theory of co-transmission [20, 25, 26]. In the presented theory, it is proved that one or several types of synaptic active molecules, the so-called co-transmitters (co-mediators), are released from one neuron. Co-transmitters have their effects on target cells and can also regulate presynaptic and postsynaptic modulation [27].

The most studied mediators capable of playing a certain signaling role in the functioning of cholinergic neurotransmission are purines, glutamic acid (glutamate), N-acetyl-aspartyl-glutamate, substance P, calcitonin gene-related peptide, nitric oxide (NO), and neurotrophins [26].

In summary, the description of the neuroanatomical and physiological features of the development of the brain in children will allow a deeper understanding of the specifics of CNS damage in sepsis.

Correct and timely diagnosis of SAE

When confirming the diagnosis of septic encephalopathy, the brain must be intact from the current infectious process in a child with sepsis [28]. Currently, some methods, both laboratory and instrumental, are used in the pediatric ICU, including neuroimaging, as well as clinical assessment of the severity of the condition using scales aimed at diagnosing and confirming septic encephalopathy, determining the tactics of patient treatment and further prognosis (Figure 9.4). However, as in adults, some methods may be difficult in pediatric patients due to the necessary sedation and/or mechanical ventilation, which can waste time for diagnosis and initiation of certain therapy [29]. It would be appropriate to consider some diagnostic methods, taking into account pediatric features.

Neurological examination

The acquaintance of the doctor with the patient begins with his examination. A patient with verified sepsis should be examined daily by a neurologist from the first day. A pediatric patient is subject to extremely close observation by a specialist due to differences in cellular metabolism, hemodynamic and respiratory profile parameters, as well as age-related characteristics of the nervous system as a whole [30]. An important task of the clinical examination of the patient is the early recognition of neurological disorders (focal or cerebral symptoms) and the topical diagnosis of the localization of disorders against the background of the course of sepsis associated with the development of complications, in particular, signs of septic encephalopathy. This largely determines the success of further therapy and improves the prognosis for life [30, 31].

Neurological examination of newborns and young children has several features that are unique to this age period. Some symptoms that are regarded as unconditionally pathological in older children and adults are normal in newborns and infants and reflect the degree of maturity of certain structures of the nervous system and the stages of functional morphogenesis [32].

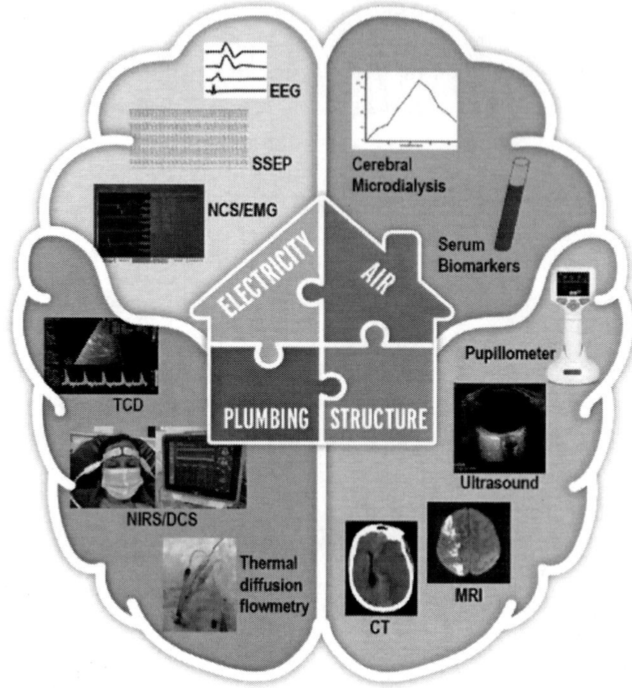

Figure 9.4 Pictorial representation of major physiologic compartments of the cranium analogous to components of a house that inform neuromonitoring. The electrical grid is represented by electroencephalography (EEG), somatosensory evoked potentials (SSEPs), nerve conduction studies (NCS), and electromyography (EMG). Plumbing pressures/perfusion is represented by cerebral blood flow assessed by transcranial Doppler (TCD), near-infrared spectroscopy (NIRS), thermal diffusion flowmetry, and jugular venous oxygen saturation (not shown). The structure is represented by automated pupillometry, optic nerve sheath ultrasound, and other neuroimaging modalities. Air/composition is signaled by serum biomarkers and cerebral microdialysis. DCS = diffuse correlation spectroscopy (Naresh Mullaguri, 2020).

In addition to topical diagnostics during a neurological examination of newborns and infants, it is important to take into account some features of the examination conditions that help to exclude possible negative emotional reactions, some exaltation of unconditioned reflexes, a clear increase in extrapyramidal manifestations: physiological muscle spasticity and tremor, for example, an examination is best done after 1–2 h after feeding, when the child is calm, in a sufficiently lit room, at an air temperature of 25–27 °C, placing the child on the changing table. In a neurological examination of premature babies, it is necessary to take into account their real age, based on the gestational age, since for these children the timing of the extinction of congenital reflexes, and psychomotor development is assessed in terms of the true age.

The examination itself includes the main points, in many respects similar to other age groups: visual observation, position, size, shape, and palpation of the head with the determination of the size of the fontanelles in children of the first year of life, trunk, limbs, the volume of spontaneous movements with an assessment of deep reflexes, the posture of the child, muscle tone, equivalence on both sides, and so on, the presence or extinction of physiological reflexes is taken into account. When assessing the consciousness of a small child, it is worth focusing on specially designed scales for infants and young children. In newborns and young children, disorders of consciousness occur more often in the form of oppression and much less often as stupefaction [9]. Stupefaction of consciousness with pronounced psychomotor agitation is observed in the most acute period in children with neuro infections, subarachnoid hemorrhages, the development of delirium, and other pathologies. However, more often they have an alternation of periods of clouding of consciousness with psychomotor agitation and its oppression. In infants, as well as in adults, the following degrees of depression of consciousness are distinguished: stunning, stupor, and coma [32].

Early neurological clinical manifestations of sepsis-associated encephalopathy in children, according to the data presented in the literature, were excitation, depression of consciousness, alternation of excitation and depression of consciousness, muscle hypotension or hypertonicity, inhibition of reflexes or hyperreflexia, the tension of the fontanel in children of the first year of life, coma, and focal or generalized convulsions [33].

It is worth focusing on one of the early clinical and neurological manifestations of septic encephalopathy – the development of agitation in children. The fact is that manifestations of agitation, or rather, the development of delirium (emergence delirium), have similar features to cognitive dysfunction: diffuse damage, accompanied by short-term disorientation or a decrease in intelligence and memory, often requiring special diagnostic methods, in other words, cognitive impairment, and have common development mechanisms [34]. If the clinician is in doubt during the assessment of a child between cognitive dysfunction, agitation, and delirium, the validated Pediatric Anesthesia Emergence Delirium (PAED) score should be used. However, such a high level of sensitivity is achieved only with the active manifestation of the clinical picture, that is, with a hyperactive form of delirium [35].

Examination of a child with sepsis in the intensive care unit should be carried out at least once a day. In children with severe neurological manifestations, an examination is carried out before and after the results of additional laboratory or instrumental studies [30, 36].

Neuroimaging methods of diagnosis of SAE

Magnetic resonance imaging

Currently, MRI is a widely used and practically universally available neuroimaging method. When visually assessing the degree of damage to the brain and its structural divisions involved in the pathological process of septic encephalopathy, the most interesting MRI modes are used: DWI (Diffusion-weighted imaging) is a modern MRI technology that makes it possible to visualize pathological changes already after five minutes after the onset of symptoms of a stroke; measured diffusion coefficient (ADC) (apparent diffusion coefficient (ADC) is a quantitative characteristic of diffusion (movement of water molecules) in tissue and is calculated from diffusion-weighted images. Fluid attenuation inversion recovery (FLAIR) mode is a sequence of inversion-recovery with a long time interval, which is used to eliminate the influence of fluid in the resulting image. Common pathognomonic patterns of damage in encephalopathy in these imaging modes are a hyperintense signal in the area of the hippocampus and the cerebral cortex [37], and some studies report diffuse foci of edema brain matter involving the basal ganglia and thalamus [37]. Also, in one of the large studies of sepsis-induced encephalopathy in the pediatric ICU, other brain lesions were identified: foci of ischemia or hemorrhage, thrombosis, PRES syndrome, or posterior reversible encephalopathy syndrome [3].

There are many mechanisms of brain damage in sepsis, both direct and indirect. Brain MRI images of patients with sepsis can in most cases be explained in terms of the pathophysiology of sepsis. Thus, cytokine-mediated cellular dysfunction has been most clearly studied, which leads to impaired permeability of the blood-brain barrier, impaired microcirculation, and imbalance of the biochemical profile, which is accompanied by edema of the brain substance and neuroinflammation [38, 39]. Dysfunction of the endothelium of the extracranial system against the background of endotoxemia can lead to disruption of the systemic coagulation link and the occurrence of foci of ischemia or hemorrhages in the brain [5, 40]. Equally important are indicators of systemic hemodynamics because when blood pressure changes, usually with sepsis, hypotension occurs more often, and cerebral blood flow and autoregulation are disturbed, which negatively affects the developing brain.

Despite the undoubted clinical and diagnostic value of this method of neuroimaging, MRI examination of the brain has some disadvantages. This is primarily due to the transportation of the patient to the MRI room. At times, not all critically ill pediatric patients with sepsis may meet the eligibility criteria for transport. Often, young children require additional sedation at the time of transport, as for them, it would seem that such a normal process can cause serious stress. Also, the performance of the study itself in children of the younger group requires anesthesia to fulfill the conditions of complete immobility [41]. In such a situation, the MRI room should be equipped with special MRI-compatible equipment for both intravenous sedation and inhalation anesthesia [42].

Currently, much attention is paid to the study of outcomes in children with sepsis and sepsis-associated encephalopathy. Some authors have identified neurological deficits in children after discharge from the ICU in the form of cognitive impairments and impaired communication skills, children were more irritable, and attention deficit disorder presents in almost all cases. It is noteworthy that all children in this study had encephalopathy-specific MRI findings for encephalopathy during their stay in the ICU [3, 43]. It should be taken into account that the degree of manifestation of neurological deficit after suffering sepsis and encephalopathy can be severe, leading to early death or the formation of persistent disability [42].

Computed Tomography

Among the existing methods for diagnosing septic encephalopathy in children, it is worth noting such a routine method as computed tomography of the brain. However, the method of computed tomography of the brain routinely used in clinical practice cannot fully reflect the degree of cerebral damage in septic encephalopathy, especially when the first clinical symptoms appear [37]. With the help of CT, it is possible to assess already severe, not always reversible, brain damage – vasogenic edema, dislocation of midline structures, massive areas of ischemia or hemorrhage, etc. [44].

In most cases, CT can be classified as an urgent neuroimaging method and a method for controlling the position of invasive neuromonitoring devices. The optimal condition in pediatric emergency care would be to have a mobile CT scanner, but at present such a high-tech resource is not available in every hospital [43].

Positron emission tomography

Early diagnosis of septic encephalopathy in patients with sepsis undoubtedly determines all aspects of medical care, including improved prognosis and quality of life in the future. Among the methods of neuroimaging, the method of positron emission tomography is gaining more and more popularity, which is of particular value for the diagnosis of early sepsis-associated encephalopathy [45]. The principle of the method is based on a change in the rate of metabolism of radiopharmaceuticals introduced into the body in the place where the most pronounced violations of cellular autoregulation occur. However, along with the high sensitivity of the method, it can be quite difficult to establish the most accurate localization of the lesion, this is especially true for the study of the brain [46]. So, in a recently published experimental animal study on the diagnosis of early sepsis-associated encephalopathy, a combination of two research methods was performed: PET with 18F-fluorodeoxyglucose and a comparison of the data obtained on changes in the metabolic rate of labeled atoms in the hippocampus, cerebellum with functional MRI. The data obtained allowed the authors to identify early disorders at the cellular level in the brain in experimental septic animal models when clinical signs have not yet appeared [46].

Both in the case of brain MRI and PET CT, there are certain requirements for pediatric patients, and in most cases, this is a decision on the necessary sedation for transportation and during the examination itself.

Non-invasive methods of diagnosis of SAE

Transcranial Dopplerography

The method of Transcranial Dopplerography (TCD) can certainly be attributed to the most mobile method of screening and dynamic monitoring in detecting insufficient blood supply to the brain, which allows you to assess the state, speed, and volume of cerebral blood flow in the most significant cerebral arteries [47]. As a rule, in the modern approach to the treatment of critically ill patients, the TCD method closely correlates with an MRI study, which reflects a comprehensive assessment of cerebral damage [48].

It is known that relative or absolute cerebral circulatory failure is a powerful damaging factor for the substance of the brain. For example, the significance of the detrimental effect of ischemia is determined by the degree and duration of a decrease in cerebral blood flow to a critical threshold, as well as the degree of functional activity during perfusion insufficiency [28, 49]. Perfusion deficiency also entails the reverse mechanism of the damaging effect – reperfusion injury in the case of revascularization of the vascular bed (thrombolysis, thrombectomy, spontaneous recanalization, etc.) [28].

With all the variety of pathogenetic variants of damage to the vascular bed of the brain, there are several diagnostically important parameters of the Doppler signal, the changes which are universal and reproducible – the direction of blood flow concerning the source of ultrasound radiation, the type of spectrum, and the value of the maximum systolic and minimum diastolic velocity. The most commonly used calculated indicators are determined by the pulsation index (PI), the circulatory resistance index (RI), and the asymmetry coefficient (KA) [28].

When analyzing the quantitative data of TCD among the pediatric group, it is important to take into account their difference from adults. The age of the child is of decisive importance, since, depending on age, changes in the morphological structure of the vascular wall occur, which ensures the active growth and development of the brain tissue of the child. During the first three years, the middle muscular layer of the arteries develops more intensively, and the vessel wall is mainly represented by a well-developed elastic membrane and developed muscle fibers [8]. With a simultaneous increase in the density of the vascular wall, there is an increase in the rate of cerebral blood flow, and, accordingly, cerebral metabolism [8]. By the end of the younger age, approximately by the age of 6 years, the number of nerve fibers in the walls of the intracranial vessels reaches a maximum (their highest concentration is in the MCA). Further, after 5–6 years, the diameter of the vessels does not change significantly, but the morphological differentiation of the arteries occurs before puberty [8]. In the pubertal period, the number of elastic fibers in the walls of the vessel increases, the lumen of the arteries increases, and their wall becomes thinner, along with this, the innervation of the vascular wall also develops intensively. Thus, when analyzing the quantitative indicators of blood flow in the cerebral arteries, it can be seen that the linear speed indicators decrease with age, but they remain slightly higher than in young people (20–39 years old). The value of RI and PI gradually increases with age, while the most significant is the change in the pulsation index (PI) [50].

The current accumulated literature data demonstrate an increase in the RI and PI indices in pediatric patients with sepsis and septic shock compared with healthy controls, and it is noteworthy that these data correlate with MRI data of the brain, where cerebral lesions are present, indicating the development of septic encephalopathy [51, 52]. Other data confirm the presence of a relationship between dynamic TCD results in critically ill patients with negative dynamics on the FOUR scale [52]. Therefore, high PI and RI scores increase the association with mortality [53]. When studying and comparing MRI data of the brain and TCD in children after sepsis and complications in the form of septic encephalopathy, a general decrease in cerebral blood flow and an increase in PI and RI due to previous ischemia or hemorrhage were revealed [37, 54].

For a more reliable analysis of TCD during the study, the specialist must take into account, in addition to the patient's age, the severity of the condition, hemodynamic profile parameters, blood pressure stability, and partial tension of carbon dioxide in the blood, since a number of these factors have a significant impact on cerebral blood flow.

Cerebral oximetry

Among the dynamic non-invasive monitoring at the patient's bedside, it is worth noting the method of cerebral oximetry. The method is based on the principle of optical spectroscopy using infrared light with a range from 650 to 1100 nm [55]. The light beam of this range easily passes through the scalp, the bones of the cranial vault, and the medulla. Para-infrared radiation is absorbed by blood hemoglobin and its reduced fraction. It is known that in the cortical regions of the brain, up to 70–85% of the volume of the vascular bed of the brain falls on venous vessels, 10–15% on arteries, and about 5–10% on capillaries; therefore, the method of cerebral oximetry allows assessing the oxidative status (saturation of hemoglobin with oxygen), mainly in the blood of cerebral venous vessels [55]. In healthy volunteers without intracranial pathology, normal values of cerebral oxygenation – saturation of hemoglobin with oxygen (rSO_2) – are in the range of 60–80%.

A decrease in volumetric blood flow in the tissue (ischemia) or a reduced oxygen content in the inflowing arterial blood (hypoxia) forms tissue oxygen deficiency [30]. It is known that one of the first compensatory mechanisms aimed at eliminating tissue oxygen deficiency is an increase in its extraction from the flowing blood [56]. The result of increased tissue oxygen extraction is a certain decrease in the content of oxyhemoglobin in the outflowing venous blood. At the same time, para-infrared spectroscopy (NIRS) reflects local oxygen saturation (rSO_2) as a dynamic balance between the delivery and consumption of oxygen by the brain tissue. The method of cerebral oximetry makes it possible to quantify this process. The measuring sensor of the cerebral oximeter is placed on the skin of the forehead at the border of the scalp. After connecting the sensor to the device, the rSO_2 indicator from the left and right hemispheres is constantly displayed on the screen. The main advantage of cerebral oximetry over other methods of assessing cerebral oxygenation is undoubtedly its non-invasiveness and safety, which is certainly very important in pediatrics, as well as the fact that the measurement of brain oxygenation occurs in real time.

In the aggregate of the numerous studies available, it is possible to determine the indicators of cerebral oxygenation in children at different ages in normal values: in children under 1 year, they are 62–64%, from 1 year to 3 years old – 70%, from 3 to 10 years old – 69.4– 69.4%, in children older than 10 years – 73.8%. It is believed that the indicators of cerebral oxygenation taken from the right and left hemispheres do not differ from each other and do not depend on the sex of the child. In children from 0 to 3 years old, there is an increase in brain oxygenation from 62.5 to 70%, and in children over 10 years old, these indicators stabilize and amount to 73.8% [55, 56].

In the study of cerebral oximetry parameters in critically ill children with sepsis and septic encephalopathy, a regular relationship with the central venous saturation index (ScvO2) was revealed. One study reported a strong relationship between high ScvO2 and low rSO2 values in deceased patients compared to those in surviving children [57]. Similar changes in ScvO2 and rSO2 correlated with changes in the EEG, as well as with the results of examining the severity of the condition using diagnostic scales. Thus, dynamic monitoring of brain tissue oxygenation fully reflects the degree of impairment of cerebral autoregulation, cerebral blood flow, brain metabolism, and the adequacy of intensive care and allows not directly determining the prognosis in children with septic encephalopathy [31].

Electroencephalography (EEG)

Perhaps there is no more perfect method for assessing the bioelectrical activity of the brain in normal and pathological conditions than an electroencephalogram. A method that reflects the functional state of the brain, since not a single action of our body, not a single thought occurs without the generation of an electrical impulse in a neuron. EEG is the most widely used method of objectifying spontaneous electrical activity of the brain in critically ill patients in anesthesiology and intensive care units of various profiles; it reflects the biological process, which is caused by the activity of many electrical generators – neurons [33, 58]. The field created by these generators is not uniform in the space of the brain and is changeable at every moment. Therefore, between two points located within the brain, there are variable potential differences that can be registered. Registration of biological potentials arising in the brain is the main task of EEG [59]. To divert potentials from these selected points, electroencephalographic electrodes are used. It is worth remembering that when conducting a study on children on the developing brain, wave activity, and interpretation of EEG results differ from those in adult patients [59]. It is known that in the first year of a child's life, there is an active maturation of new neurons, thus they are in excess [8]. In this regard, in children in the first year of life, increased high-amplitude waves can be recorded, which alternate with low-amplitude ones, as well as different in frequency and morphology (Figure 9.4). So, for example, some authors show strong functional connections according to EEG data in the frontal and parietal-occipital regions in newborns with a predominance of theta and alpha rhythms [60] with a gradual differentiation from more mature structures to the least mature as the child grows and develops.

When it is necessary to verify septic encephalopathy using an electroencephalogram, it is worth paying attention to the following data when deciphering it: a slowdown in alpha activity and an increase in theta activity in children may indicate cortical dysfunction, often observed in encephalopathy [4], slow delta activity may indicate damage to deeper brain structures [4], and the presence of burst-suppression cycles raises serious concerns about the severity and prognosis in septic encephalopathy [28]. Some drugs used for sedation and relaxation in the ICU in critically ill patients may interfere with reliable EEG analysis. These drugs include a group of muscle relaxants, benzodiazepines. In this case, to perform an EEG, it is necessary to stop the administration of these drugs and wait for a period of complete elimination. This procedure is difficult in young children, especially those who require mechanical ventilation.

Invasive methods of diagnosis of SAE

Dynamic monitoring of intracranial pressure

Monitoring of intracranial pressure (ICP) is commonly used as an assessment and to maintain adequate cerebral perfusion pressure (CPP), calculated as the difference between mean arterial pressure (MAP) and ICP [30]. This method is very informative in extremely severe patients with impaired consciousness, in a coma, or patients in deep sedation and relaxation, when the possibilities of transportation for a more detailed diagnosis of cerebral damage are limited [61].

Normal ICP in children of the older group and adults does not exceed 15 mm Hg, in young children – does not exceed 7 mm Hg, in newborns – 6 mm Hg. With dynamic monitoring of ICP, it is important to qualitatively assess the waveform that is displayed on the monitor screen for measuring ICP in real time. Types of waves have their names and origins.

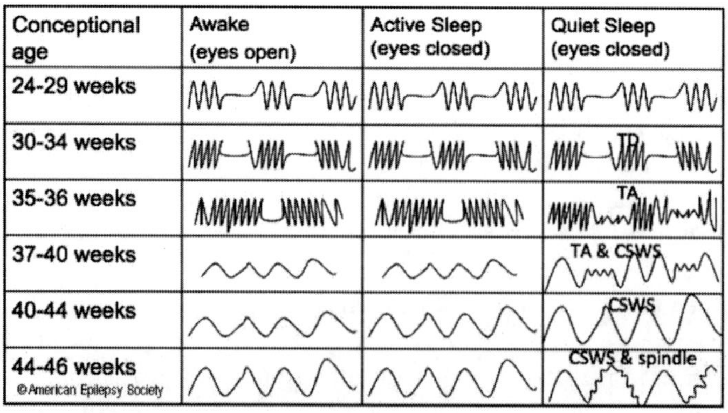

Figure 9.5 Normal EEG of the neonatal period in the state of sleep and wakefulness (Britton J. W., 2016).

The normal forms of the curves include ICP pulse waves, the frequency of which corresponds to the pulse rate, ICP respiratory waves, the frequency of which corresponds to the respiratory rate, and vasogenic waves of intracranial pressure – a physiological phenomenon whose nature is poorly understood. They are smooth rises in intracranial pressure by 10–20 mm Hg, from the basal level, followed by a smooth return to the original numbers. The pathological types of the curve include the presence of B-waves – conditionally pathological slow waves of intracranial pressure with an amplitude of 1–5 mm Hg, a period of 20 seconds to 3 minutes, their frequency is increased in hydrocephalus, however, the specificity of B-waves for the diagnosis of hydrocephalus is low; plateau waves are pathological waves of intracranial pressure, represent sudden fast long-term, for several tens of minutes, increases in intracranial pressure up to 50–100 mm Hg followed by a rapid return to baseline. Unlike vasogenic waves, at the height of plateau waves, there is no direct relationship between intracranial pressure and the amplitude of its pulse fluctuations, and sometimes even reverses, cerebral perfusion pressure decreases, and autoregulation of cerebral blood flow is disturbed. Plateau waves indicate an extreme depletion of mechanisms for compensating for increased intracranial pressure, as a rule, they are observed only with intracranial hypertension [61].

Much literature data indicate a correlation between intracranial hypertension with adverse neurological outcomes or high mortality [62]. Probably, this correlation may come from the fact that often high ICP is a delayed marker of parenchymal damage.

Along with the informativeness and dynamism of the method, it is worth remembering the complications associated with the invasiveness of the technique, as a rule; this is the addition of an infection, liquorrhea, migration of the ICP sensor, and others.

Currently, together with ICP, monitoring of cerebral autoregulation is also carried out. The parameter is calculated based on the indicators of ICP and blood pressure; however, its information content is very valuable. In children, cerebral autoregulation of cerebral blood flow is maintained by a change in vascular resistance in response to an increase or decrease in mean arterial pressure. Therefore, when conducting a test with a deliberate change in blood pressure or intentional hyperventilation to assess cerebral autoregulation, a change in cerebral blood flow can be assumed [63]. Impairment of cerebral autoregulation makes the damaged brain unable to maintain a constant cerebral blood flow in response to changes in systemic hemodynamics.

Other methods for diagnosis of septic encephalopathy

Automatic pupillometry

Pupil size and impaired pupillary response to light with size changes have a direct neurophysiological relationship with changes in intracranial volume [64].

Somatosensory evoked potentials (SSEPs) are CNS responses elicited by stimulation of peripheral nerves, usually the median, ulnar, or posterior tibial nerves, to detect a focal lesion, the relationship of the cortex, and subcortical structures [65].

Biomarkers

Determination of biological markers in blood serum is routinely used in every patient in the intensive care unit. To determine the degree of damage to the medulla, the three most studied markers are most often determined: NSE, S100B, and GFAP [36].

Neuron-specific enolase (NSE)

NSE is an intracellular enzyme of mature neurons in the brain and peripheral nervous system. The level of NSE increases in the blood and cerebrospinal fluid when neurons are damaged, as is observed in neurodegenerative diseases (Alzheimer's disease, dementia, etc.), hypoxia, and brain injuries [66]. It also has a high prognostic value, since its elevated level indicates the ongoing process of neuronal destruction and a high probability of an unfavorable neurological outcome. In this case, the rate of increase in the concentration of the marker in the blood is of great importance [66]. There are also studies in children proving the relationship between NSE and glial fibrillar acidic protein with the development of septic encephalopathy [67].

In a relatively recent study, the authors demonstrated clinical and prognostic significance for the development of encephalopathy at high values of cord blood NSE levels in newborns with sepsis [68].

Glial fibrillar acidic protein (GFAP)

It is an intermediate filament protein and is part of the glial cells – astrocytes. It performs a supporting function, being part of the cytoskeleton of cells; in addition, it takes part in cell movement and communication, as well as in the functioning of the blood-brain barrier. It is a highly specific protein and is found only in the brain. GFAP stimulates white matter vascularization through the induction effect of astrocytes on endothelial cells. Myelin synthesis also depends on the acidic protein content [69]. In addition, with the help of GFAP, the processes of mitosis of astrocytes proceed, which is of exceptional importance in brain damage of any origin. Elevated concentrations of GFAP in the blood and cerebrospinal fluid indicate a violation of the integrity of the astrocyte membranes and suggest BBB dysfunction and subsequent neuronal death [69]. Modern studies have demonstrated the high significance of GFAP elevation and deterioration for prognosis in patients with septic encephalopathy [70].

Protein S100-ß

It is a neurospecific marker and increases with damage to the neurovascular unit of various etiologies (hypoxic, ischemic, traumatic, neurotoxic). Although it is impossible to determine the etiology of damage to the nervous tissue by its indicators, it has a high diagnostic significance due to several distinctive features: it is easily detected in the blood serum, while its minimum amount is required, in addition, it is also found in the cerebrospinal fluid (which is even more reliable). It should also be noted that the S100-ß protein has a high prognostic value, increasing even with minimal brain damage, long before clinical or instrumental signs of cerebral damage, and correlates with the extent of damage [70].

Clinical case

Patient K. (female), 12-year-old, was admitted to the ICU with electrical trauma and cata-trauma as a result of a fall on an electric train, multiple bruises of soft tissues, a fracture of the right femur with displacement, facial burns, and a fracture of the bones of the cranial vault without displacement of fragments. In the ICU, after the surgical intervention of osteosynthesis of the femur with repositioning of fragments, neurovegetative stabilization, and artificial lung ventilation was performed.

On the second day of stay in the ICU, an MRI study of the brain was performed, where no signs of focal lesions of the GM were found.

On the fifth day, a clinical picture of sepsis developed, confirmed by laboratory data (the levels of CRP and PCT biomarkers in the blood serum were high), and the source of infection was identified. Antibacterial therapy was started taking into account the sensitivity of microorganisms and intensive therapy for sepsis according to the severity of the patient's condition due to multiple organ dysfunction.

On the 13th day from admission (day 9 from diagnosed sepsis), a repeated MRI study of the brain revealed a symmetrical lesion of the basal nuclei of both hemispheres of the brain, signs of emerging cerebral edema (Figure 9.6a, b, c, d, e).

When EEG was recorded on the ninth day from the development of sepsis in a patient who was under conditions of neurovegetative stabilization, convincing data were obtained on persistent epileptic status with recorded fast-wave dysrhythmia of background activity and ictal/interictal epileptiform activity, represented by spike/polyspike discharges (Figure 9.7a, b). Also, bursts of the "high-frequency" beta rhythm were periodically recorded laterally in the left hemisphere (Figure 9.7c, d). Anticonvulsants were connected to therapy.

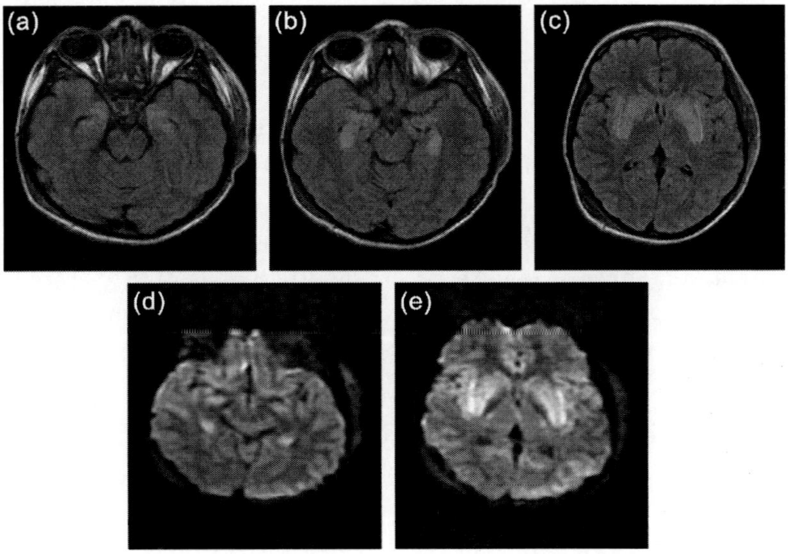

Figure 9.6 Sepsis-associated encephalopathy. MRI of the brain of patient K., 12-year-old, on the ninth day after sepsis starting in the ICU, axial projection, FLAIR IP (a–c), DWI (d, e). Diffuse changes in the increased intensity of the MR signal are revealed in the subcortical nuclei, heads, and bodies of the hippocampus (a–c), on diffusion-weighted images (b 1000) the described zones also have an increased intensity of the MR signal (d, e). Bruising of the soft tissues of the temporal region on the left and the occipital region on the right.

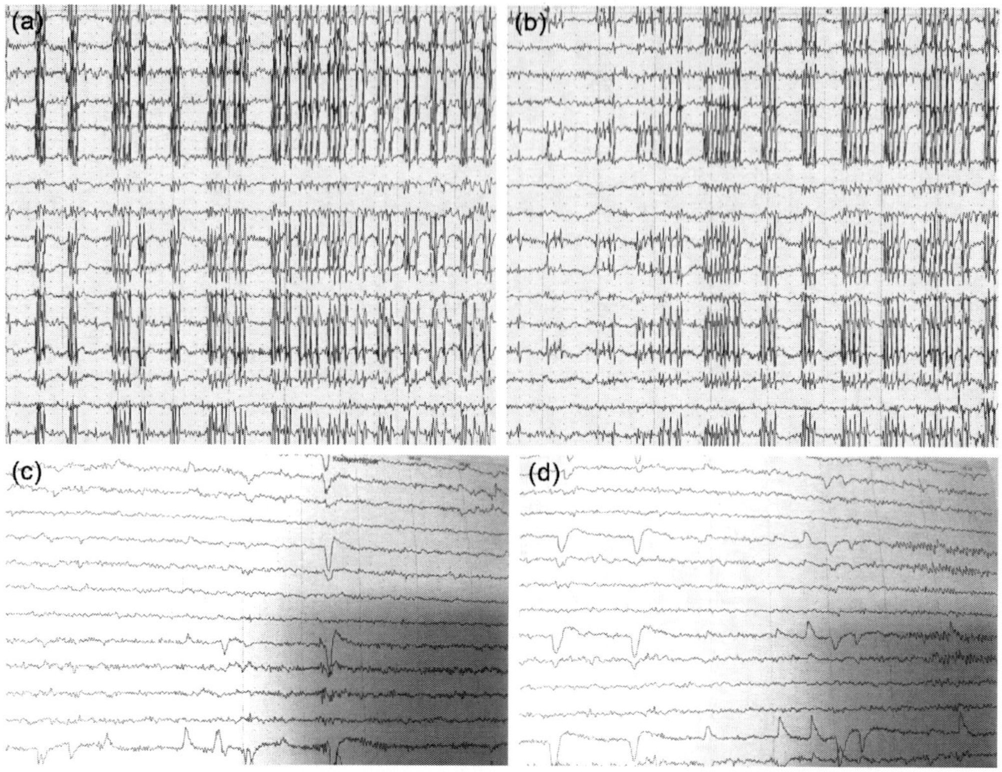

Figure 9.7 EEG patterns of patient K., 12-year-old, on the ninth day of sepsis. The patient is under conditions of neurovegetative stabilization (sodium thiopental 4 mg/kg/h; fentanyl 1.0 mcg/kg/h; clonidine 0.15 mcg/kg/h).

Against the background of complex intensive care for sepsis on the 33rd day, the girl was transferred to the specialized department in a state of moderate severity. According to the EEG data, no epileptic activity was recorded against the background of taking anticonvulsants. Data for cognitive deficits were not noted. After 2.5 years, the patient was called to the clinic for examination. Development corresponds to the age of 15, school performance is good, and there is no cognitive deficit. During the time that has passed since the injury, two children were born in the family; the girl is actively involved in caring for her brother and sister. Control MRI examination of the brain did not reveal any changes (Figure 9.8a, b, c, d, e).

EEG control showed no epileptiform activity, and anticonvulsant therapy was discontinued.

Conclusion

In summary, sepsis-associated encephalopathy in pediatric practice, as well as in adults, is an early sign of a systemic infection when the source of infection is verified outside the central nervous system, and cognitive impairments from agitation to impaired consciousness in

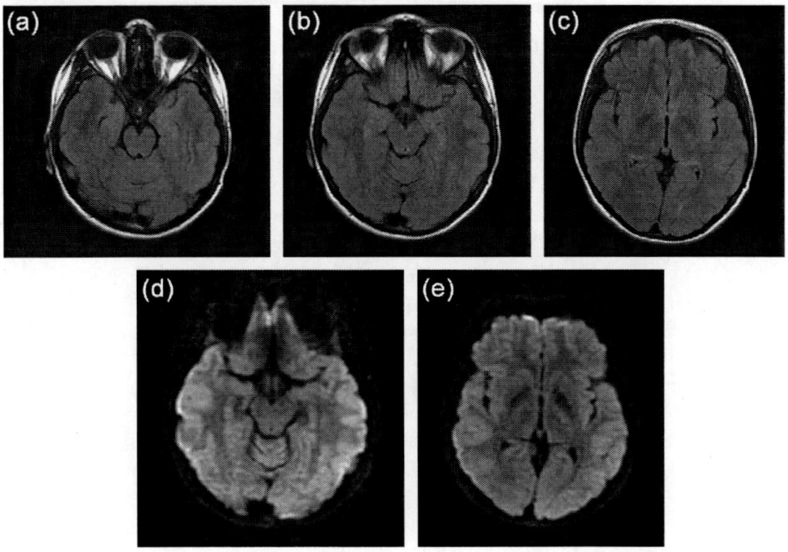

Figure 9.8 Brain MRI, axial view, FLAIR IP (a–c), DWI (d, e). A complete regression of previously identified changes in SAE is revealed.

the form of delirium and coma play a leading role in the structure early multiple organ dysfunction in sepsis. Taking into account the peculiarities of the development and maturation of the nervous system described in this chapter, the nervous system of young children is probably most susceptible to structural and functional changes in the long-term program due to impaired synaptogenesis and myelination of nerve tracts, activation of neuronal apoptosis, etc. Neuroplasticity of the child's brain and its compensatory opportunities allow us to observe in clinical practice successful long-term results in the form of complete recovery after sepsis and SAE, as in the clinical example given in this chapter.

Conflict of interest: The authors declare that there is no conflict of interest.
Acknowledgments: The authors of the chapter express their gratitude to the colleagues of the Children's Regional Hospital of St. Petersburg for providing data and illustrative material for the clinical case, as well as to Elena G. Potemkina, Radiologist, Doctor of Medical Sciences, for preparing these data for publication.

References

1. Pandharipande PP, Girard TD, Jackson JC, et al. Long-term cognitive impairment after critical illness. *New England Journal of Medicine*. 2013;369(14):1306–1316. DOI: 10.1056/nejmoa1301372.
2. Catarina AV, Branchini G, Bettoni L, De Oliveira JR, Nunes FB. Sepsis-associated encephalopathy: From pathophysiology to progress in experimental studies. *Molecular Neurobiology*. 2021;58(6):2770–2779. DOI: 10.1007/s12035-021-02303-2.
3. Becker AE, Teixeira SR, Lunig NA, et al. Sepsis-related brain MRI abnormalities are associated with mortality and poor neurological outcome in pediatric sepsis. *Pediatric Neurology*. 2022;128:1–8. DOI: 10.1016/j.pediatrneurol.2021.12.001.

4. Nwafor DC, Brichacek AL, Mohammad AS, et al. Targeting the blood-brain barrier to prevent sepsis-associated cognitive impairment. *Journal of Central Nervous System Disease*. 2019;11:1179573519840652. Published 2019 Apr 9. DOI: 10.1177/1179573519840652.
5. Orhun G, Esen F, Özcan PE, et al. Neuroimaging findings in sepsis-induced brain dysfunction: Association with clinical and laboratory findings. *Neurocritical Care*. 2019;30(1):106–117. DOI: 10.1007/s12028-018-0581-1.
6. Yang Y, Liang S, Geng J, et al. Development of a nomogram to predict 30-day mortality of patients with sepsis-associated encephalopathy: A retrospective cohort study. *Journal of Intensive Care*. 2020;8:45. Published 2020 Jul 2. DOI: 10.1186/s40560-020-00459-y.
7. Chen J, Shi X, Diao M, et al. A retrospective study of sepsis-associated encephalopathy: Epidemiology, clinical features, and adverse outcomes. *BMC Emergency Medicine*. 2020;20(1):77. Published 2020 Oct 6. DOI: 10.1186/s12873-020-00374-3.
8. Lagercrantz H, Hanson MA, Ment LR, Peebles DM. *The Newborn Brain*. Cambridge: Cambridge University Press; 2010.
9. Wolpert L. *Principles of Development*. 6th ed. Oxford: Oxford University Press; 2019.
10. Wolpert L. *The Triumph of the Embryo*. Mineola, NY: Dover Publications; 2008.
11. Herlenius E, Lagercrantz H. Development of neurotransmitter systems during critical periods. *Experimental Neurology*. 2004;190:8–21. DOI: 10.1016/j.expneurol.2004.03.027.
12. Sanes DH, Thomas A, Reh WA. *Development of the Nervous System*. San Diego: Academic Press; 2000.
13. Mullor JL, Sánchez P, Ruiz I Altaba A. Pathways and consequences: Hedgehog signaling in human disease. *Trends in Cell Biology*. 2002;12(12):562–569. DOI: 10.1016/s0962-8924(02)02405-4.
14. Kostović I, Judas M. The development of the subplate and thalamocortical connections in the human fetal brain. *Acta Paediatrica*. 2010;99(8):1119–1127. DOI: 10.1111/j.1651-2227.2010.01811.x.
15. Diamond A, Briand L, Fossella J, Gehlbach L. Genetic and neurochemical modulation of prefrontal cognitive functions in children. *The American Journal of Psychiatry*. 2004;161(1):125–132. DOI: 10.1176/appi.ajp.161.1.125.
16. Rakic P. Neurogenesis in adult primate neocortex: An evaluation of the evidence. *Nature Reviews: Neuroscience*. 2002;3(1):65–71. DOI: 10.1038/nrn700.
17. Parnavelas J, Stirling V, Stern C. *The Making of the Nervous System*. Harlow: Longman Higher Education; 1993.
18. Bourgeois JP. Synaptogenesis, heterochrony, and epigenesis in the mammalian neocortex. *Acta Paediatrica*. 1997;422:27–33. DOI: 10.1111/j.1651-2227.1997.tb18340.x.
19. Brigadski T, Leßmann V. The physiology of regulated BDNF release. *Cell Tissue Research [Internet]*. 2020;382(1):15–45. DOI: 10.1007/s00441-020-03253-2.
20. Serra R. Matrix metalloproteinases in health and disease. *Biomolecules [Internet]*. 2020;10(8):1138. DOI: 10.3390/biom10081138.
21. Stjarne L. *Chemical Neurotransmission*. San Diego: Academic Press; 1981.
22. Williams GV, Goldman-Rakic PS. Modulation of memory fields by dopamine D1 receptors in the prefrontal cortex. *Nature [Internet]*. 1995;376(6541):572–575. DOI: 10.1038/376572a0.
23. Oh J, Petersen C, Walsh CM, Bittencourt JC, Neylan TC, Grinberg LT. The role of co-neurotransmitters in sleep and wake regulation. *Molecular Psychiatry*. 2019;24(9):1284–1295. DOI: 10.1038/s41380-018-0291-2.
24. Ashwal S, editor. *Child Neurology: Its Origins, Founders, Growth, and Evolution*. 2nd ed. San Diego: Academic Press; 2021.
25. Burnstock G. Cotransmission in the autonomic nervous system. *Handbook of Clinical Neurology*. 2013;117:23–35. DOI: 10.1016/B978-0-444-53491-0.00003-1.
26. Svensson E, Apergis-Schoute J, Burnstock G, Nusbaum MP, Parker D, Schiöth HB. General principles of neuronal co-transmission: Insights from multiple model systems. *Frontiers in Neural Circuits*. 2019;12:117. Published 2019 Jan 21. DOI: 10.3389/fncir.2018.00117
27. Svensson E, Williams MJ, Schiöth HB. Neural cotransmission in spinal circuits governing locomotion. *Trends in Neurosciences*. 2018;41(8):540–550. DOI: 10.1016/j.tins.2018.04.007.

28. Czempik PF, Gąsiorek J, Bąk A, Krzych ŁJ. Ultrasonic assessment of optic nerve sheath diameter in patients at risk of sepsis-associated brain dysfunction: A preliminary report. *International Journal of Environmental Research and Public Health*. 2020;17(10):3656. Published 2020 May 22. DOI: 10.3390/ijerph17103656.
29. Huang L, Peng S, Li R, Xie D, Huang D. Fulminant encephalopathy in a child with hyperferritinemic sepsis: A case report. *BMC Neurology*. 2020;20(1):73. Published 2020 Mar 2. DOI: 10.1186/s12883-020-01661-z.
30. Rajagopalan S, Sarwal A. Neuromonitoring in critically ill patients. *Critical Care Medicine*. 2023;51(4):525–542. DOI: 10.1097/CCM.0000000000005809.
31. Laws JC, Jordan LC, Pagano LM, Wellons JC 3rd, Wolf MS. Multimodal neurologic monitoring in children with acute brain injury. *Pediatric Neurology*. 2022;129:62–71. DOI: 10.1016/j.pediatrneurol.2022.01.006.
32. Postelnicu R, Evans L. Monitoring of the physical exam in sepsis. *Current Opinion in Critical Care*. 2017;23(3):232–236. DOI: 10.1097/MCC.0000000000000403.
33. Chen Y, Hu Y, Li X, et al. Clinical features and factors associated with sepsis-associated encephalopathy in children: Retrospective single-center clinical study. *Frontiers in Neurology*. 2022;13:838746. Published 2022 May 16. DOI: 10.3389/fneur.2022.838746.
34. Chung HY, Wickel J, Brunkhorst FM, Geis C. Sepsis-associated encephalopathy: From delirium to dementia? *Journal of Clinical Medicine*. 2020;9(3):703. DOI: 10.3390/jcm9030703.
35. Alvarez RV, Palmer C, Czaja AS, et al. Delirium is a common and early finding in patients in the pediatric cardiac intensive care unit. *The Journal of Pediatrics*. 2018;195:206–212.
36. Zhu J, Zhang M, Han T, et al. Exploring the biomarkers of sepsis-associated encephalopathy (SAE): Metabolomics evidence from gas chromatography-mass spectrometry. *BioMed Research International*. 2019;2019:2612849. DOI: 10.1155/2019/2612849.
37. Sanz D, D'Arco F, Robles CA, Brierley J. Incidence and pattern of brain lesions in pediatric septic shock patients. *The British Journal of Radiology*. 2018;91(1084):20170861. DOI: 10.1259/bjr.20170861.
38. Ehlenbach WJ, Sonnen JA, Montine TJ, Larson EB. Association between sepsis and microvascular brain injury. *Critical Care Medicine*. 2019;47(11):1531–1538. DOI: 10.1097/CCM.0000000000003924.
39. Barbosa-Silva MC, Lima MN, Battaglini D, et al. Infectious disease-associated encephalopathies. *Critical Care*. 2021;25(1):236. DOI: 10.1186/s13054-021-03659-6.
40. Tauber SC, Djukic M, Gossner J, Eiffert H, Brück W, Nau R. Sepsis-associated encephalopathy and septic encephalitis: An update. *Expert Review of Anti-Infective Therapy*. 2021;19(2):215–231. DOI: 10.1080/14787210.2020.1812384.
41. Johnson KL, Cochran J, Webb S. Lower-dose propofol use for MRI: A retrospective review of a pediatric sedation team's experience. *Pediatric Emergency*. 2021;37(11):700–706. DOI: 10.1097/PEC.0000000000002289.
42. Killian EY, Farris RWD, Watson RS, Dervan LA, Zimmerman JJ. Health-related quality of life among survivors of pediatric sepsis. *Pediatric Critical Care Medicine*. 2019;20(6):501–509. DOI: 10.1097/PCC.0000000000001886.
43. Cho SM, Wilcox C, Keller S, et al. Assessing the safety and feasibility of bedside portable low-field brain magnetic resonance imaging in patients on ECMO (SAFE-MRI ECMO study): Study protocol and first case series experience. *Critical Care*. 2022;26(1):119. DOI: 10.1186/s13054-022-03990-6.
44. Kochanek PM, Tasker RC, Carney N, et al. Guidelines for the management of pediatric severe traumatic brain injury, third edition: Update of the brain trauma foundation guidelines, executive summary. *Neurosurgery*. 2019;84(6):1169–1178. DOI: 10.1093/neuros/nyz051.
45. Feng T, Zhao Y, Shi H, et al. Total-body quantitative parametric imaging of early kinetics of ^{18}F-FDG. *Journal of Nuclear Medicine*. 2021;62(5):738–744. DOI: 10.2967/jnumed.119.238113.
46. Zhu T, Jiang J, Xiao Y, et al. Early diagnosis of murine sepsis-associated encephalopathy using dynamic PET/CT imaging and multiparametric MRI. *Molecular Imaging and Biology*. 2022;24(6):928–939. DOI: 10.1007/s11307-022-01743-z.

47. Algebaly H, ElSherbini S, Galal A, Hamdi R, Baz A, Elbeleidy A. Transcranial doppler can predict development and outcome of sepsis-associated encephalopathy in pediatrics with severe sepsis or septic shock. *Frontiers in Pediatrics.* 2020;8:450. DOI: 10.3389/fped.2020.00450.
48. Blanco P, Blaivas M. Applications of transcranial color-coded sonography in the emergency department. *Journal of Ultrasound in Medicine: Official Journal of the American Institute of Ultrasound in Medicine.* 2017;36(6):1251–1266. DOI: 10.7863/ultra.16.04050.
49. Crippa IA, Subirà C, Vincent JL, et al. Impaired cerebral autoregulation is associated with brain dysfunction in patients with sepsis. *Critical Care: The Official Journal of the Critical Care Forum.* 2018;22(1):327. DOI: 10.1186/s13054-018-2258-8.
50. Bode H. *Pediatric Applications of Transcranial Doppler Sonography.* New York: Springer; 2014.
51. Gorgis N, Asselin JM, Fontana C, Heidersbach RS, Flori HR, Ward SL. Evaluation of the association of early elevated lactate with outcomes in children with severe sepsis or septic shock. *Pediatric Emergency Care.* 2019;35(10):661–665. DOI: 10.1097/PEC.0000000000001021.
52. Choi SJ, Ha EJ, Jhang WK, Park SJ. Elevated central venous pressure is associated with increased mortality in pediatric septic shock patients. *BMC Pediatrics.* 2018;18(1):58. DOI: 10.1186/s12887-018-1059-1.
53. Nyirasafari R, Corden MH, Karambizi AC, et al. Predictors of mortality in a pediatric intensive care unit in Kigali, Rwanda. *Pediatrics and International Child Health.* 2017;37(2):109–115. DOI: 10.1080/20469047.2016.1250031.
54. Sandquist MK, Clee MS, Patel SK, et al. High frequency of neuroimaging abnormalities among pediatric patients with sepsis who undergo neuroimaging. *Pediatric Critical Care Medicine.* 2017;18(7):607–613. DOI: 10.1097/PCC.0000000000001173.
55. Viderman D, Abdildin YG. Near-infrared spectroscopy in neurocritical care: A review of recent updates. *World Neurosurgery.* 2021;151:23–28. DOI: 10.1016/j.wneu.2021.04.054.
56. R M, Bansal A. Multimodal neuromonitoring in pediatric neurocritical care: Current perspectives. *Indian Journal of Pediatrics.* 2023;90(3):261–271. DOI: 10.1007/s12098-022-04415-6.
57. Guo J, Cheng Y, Wang Q, Su J, Cui L, Jin Z. Changes of $rScO_2$ and $ScvO_2$ in children with sepsis-related encephalopathy with different prognoses and clinical features. *Experimental and Therapeutic Medicine.* 2019;17(5):3943–3948. DOI: 10.3892/etm.2019.7451.
58. Hu DK, Goetz PW, To PD, et al. Evolution of cortical functional networks in healthy infants. *Frontiers in Network Physiology.* 2022;2:893826. DOI: 10.3389/fnetp.2022.893826.
59. Boersma M, Smit DJ, de Bie HM, et al. Network analysis of resting state EEG in the developing young brain: Structure comes with maturation. *Human Brain Mapping.* 2011;32(3):413-425. DOI: 10.1002/hbm.21030.
60. Tóth B, Urbán G, Háden GP, et al. Large-scale network organization of EEG functional connectivity in newborn infants. *Human Brain Mapping.* 2017;38(8):4019–4033. DOI: 10.1002/hbm.23645.
61. Kofke WA, Rajagopalan S, Ayubcha D, et al. Defining a taxonomy of intracranial hypertension: Is ICP more than just a number? *Journal of Neurosurgical Anesthesiology.* 2020;32(2):120–131. DOI: 10.1097/ANA.0000000000000609.
62. Rajajee V, Fontana RJ, Courey AJ, Patil PG. Protocol-based invasive intracranial pressure monitoring in acute liver failure: Feasibility, safety, and impact on management. *Critical Care (London, England).* 2017;21(1):178. DOI: 10.1186/s13054-017-1762-6.
63. Silverman A, Petersen NH. Physiology, cerebral autoregulation. In: *StatPearls.* Treasure Island (FL): StatPearls Publishing; March 15, 2023.
64. Bower MM, Sweidan AJ, Xu JC, Stern-Neze S, Yu W, Groysman LI. Quantitative pupillometry in the intensive care unit. *Journal of Intensive Care Medicine.* 2021;36(4):383–391. DOI: 10.1177/0885066619881124.
65. Koenig MA, Kaplan PW. Clinical applications for EPs in the ICU. *Journal of Clinical Neurophysiology: Official Publication of the American Electroencephalographic Society.* 2015;32(6):472–480. DOI: 10.1097/WNP.0000000000000215.
66. Luescher T, Mueller J, Isenschmid C, et al. Neuron-specific enolase (NSE) improves clinical risk scores for prediction of neurological outcome and death in cardiac arrest patients: Results from a prospective trial. *Resuscitation.* 2019;142:50–60. DOI: 10.1016/j.resuscitation.2019.07.003.

67. Zhang LN, Ai YH, Gong H, et al. Expression and role of neuroglobin in rats with sepsis-associated encephalopathy. *Critical Care Medicine*. 2014;42(1):12–21. DOI: 10.1097/CCM.0b013e3182a63b1a.
68. El Shimy MS, El-Raggal NM, El-Farrash RA, et al. Cerebral blood flow and serum neuron-specific enolase in early-onset neonatal sepsis. *Pediatric Research*. 2018;84(2):261–266. DOI: 10.1038/s41390-018-0062-4.
69. Yan S, Gao M, Chen H, Jin X, Yang M. Expression level of glial fibrillary acidic protein and its clinical significance in patients with sepsis-associated encephalopathy. *Zhong Nan Da Xue Xue Bao Yi Xue Ban*. 2019;44(10):1137–1142. DOI: 10.11817/j.issn.1672-7347.2019.190180.
70. Wu L, Feng Q, Ai ML, et al. The dynamic change of serum S100B levels from day 1 to day 3 is more associated with sepsis-associated encephalopathy. *Scientific Reports*. 2020;10(1):7718. DOI: 10.1038/s41598-020-64200-3.

Chapter 10

Therapeutic tactics in sepsis-associated encephalopathy: present and prospects

Irina A. Savvina[1,2,3*], MD., Ph.D., Kristina M. Bykova[1], MD., Victoria I. Gurskaya[1], MD., Ph.D.

[1] Department of Anesthesiology and Intensive Care, Almazov National Medical Research Centre of Ministry of Health Care of Russian Federation, Saint Petersburg, Russian Federation

[2] Department of Pathomorphology of Nervous System, Russian Polenov Scientific Research Neurosurgical Institute – the branch of Almazov National Medical Research Centre of Ministry of Health Care of Russian Federation, Saint Petersburg, Russian Federation

[3] Department of Anesthesiology and Intensive Care named after V.L. Vanevskiy of the North-Western State Medical University named after Ilya I. Mechnikov of the Ministry of Health of Russian Federation, St. Petersburg, Russian Federation

Abstract

Currently, there is no evidence-based treatment for sepsis-associated encephalopathy. Only etiopathogenetic therapy for sepsis remains an effective way to treat both sepsis and its consequences. It is important to remember that there are no small things to treat a severe patient, and only comprehensive personalized therapy with a multidisciplinary approach will help to preserve not only the patient's life but also improve the quality of life.

Keywords: sepsis-associated encephalopathy, eCASH, melatonin, dexmedetomidine, neurovegetative stabilization, selenium

Introduction

Sepsis-associated encephalopathy (SAE) begins as a reversible complication during sepsis but can develop into irreversible long-term cognitive impairment affecting functional ability,

* Corresponding author: Irina A. Savvina, Professor, MD., Ph.D.
e-mail address: irinasavvina@mail.ru

Editor: Irina A. Savvina, Natalia V. Beloborodova and Tatyana N. Trofimova
In: Sepsis-Associated Encephalopathy
ISBN: 979-8-89113-178-1

verbal learning, and memory, resulting in reduced quality of life and ability to return to work after an intensive care unit stay.

Even though the incidence of SAE, according to some sources, reaches 70% in patients with sepsis, there is currently no effective treatment for this condition [1] except for the treatment of the septic process itself. Comprehensive diagnostics help identify organic pathological changes in the brain and further make them functionally reversible.

Despite significant advances in sepsis treatment, SAE is still associated with high mortality and the development of gross cognitive impairment. Detectable changes prove that the course of the septic process causes not only functionally reversible but also organic pathological changes in the brain resulting from impaired functions of the blood-brain barrier, which can serve as an applied point for the development of treatments for SAE.

Basic etiopathogenetic principles of therapy

There are well-known international guidelines for the treatment of sepsis and septic shock (2016) – III International consensus on the definition of sepsis and septic shock (Sepsis-3), which were adopted in 2016 by the Society of Critical Care Medicine and the European Society of Intensive Care Medicine [2]. They include all the main areas of sepsis therapy: antibacterial therapy, sanitation of the source of infection, infusion therapy, vasoactive drugs, corticosteroids, blood components, immunoglobulins, hemosorption, anticoagulants, mechanical ventilation, sedation and analgesia, glucose control, renal replacement therapy, bicarbonate infusion, venous prophylaxis thromboembolism, prevention of steroid ulcers, and nutrition.

Several studies have found different ways to improve day-to-day care in the intensive care unit. Vincent et al. (2016) proposed a model designated by the acronym eCASH – early Comfort using Analgesia, minimal Sedatives, and maximal Humane care, which includes a set of interventions aimed at providing patient comfort with minimal sedation, optimal analgesia, and maximum care for the person [3]. This approach emphasizes optimizing pain relief to avoid deep sedation, which is one of the most important risk factors for delirium, focusing on early mobilization and improving sleep. In addition, this model aims to improve the participation of the patient's family through measures such as the open concept of the intensive care unit and the implementation of an active family and visitor presence in the day-to-day operations of the intensive care unit. These measures underpin a new patient-centered ICU concept that aims to prevent neurological, emotional, and functional impairment by improving day-to-day care (Figure 10.1).

Managing pain with effective analgesia is a top priority when implementing the eCASH concept. For example, the use of paracetamol may reduce the overall opioid burden and associated side effects [4]. Administration of additional analgesics such as lidocaine, alpha-2 agonists, and low-dose ketamine should be considered early if the need for opioids increases. It has been suggested that in the context of invasive mechanical ventilation, both ketamine and alpha-2 agonists provide an opioid-sparing effect with moderate sedation in patients requiring both pain relief and sedation [5, 6].

It is important to emphasize that the group of sepsis patients admitted to intensive care units must be treated in all already known ways to improve long-term outcomes after admission to the intensive care unit (Figure 10.2).

Non-drug methods, including music therapy and relaxation techniques, may be opioid-sparing and enhance analgesia [7]. These options are safe but not reliable ways.

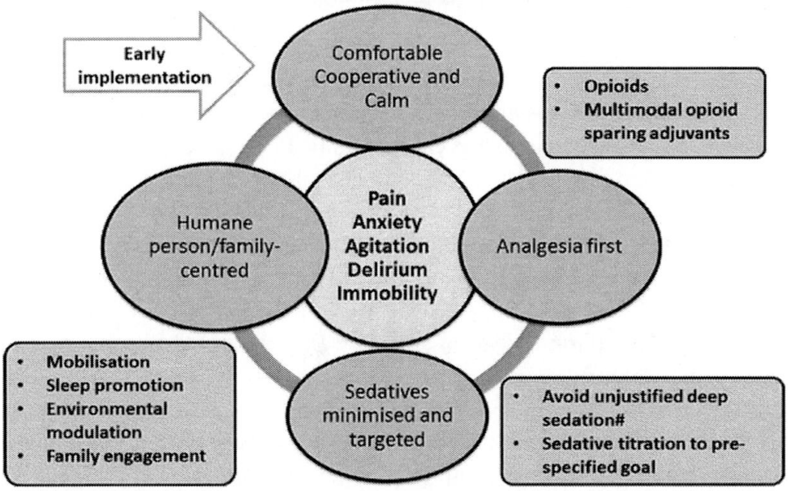

Figure 10.1 eCASH concept: early implementation to treat and prevent pain, anxiety, arousal, delirium, and immobility, and facilitate patient care (Vincent JL et al., 2016).

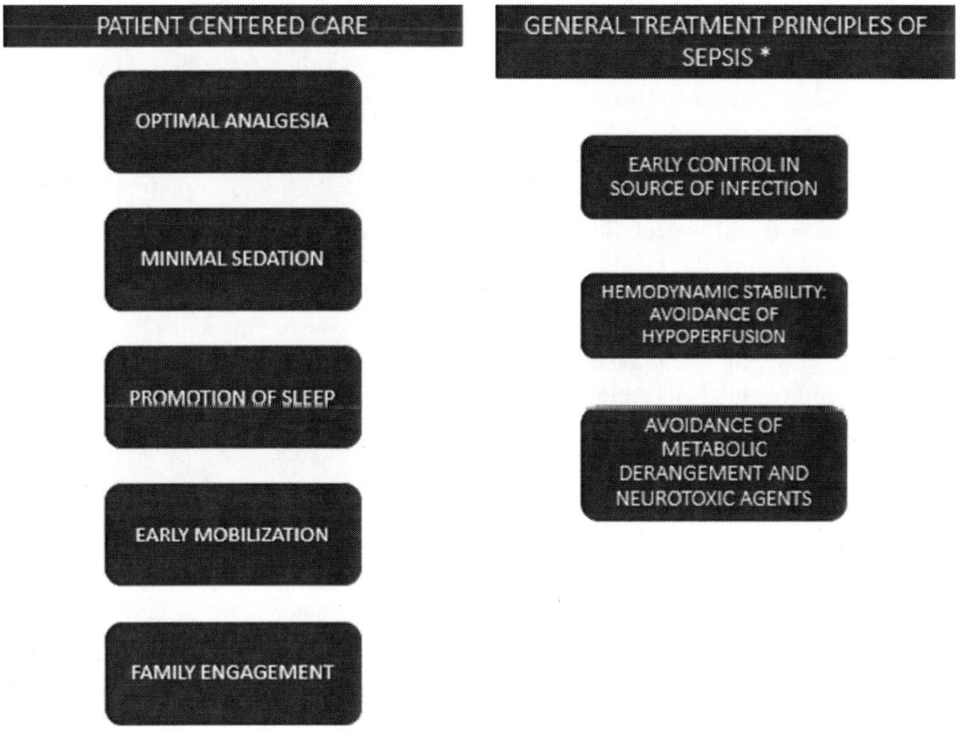

Figure 10.2 Strategies to prevent long-term cognitive impairment caused by sepsis.

Various data indicate a consistent and strong association between early deep sedation and poor long-term outcomes, including mortality, cognitive decline, and psychological complications [8–10]. Several interventions [11] have been proposed to address this problem, and the transition to mild sedation has been strongly recommended in guidelines on pain, arousal, and delirium [12], as well as in the published German manual on delirium, analgesia, and sedation [13]. But the experience of controlled studies suggests that deep sedation is still common in the intensive care unit [14, 15]. Ideally, the patient may be awake to maintain eye contact, communicate with caregivers and family members, and participate in physical and/or occupational therapy, but is allowed to fall asleep when not distracted. This condition, generally equivalent to the Richmond Sedation Scale (RASS) -1/0 [16], was associated with a favorable effect on some clinical outcomes [12]. A pilot study demonstrated the successful use of targeted early mild sedation using dexmedetomidine as the primary sedative [10]. Similarly, in a study comparing dexmedetomidine and midazolam sedation for mild sedation, dexmedetomidine sedation was associated with a lower frequency of delirium and a shorter time with invasive mechanical ventilation [17]. Comparative studies of propofol and dexmedetomidine are mixed [18]; therefore, any of these drugs can be used when targeted mild sedation is required.

Agitation in critically ill patients can be caused by many factors, including pain, delirium, anxiety, drug withdrawal syndrome, and discomfort arising from poor synchronization with a ventilator or bowel dysfunction. Emphasis should be placed on diagnosing the cause of arousal rather than simply treating symptoms that may lead to unnecessary re-sedation. Optimal pain management should also be considered as the main cause of agitation and treated with a focus on effective pain management rather than masking signs of agitation. Attention should also be paid to concomitant factors of brain dysfunction, such as decreased cerebral perfusion, severe hypoxemia, high temperature, electrolyte imbalance, sleep disturbance, and medication that causes hallucinations. Short-term sedation may be required during the treatment of these disorders [3].

The sleep of many patients in the intensive care unit is unsatisfactory and potentially adverse, and poor sleep has been identified in some studies as a risk factor for delirium [19, 20]. Restoring more normal sleep can be a therapeutic target in the intensive care unit, although it is currently difficult to determine whether this is an advantage in itself or a substitute for other changes [21]. Improving a patient's sleep can be justified as a matter of quality of treatment, with non-drug methods representing a natural starting point. The use of "sleep bundles," which include maintaining regular sleep and wake rhythms, reducing night lighting, noise, and grooming episodes, and the use of earplugs and music, may be beneficial [7, 22].

Adjuvant therapy of sepsis-associated encephalopathy

A double-blind, randomized, placebo-controlled study on the efficacy and safety of intravenous melatonin in surgical patients with severe sepsis admitted to the intensive care unit found a reduction in redox status in melatonin-treated patients over 5 days of treatment compared to placebo-treated patients, and reduced days of hospital stay. Intravenous administration of melatonin improved the course of the disease in surgical patients with severe sepsis without causing side effects [23]. In another study, a suitable dose of melatonin was determined for intravenous administration and was 20 mg at a dosing interval of 8 hours in patients with sepsis, although higher doses of 50 mg of melatonin did not have any side effects and were tolerated well enough

[24]. One recent pilot single-center randomized controlled trial of patients with septic shock treated with melatonin demonstrated the potential benefit of reducing the number of days with mechanical ventilation and reducing the number of days with vasopressors compared to the placebo group [25]. Also, some researchers propose the use of melatonin as adjuvant therapy in the treatment of neonatal sepsis in both preterm and full-term newborns, in addition to traditional treatment, and attribute this to improved clinical and laboratory results [26, 27].

The researchers propose additional treatment with Drotrecogin alpha (activated) (DrotAA), a human recombinant form of activated protein C that reduces mortality in patients with severe organ failure caused by sepsis [28]. A group of patients with sepsis was shown to have lower S100B values at 64 hours and 96 hours compared to a group of septic patients without receiving DrotAA [29].

Clinical studies have shown that α2-adrenoagonist dexmedetomidine reduces mortality in patients with sepsis. The neuroprotective effects of dexmedetomidine have also been demonstrated in an experimental model of sepsis [30]. According to the data obtained, dexmedetomidine caused a correction of a peripheral shift of activated T-helpers and reduced the level of pro-inflammatory cytokines in the hippocampus, stopped the manifestations of cognitive impairment by restoring the selective permeability of the blood-brain barrier (BBB), and reduced neuroinflammation [30]. Administration of atipamezole (α2-adrenoblocker, dexmedetomidine antagonist) prevented the protective effect of dexmedetomidine [30].

In previous studies, it was shown that Inosine + Nicotinamide + Riboflavin + Succinic Acid has a neuronal cytoprotective effect and contributes to the activation of aerobic glycolysis and stimulation of the synthesis of gamma-aminobutyric acid in neurons. The correction of cognitive disorders with Inosine + Nicotinamide + Riboflavin + Succinic Acid administration seems to be carried out by optimizing neuronal intracellular metabolism and neurotransmission mechanisms, increasing the resistance of nerve and glial cell membranes to ischemia against the background of septic encephalopathy [31]. An important circumstance is the proactive administration of Inosine + Nicotinamide + Riboflavin + Succinic Acid in the absence of neurological symptoms in verified sepsis.

One potential way to manage a dysregulated host response to infection is to modulate the redox state of glutathione using the glutoxime preparation. In the Russian Federation, glutoxime is approved as a drug for immunological correction. Reduced glutathione is considered one of the most important neutralizers of reactive oxygen species, and its ratio to oxidized glutathione can be used as a marker of oxidative stress. In the study of Kobeliatsky Yu. et al. (2021) administration of glutoxime as adjunctive therapy in sepsis patients did not affect ICU mortality, so the use of glutoxime may be proposed as adjuvant therapy in septic patients to reduce the risk of cognitive impairment [32].

Low levels of selenium (Se) and glutathione peroxidase (GSHPx), a key selenoenzyme, have been reported in systemic inflammatory response syndrome (SIRS) and sepsis, both of which are associated with high mortality. The addition of selenium had a mixed effect on the outcome. High-dose Se supplementation did not affect mortality, but the strong downward trend in mortality in patients with SIRS requires further studies in this population [33]. One study tested the hypothesis that treatment with sodium Na-selenite expression could reduce oxidative stress and increase plasma antioxidant content while modulating leukocyte antigen expression in severe sepsis. Selenite is a well-known cofactor of glutathione peroxidase and other antioxidant enzymes. The proposed treatment regimen with Na-selenite successfully restored selenium deficiency in patients with severe sepsis, but there was no effect of therapy modulating

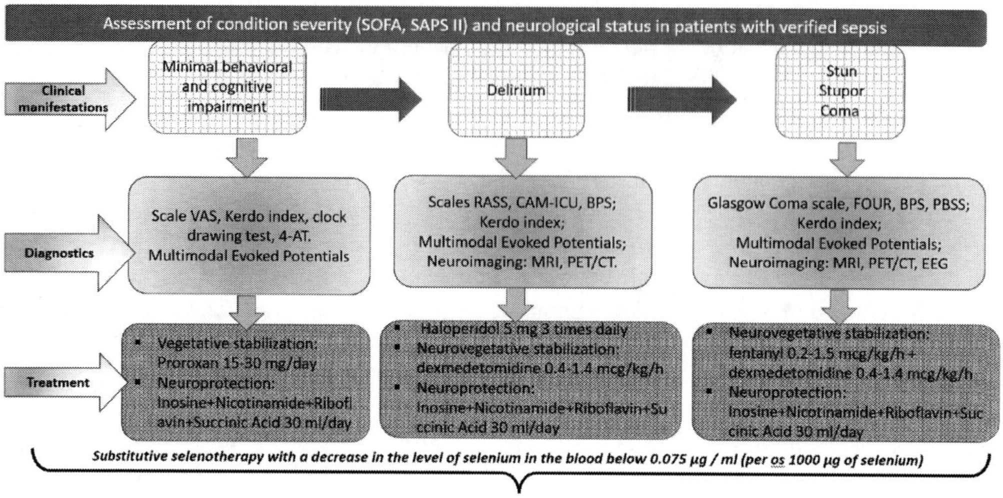

Figure 10.3 Algorithm treatment in patients with sepsis-associated encephalopathy.

the expression of antioxidant and leukocyte antigens [34]. High-dose Se replacement therapy in patients with SIRS/sepsis increased plasma levels of Se and GPx but did not reduce mortality. Inflammatory markers were reduced equally in both groups [35].

We propose to separate SAE therapy depending on clinical manifestations according to neurological examination using scales and neurophysiological examination: (1) minimal behavioral and cognitive impairment, (2) with delirium, (3) stunning, sopor, and coma. From the first day, all patients should receive proactive neurometabolic therapy Inosine + Nicotinamide + Riboflavin + Succinic Acid at high doses (30 mL/day) for 7 days. Patients without delirium with minimal cognitive and behavioral disorders should be prescribed proroxan at a dose of 15–30 mg/day as a vegetostabilizing component of therapy. Patients diagnosed with delirium should be treated with haloperidol. Neurovegetative stabilization with dexmedetomidine at a dose of 0.1 µg/kg/h should be a mandatory component of intensive care of sepsis-associated encephalopathy with delirium manifestations (Figure 10.3). The effectiveness of the therapy should be assessed by clinical and neurophysiological methods of examination: absence of seizures and increased muscle tone, "0" points on the RASS scale, absence of delirium on the CAM-ICU scale, and 4-AT test, Kerdo index close to "0," normalization of rhythms according to electroencephalography (EEG), change in amplitude data, interstitial intervals, and latencies from multimodal evoked potentials.

Therapeutic tactics of acute cerebral injury in sepsis in the structure of multi-organ dysfunction should include proactive neurometabolic therapy against the background of neurovegetative stabilization, the structure and depth of which is determined by the severity of brain damage, taking into account neurological disorders and neurophysiological monitoring data.

Animal studies

To study the treatment of septic encephalopathy, the most commonly used model of cecum ligation and perforation. This model is well known in the international literature for reproducing polymicrobial sepsis and allows inducing different degrees of severity, similar to what occurs in humans. This model is also effective for studying neurological dysfunction during and after sepsis [36].

In an animal experiment, many drugs for the therapy of SAE were studied. Thus, a study in mice with sepsis examined the effect of mirtazapine (an antidepressant – an antagonist of central presynaptic α2-adrenergic receptors, the effect of which leads to an increase in central noradrenergic and serotonergic activity) on the function of the BBB. Mice showed increased BBB permeability, high concentration of proinflammatory factors in brain tissues, and decreased ZO-1. When mirtazapine was administered, all these negative effects were reduced. Mirtazapine had a protective effect on the increased permeability of endothelial cells by enhancing the transcription factor NF- κB [37].

Selegiline, a selective and irreversible type B monoamine oxidase inhibitor, has been used to treat nervous disorders. In a study by Pu, Qian, et al., selegiline has been shown to have a protective ability against impaired BBB in both in vivo and in vitro experiments. When treated with selegiline, the integrity of the BBB was maintained, and the expression of tight contact proteins increased. In addition, selegiline has been found to inhibit the production of pro-inflammatory cytokines TNFα and IL-1β [38].

One study looked at the therapeutic effect of umbilical cord mesenchymal stem cells in a model of sepsis mice. The results showed that the production of pro-inflammatory cytokines (IL-1,6; TNFα and others) decreased with the use of umbilical cord mesenchymal cells. In addition, umbilical cord mesenchymal stem cells inhibited lipopolysaccharide-induced cellular apoptosis and damage to cortical neurons [39]. Mesenchymal stem cells have great immunomodulatory potential, so their use in clinical and preclinical studies in various diseases, including central nervous system (CNS) diseases, has increased over the past decade. Mesenchymal cells are involved in neuroinflammation processes, leading to improved survival and reduced behavioral disorders [40].

Also, a study in mice demonstrated the participation of cyclophilin-D in the link of the pathogenesis of SAE associated with an increase in mitochondrial permeability and, as a result, with a decrease in the production of free radicals, the protection of mitochondrial and cellular functions [41].

The mouse study examined the protective effect of memantine (an NMDA- receptor antagonist) on the long-term effects of sepsis in the brain. Evidence suggests that early treatment of septic mice with memantine may reduce brain inflammation and oxidative damage and prevent the long-term behavioral consequences of sepsis [42].

Hydrogen plays a protective role in various diseases; however, the detailed mechanism of action caused by hydrogen remains unclear. The purpose of one of the studies was to study the effect of hydrogen on SAE in vitro and in vivo, as well as the mechanism of action of hydrogen in mitochondrial dynamics and its function in astrocytes and microglia. Hydrogen improved damaged cells and mitochondrial quality, which was associated with HO-1 expression stimulated by the Nrf2/YY1 complex in vitro. Thus, hydrogen treatment may be a novel treatment for SAE [43].

In a study by Yi et al., glucagon-like peptide-1 (GLP-1R) was found to be activated in the microglia of septic mice [44]. Activation of GLP-1R with liraglutide can inhibit endoplasmic reticulum stress and its associated inflammatory response, as well as lipopolysaccharide-triggered apoptosis. In vivo, experiments confirmed the benefits of liraglutide in regulating microglial activation, inflammation, and apoptosis in the hippocampus of sepsis mice. In addition, survival and cognitive dysfunction of mice with sepsis also improved after liraglutide administration [44].

Conclusion

The short and long-term neurological consequences of severe infection have been extensively investigated. We know that the pathophysiology of EPSS is multifactorial, and its clinical diagnosis is confirmed by special diagnostic tools, which significantly complicates its recognition in linear intensive care units and multidisciplinary hospital departments.

In the absence of specific therapy, the general principles of sepsis treatment should be applied, and neurotoxic agents and metabolic disorders should be avoided along with early physical rehabilitation to reduce the risk of subsequent neurodegeneration [45].

There is no conflict of interest.

References

1. Zhao L, Li Y, Wang Y, et al. Non-hepatic hyperammonemia: A potential therapeutic target for sepsis-associated encephalopathy. *CNS & Neurological Disorders Drug Targets*. 2022;21(9):738–751. doi:10.2174/1871527321666211221161534.
2. Rhodes A, Evans LE, Alhazzani W, et al. Surviving sepsis campaign: International guidelines for management of sepsis and septic shock: 2016. *Critical Care Medicine*. 2017;45(3):486–552. doi:10.1097/CCM.0000000000002255.
3. Vincent JL, Shehabi Y, Walsh TS, et al. Comfort and patient-centered care without excessive sedation: The eCASH concept. *Intensive Care Medicine*. 2016;42(6):962–971. doi:10.1007/s00134-016-4297-4.
4. Dahl JB, Nielsen RV, Wetterslev J, et al. Post-operative analgesic effects of paracetamol, NSAIDs, glucocorticoids, gabapentinoids, and their combinations: A topical review. *Acta Anaesthesiologica Scandinavica*. 2014;58(10):1165–1181. doi:10.1111/aas.12382.
5. McGuinness SK, Wasiak J, Cleland H, et al. A systematic review of ketamine as an analgesic agent in adult burn injuries. *Pain Medicine (Malden, Mass.)*. 2011;12(10):1551–1558. doi:10.1111/j.1526-4637.2011.01220.x.
6. Patel A, Davidson M, Tran MC, et al. Dexmedetomidine infusion for analgesia and prevention of emergence agitation in children with obstructive sleep apnea syndrome undergoing tonsillectomy and adenoidectomy. Anesthesia and Analgesia. 2010;111(4):1004–1010. doi:10.1213/ANE.0b013e3181ee82fa.
7. Beaulieu-Boire G, Bourque S, Chagnon F, Chouinard L, Gallo-Payet N, Lesur O. Music and biological stress dampening in mechanically-ventilated patients at the intensive care unit ward-a prospective interventional randomized crossover trial. *Journal of Critical Care*. 2013;28(4):442–450. doi:10.1016/j.jcrc.2013.01.007.
8. Brummel NE, Jackson JC, Pandharipande PP, et al. Delirium in the ICU and subsequent long-term disability among survivors of mechanical ventilation. *Critical Care Medicine*. 2014;42(2):369–377. doi:10.1097/CCM.0b013e3182a645bd.
9. Balzer F, Weiß B, Kumpf O, et al. Early deep sedation is associated with decreased in-hospital and two-year follow-up survival. *Critical Care (London, England)*. 2015;19(1):197. Published 2015 Apr 28. doi:10.1186/s13054-015-0929-2.
10. Shehabi Y, Chan L, Kadiman S, et al. Sedation depth and long-term mortality in mechanically ventilated critically ill adults: A prospective longitudinal multicentre cohort study. *Intensive Care Medicine*. 2013;39(5):910–918. doi:10.1007/s00134-013-2830-2.
11. Hughes CG, Girard TD, Pandharipande PP. Daily sedation interruption versus targeted light sedation strategies in ICU patients [published correction appears in Crit Care Med. 2013 Nov;41(11):e400]. *Critical Care Medicine*. 2013;41(9 Suppl 1):S39–S45. doi:10.1097/CCM.0b013e3182a168c5.
12. Barr J, Fraser GL, Puntillo K, et al. Clinical practice guidelines for the management of pain, agitation, and delirium in adult patients in the intensive care unit. *Critical Care Medicine*. 2013;41(1):263–306. doi:10.1097/CCM.0b013e3182783b72.

13. DAS-Taskforce 2015, Baron R, Binder A, et al. Evidence and consensus-based guidelines for the management of delirium, analgesia, and sedation in intensive care medicine. Revision 2015 (DAS-Guideline 2015) - short version. *GMS German Medical Science*. 2015;13:Doc19. Published 2015 Nov 12. doi:10.3205/000223.
14. Page VJ, Ely EW, Gates S, et al. Effect of intravenous haloperidol on the duration of delirium and coma in critically ill patients (Hope-ICU): a randomized, double-blind, placebo-controlled trial [published correction appears in Lancet Respir Med. 2013 Oct;1(8):592]. *The Lancet: Respiratory Medicine*. 2013;1(7):515–523. doi:10.1016/S2213-2600(13)70166-8.
15. TEAM Study Investigators, Hodgson C, Bellomo R, et al. Early mobilization and recovery in mechanically ventilated patients in the ICU: A bi-national, multi-center, prospective cohort study. *Critical Care*. 2015;19(1):81. Published 2015 Feb 26. doi:10.1186/s13054-015-0765-4.
16. Ely EW, Truman B, Shintani A, et al. Monitoring sedation status over time in ICU patients: Reliability and validity of the Richmond Agitation-Sedation Scale (RASS). *JAMA*. 2003;289(22):2983–2991. doi:10.1001/jama.289.22.2983.
17. Riker RR, Shehabi Y, Bokesch PM, et al. Dexmedetomidine vs midazolam for sedation of critically ill patients: A randomized trial. *JAMA*. 2009;301(5):489–499. doi:10.1001/jama.2009.56.
18. Jakob SM, Ruokonen E, Grounds RM, et al. Dexmedetomidine vs midazolam or propofol for sedation during prolonged mechanical ventilation: two randomized controlled trials. *JAMA*. 2012;307(11):1151–1160. doi:10.1001/jama.2012.304.
19. Zhang WY, Wu WL, Gu JJ, et al. Risk factors for postoperative delirium in patients after coronary artery bypass grafting: A prospective cohort study. *Journal of Critical Care*. 2015;30(3):606–612. doi:10.1016/j.jcrc.2015.02.003.
20. Kamdar BB, Niessen T, Colantuoni E, et al. Delirium transitions in the medical ICU: Exploring the role of sleep quality and other factors. *Critical Care Medicine*. 2015;43(1):135-141. doi:10.1097/CCM.0000000000000610.
21. Weinhouse GL. Delirium and sleep disturbances in the intensive care unit: Can we do better? *Current Opinion in Anaesthesiology*. 2014;27(4):403–408. doi:10.1097/ACO.0000000000000093.
22. Patel J, Baldwin J, Bunting P, Laha S. The effect of a multicomponent multidisciplinary bundle of interventions on sleep and delirium in medical and surgical intensive care patients. *Anesthesia*. 2014;69(6):540–549. doi:10.1111/anae.12638.
23. Mansilla-Roselló A, Hernández-Magdalena J, Domínguez-Bastante M, et al. A phase II, single-center, double-blind, randomized placebo-controlled trial to explore the efficacy and safety of intravenous melatonin in surgical patients with severe sepsis admitted to the intensive care unit. *Journal of Pineal Research*. 2023;74(2):e12845. doi:10.1111/jpi.12845.
24. Galley HF, Allen L, Colin PJ, Galt SP, Webster NR. Dose assessment of melatonin in sepsis (DAMSEL2) study: Pharmacokinetics of two doses of oral melatonin in patients with sepsis. *Journal of Pineal Research*. 2022;73(4): e12830. doi:10.1111/jpi.12830.
25. Taher A, Shokoohmand F, Abdoli E, Mohammadi Y, Mehrpooya M. A pilot study on the melatonin treatment in patients with early septic shock: Results of a single-center randomized controlled trial. *Irish Journal of Medical Science*. 2022;191(4):1913–1924. doi:10.1007/s11845-021-02758-1.
26. El-Gendy FM, El-Hawy MA, Hassan MG. The beneficial effect of melatonin in the treatment of neonatal sepsis. *The Journal of Maternal-Fetal & Neonatal Medicine: The Official Journal of the European Association of Perinatal Medicine, The Federation of Asia and Oceania Perinatal Societies, The International Society of Perinatal Obstetricians*. 2018;31(17):2299–2303. doi:10.1080/14767058.2017.1342794.
27. El Frargy M, El-Sharkawy HM, Attia GF. Use of melatonin as an adjuvant therapy in neonatal sepsis. *Journal of Neonatal-Perinatal Medicine*. 2015;8(3):227–232. doi:10.3233/NPM-15814072.
28. Lyseng-Williamson KA, Perry CM. Drotrecogin alfa (activated). *Drugs*. 2002;62(4):617–632. doi:10.2165/00003495-200262040-00006.
29. Spapen H, Nguyen DN, Troubleyn J, Huyghens L, Schiettecatte J. Drotrecogin alfa (activated) may attenuate severe sepsis-associated encephalopathy in clinical septic shock. *Critical Care (London, England)*. 2010;14(2):R54. doi:10.1186/cc8947.
30. Tian M, Wang W, Wang K, et al. Dexmedetomidine alleviates cognitive impairment by reducing blood-brain barrier interruption and neuroinflammation via regulating Th1/Th2/Th17 polarization in

an experimental sepsis model of mice. *International Immunopharmacology.* 2021;101(Pt B):108332. doi:10.1016/j.intimp.2021.108332.

31. Savvina IA, Cherebillo VY, Zabrodskaya YM, et al. Intraoperatsionnaia profilaktika lokal'nogo ishemicheskogo povrezhdeniia golovnogo mozga u neĭrokhirurgicheskikh patsientov s tserebral'noĭ anevrizmoĭ [The intraoperative prophylaxis of local ischemical brain damage in neurosurgical patients with cerebral aneurysm]. *Khirurgiia (Mosk).* 2019;(5):57–63. doi:10.17116/hirurgia201905157.
32. Kobelyackij YU, Mal'ceva LA, Mosencev NF, Lisnichaya VN. Glutoxym as modulator of redox state of glutathione in septic patients with encephalopathy. *Medicina neotlozhnyh sostoyanij.* 2018; 4(91):104–108. doi: 10.22141/2224-0586.4.91.2018.137866.
33. Brodska H, Valenta J, Malickova K, Kohout P, Kazda A, Drabek T. Biomarkers in critically ill patients with systemic inflammatory response syndrome or sepsis supplemented with high-dose selenium. *Journal of Trace Elements in Medicine and Biology: Organ of the Society for Minerals and Trace Elements (GMS).* 2015;31:25–32. doi:10.1016/j.jtemb.2015.02.005.
34. Woth G, Nagy B, Mérei Á, et al. The effect of Na-selenite treatment on the oxidative stress-antioxidants balance of multiple organ failure. *Journal of Critical Care.* 2014;29(5). doi:10.1016/j.jcrc.2014.04.010.
35. Valenta J, Brodska H, Drabek T, Hendl J, Kazda A. High-dose selenium substitution in sepsis: a prospective randomized clinical trial. *Intensive Care Medicine.* 2011;37(5):808–815. doi:10.1007/s00134-011-2153-0.
36. Savi FF, de Oliveira A, de Medeiros GF, et al. What animal models can tell us about long-term cognitive dysfunction following sepsis: A systematic review. *Neuroscience & Biobehavioral Reviews.* 2021;124:386–404. doi:10.1016/j.neubiorev.2020.12.005.
37. Pu Y, Zhao L, Xi Y, Xia Y, Qian Y. The protective effects of Mirtazapine against lipopolysaccharide (LPS)-induced brain vascular hyperpermeability. *Bioengineered.* 2022;13(2):3680–3693. doi:10.1080/21655979.2021.2024962.
38. Pu Y, Qian F, Guo J, Sha Y, Qian Y. Selegiline protects against lipopolysaccharide (LPS)-induced impairment of the blood-brain barrier through regulating the NF-κB/MLCK/p-MLC signaling pathway. *Neurotoxicity Research.* 2022;40(1):267–275. doi:10.1007/s12640-021-00448-5.
39. Zhang Z, Wang L, Li F, et al. Therapeutic effects of human umbilical cord mesenchymal stem cell on sepsis-associated encephalopathy in mice by regulating PI3K/AKT pathway. *Journal of Integrative Neuroscience.* 2022;21(1):38. doi:10.31083/j.jin2101038.
40. Lima MN, Barbosa-Silva MC, Maron-Gutierrez T. New perspectives for mesenchymal stromal cells as adjuvant therapy for infectious disease-associated encephalopathies. *Neural Regeneration Research.* 2022;17(1):48–52. doi:10.4103/1673-5374.314292.
41. Kobayashi T, Uchino H, Elmér E, et al. Disease outcome and brain metabolomics of cyclophilin-D knockout mice in sepsis. *International Journal of Molecular Sciences.* 2022;23(2):961. Published 2022 Jan 16. doi:10.3390/ijms23020961.
42. Bardaghi Z, Rajabian A, Beheshti F, Arabi MH, Hosseini M, Salmani H. Memantine, an NMDA receptor antagonist, protected the brain against the long-term consequences of sepsis in mice. *Life Sciences.* 2023;323:121695. doi:10.1016/j.lfs.2023.121695.
43. Zhang Y, Chen J, Wu H, et al. Hydrogen regulates mitochondrial quality to protect glial cells and alleviates sepsis-associated encephalopathy by Nrf2/YY1 complex promoting HO-1 expression. *International Immunopharmacology.* 2023;118:110009. doi:10.1016/j.intimp.2023.110009.
44. Yi H, Duan Y, Song R, et al. Activation of glucagon-like peptide-1 receptor in microglia exerts protective effects against sepsis-induced encephalopathy via attenuating endoplasmic reticulum stress-associated inflammation and apoptosis in a mouse model of sepsis. *Experimental Neurology.* 2023;363:114348. doi:10.1016/j.expneurol.2023.114348.
45. Della Giovampaola M, Cavalli I, Mascia L. Neuropsychological outcome of critically ill patients with severe infection. *Biomedicines.* 2022;10(3):526. Published 2022 Feb 23. doi:10.3390/biomedicines10030526.

Chapter 11

Pathomorphology of sepsis-associated encephalopathy

Natalia V. Bodareva*, MD, Ph.D.,
Yulia M. Zabrodskaya, MD., Ph.D.
Research laboratory of the pathology of the nervous system, Almazov National Research Medical Centre, Saint Petersburg, Russian Federation

Abstract

The chapter presents pathomorphological changes in the central and autonomic nervous systems in sepsis. These changes are mainly the result of hypoxia and systemic inflammatory response to generalized infection and characterize septic encephalopathy. Structural changes of the microcirculatory bed, white matter, neurons, and glia, as well as pathological conditions that are a morphological substrate of sepsis-associated encephalopathy, are described. Special attention is paid to the structural changes of the autonomic nervous system (ANS) that characterize autonomic distress syndrome and ANS insufficiency in sepsis. The chapter is illustrated with microphotographs from the authors' archives.

Keywords: sepsis, encephalopathy, vegetative distress syndrome, brain, central nervous system, autonomic nervous system, encephalitis, brain edema, pathomorphology

Introduction

Pathomorphological changes in brain structures in patients with septic encephalopathy have a common feature characteristic of generalized infection with various etiopathogenetic factors (Savvina 2017; Rudnov, and Kulabuhov 2016; Salomão et al. 2019; Aliev 2021; Barbosa-Silva et al. 2021; Rello, and Leblebicioglu 2016). These changes are mainly the result of hypoxia and a systemic inflammatory reaction (Sonneville et al. 2013; Serafim, Gomes, and Salluh 2018). Behavioral and vegetative reactions hidden from consciousness are realized through functional systems formed in accordance following the needs, in which the ANS acts only as a component performing an organizing trophic function, along with endocrine and other anatomical and

* Corresponding author: Natalia V. Bodareva MD, Ph.D.,
e-mail address: bodarevane@mail.ru

Editor: Irina A. Savvina, Natalia V. Beloborodova and Tatyana N. Trofimova
In: Sepsis-Associated Encephalopathy
ISBN: 979-8-89113-178-1

physiological systems (Savvina 2017; Medvedev 2005; Fairchild et al. 2011; Mayr 2010). These are temporary connections that are formed as needed (Anokhin 2008; Mal'ceva, and Bazilenko 2015; Rello, and Leblebicioglu 2016; Purkayastha, Stokes, and Bell 2019; Savvina, Petrova, and Zabrodskaya 2021). The pathomorphology of sepsis-associated encephalopathy should be considered in the relationship between the central nervous system and the ANS, as places of least resistance in the body system as a whole (Medvedev 2005; Reale, and Costantini 2021).

Morphological changes of the brain in sepsis

Vascular changes. The vessels of the microcirculatory bed are the most susceptible to changes, which in the case of generalized infection plays a significant role (Bodareva, Zabrodskaya, and Savvina 2021; Savvina 2017; Singer et al. 2016; Vincent, Sakr, and Sprung 2006).

Histological examination of the vascular walls shows dystrophic and necrobiotic changes in the cellular elements of the wall. Lipoidosis occurs, which accumulates in the walls of capillaries, locally, in far-reaching cases is irreversible (Czempik, Pluta, and Krzych 2020) (**Fig. 11.1A**).

Microscopic examination reveals changes in the form of an increase in the size of endotheliocytes, their decomplexation, and pyknosis of nuclei. Generalized infection is characterized by the process of exfoliation (desquamation) of the endothelium as a result of destructive changes occurring in the vascular wall (**Fig. 11.1B**). On some walls of blood vessels, the process of proliferation occurs with the formation of small lumpy elements, which is characteristic of the reactive inflammatory process (Zakkar 2009). A commonwealth reaction is observed involving adventitia and the process of perivasculitis is triggered. In the early stages (3–4 days)

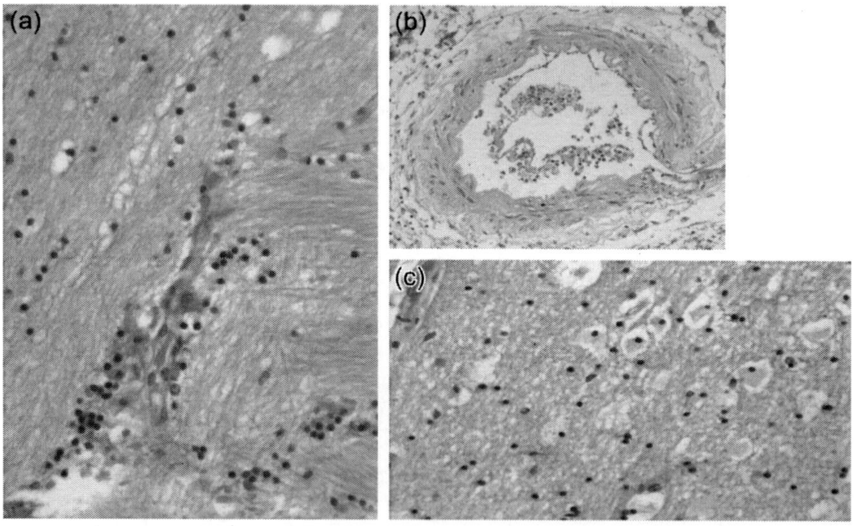

Figure 11.1 Vessel and the initial manifestations of septic leukomalacia white matter.

A – Intracerebral vessel endotheliitis. H&E. x400

B – Cerebral artery endotheliitis with desquamation of the endothelium. H&E x200

C – Macrophage transformation of microgliosis in the zone of resorption of necrotic leukomalacia. H&E x400.

of sepsis that has arisen, leukocyte-lymphocytic infiltration can be histologically detected, in later periods (5–7 days) scattered lymphocytes located perifocal in perivascular zones are more often observed (Bodareva, Zabrodskaya, and Savvina 2021; Burgaletto et al. 2020; Brinkhoff et al. 2019).

In vessels with a long-term generalized infection, there are limited spaces or scattered areas with fibrinoid necrosis. Total necrobiotic processes in the walls of blood vessels are usually not widespread. They are local in nature. In fact, morphological characteristics of changes in blood vessels have the same characteristics as in other pathological processes characterized by inflammation (Unsinger 2010; Brinkhoff et al. 2019).

Hemorrhages. Early changes were characterized by circulatory disorders accompanied by paralytic vascular hyperemia, often with hemorrhages in the perivascular zones (Cai 2010). It is characterized by the development of stagnation, the formation of blood clots mainly in the vessels of the microcirculatory bed and medium caliber, and the formation of capillary aneurysms and hemorrhages with the impregnation of the vessel wall is noted. The edematous-hemorrhagic process of various degrees of damage of the brain substance with a meager leukocyte reaction was diffuse and had a different prescription (**Fig. 11.2**).

With lightning-fast fatal forms of sepsis with the development of multiple organ failure, hemorrhagic necrotic, fibrinous lesions mainly occurred, with the development of severe perivasculitis, phlebitis, periphlebitis, arteritis, and periarteritis with the development of irreversible necrotic changes in the substance of the brain with an increase in the lesion area (Saharov et al. 2019). Thrombosis is more common in the sinuses of the dura mater with the spread of multiple hemorrhages in the cerebral cortex and subcortical white matter, as well as thrombosis of subependymal veins with paraventricular hemorrhages. Usually, this process is accompanied by massive hemorrhage into the brain, as well as subarachnoid hemorrhages (Serebryanaya, and Yakuceni 2020; Singer et al. 2016; Vincent, Sakr, and Sprung 2006).

Meningoencephalitis and encephalopathy. The combination of inflammatory changes of different composition and magnitude (with exudative, serous, purulent, and mixed) creates a

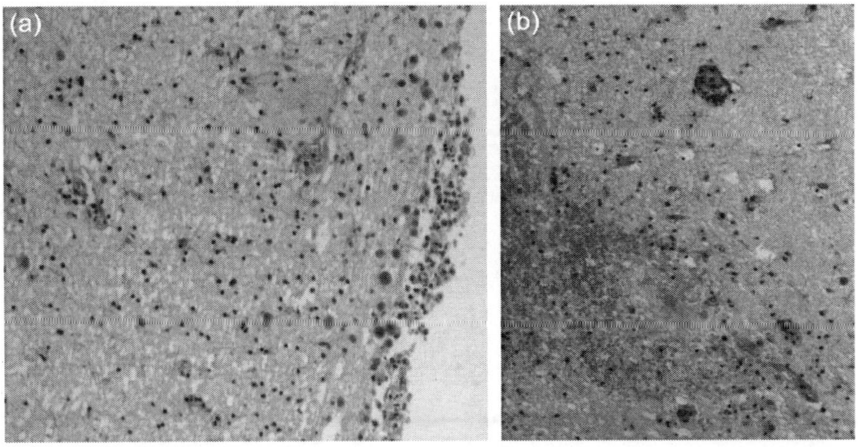

Figure 11.2 White matter in septic encephalopathy.

A – Leukocytosis and destructive thrombomicrovasculitis. H&E x200.

B – Secondary hemorrhage in sepsis. The vessels of the microvasculature with leukocytosis, eritrostasis, and diapedetic hemorrhages in the zone of necrosis. H&E x400.

classic picture of "septic" brain damage involving both soft and dura mater in the pathological process, with the development of meningoencephalitis and encephalopathy (Seymour et al. 2019; Tian et al. 2019; Savvina et al. 2017) (**Fig. 11.3**).

In the large hemispheres around the horns of the lateral ventricles, there is a loss of the ependymal lining, which leads to subependymal astrocytic gliosis and the spread of cerebrospinal fluid over the entire thickness of the white matter. There is marked perivascular and pericellular edema, which is diffused with the capture of deeper sections of the white matter, including the mastoids, hippocampus, and hypothalamus (Medvedev, and Rejnus 1989) (**Figs. 11.4, 11.5**). This process is more pronounced in the frontal lobes, mainly in the areas covering the anterior horns of the lateral ventricles (**Fig. 11.6**). Toward the cerebral cortex the intensity of the edema decreases (Gulyaeva 2017; Mayr et al. 2010).

Multifocal necrotizing leukoencephalopathy has been described among patients with septic shock, and it is characterized by intense expression of proinflammatory cytokines and apoptosis of neurons in the bridge of the brain (**Fig. 11.7**). Oligodendrocytes play a central role in the development of periventricular leukomalacia, characteristic of CNS damage in sepsis and hypoperfusion (Griesbach, and Hovda 2015; Varinthra et al. 2021) (**Fig. 11.1C**). Moreover, in cases of septic encephalopathy, along with ischemic changes, hemorrhages in the brain are noted. Diffuse changes are combined with focal ones in the form of deep (lacunar) infarcts at different stages of the organization, which depends on the age of occurrence of the local inflammatory process, which resulted in generalized infection (Mayr et al. 2010). These changes prevail in the frontal and temporal lobes, in the area of the mastoid nuclei. Depending on the prevalence of white matter lesions, there is the development of external and internal hydrocephalus (Rello, and Leblebicioglu 2016).

Reactive and destructive changes are observed in the neurons of the cortex and subcortical formations of the brain, the deposition of lipofuscin in neurons is detected in some neurons (**Fig. 11.8**). Areas with diffuse demyelination, mainly in periventricular areas, and cellular gliosis were detected in the white matter. In the myelin fibers swelling and adhesion of lamellae were

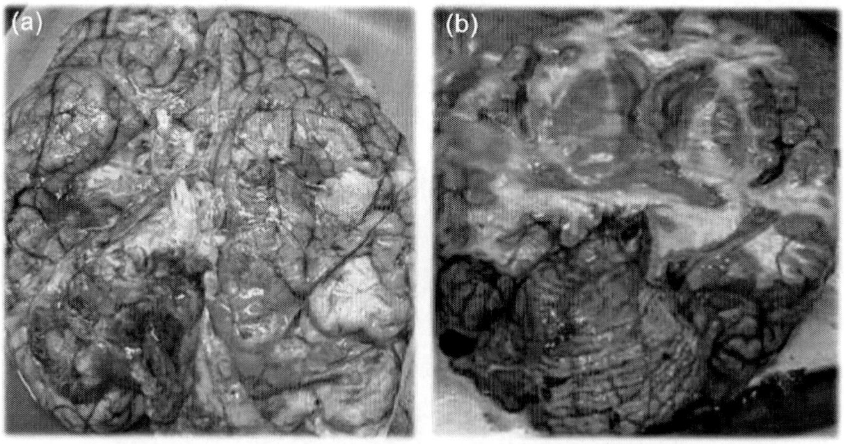

Figure 11.3 Macropreparation of the brain in sepsis.

A – Inflammatory injection of vessels pia mater.

B – Purulent ventriculitis.

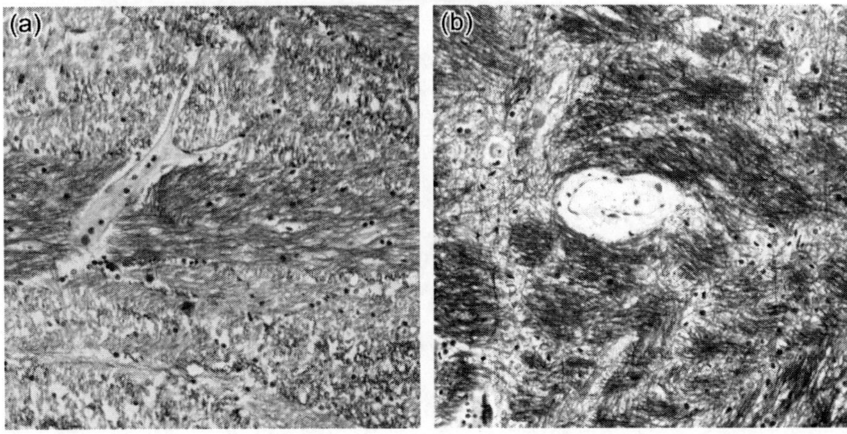

Figure 11.4 Change changes in myelin fibers in the edema zone. Spielmeyer staining x200.

A – Weak diffuse staining of myelin fibers.

B – Focal demyelination, fragmentation of myelin fibers.

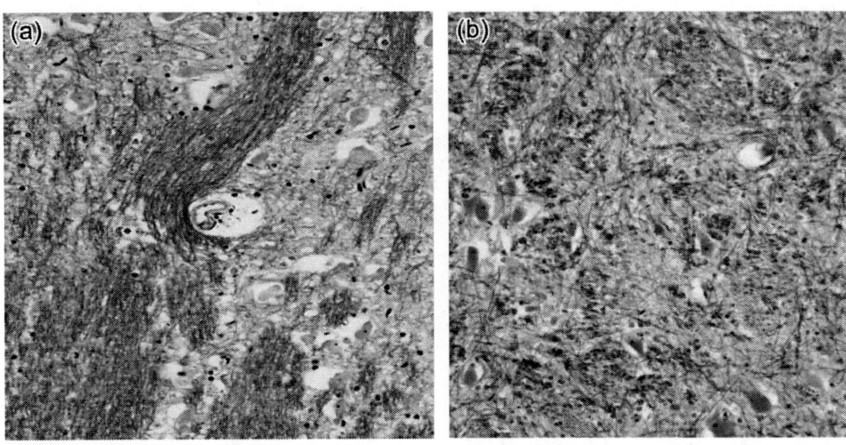

Figure. 11.5 Changes in myelin fibers in the zone with perivascular and pericellular edema. Spielmeyer staining x200.

A – Alternation of swollen and fragmented myelin fibers.

B – Necrobiotic changes in myelin fibers with fragmentation and gluing.

combined (**Fig. 11.9**). Axial cylinders disappear in individual fibers, and only a thin myelin sheath remains, represented by fused lamellae. In some myelin fibers, pronounced changes in axons persist with the decay of axial cylinders. Gliosis was widespread throughout, regardless of the structures of the brain, surrounding the structures of the brain with the most pronounced damage (Griesbach, and Hovda 2015; Gulyaeva N.V. 2017) (**Fig. 11.10**).

There are 10–15 times more macroglial cells in the central nervous system than neurons. It is considered that these cells are involved in the process of maintaining the trophic of neurons, ensuring the plasticity of the nervous system, and assisting in interneuronal integration and

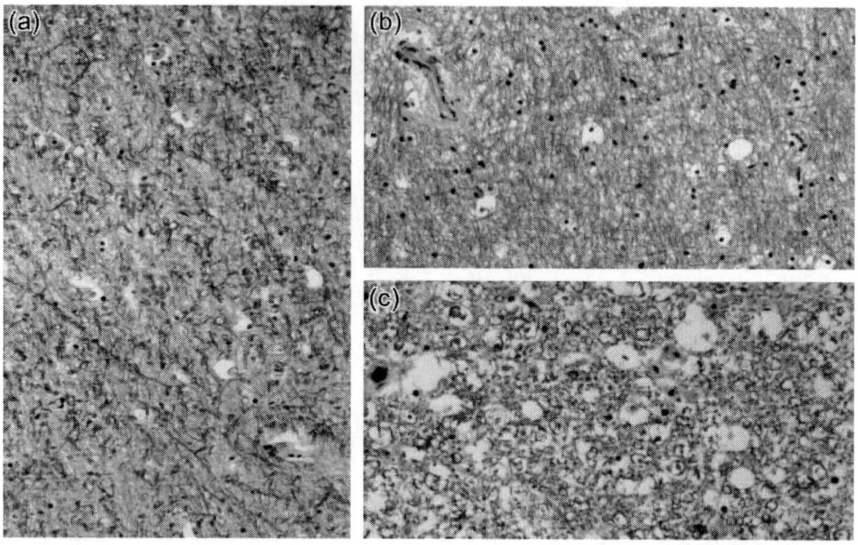

Figure 11.6 Spongiose degeneration of the white matter of the brain. Spielmeyer staining x200.

A – Pronounced rarefaction of myelin tissue, remnants of fragments of myelin fibers.

B – Rarefaction and thinning of myelin fibers. The appearance of drainage forms of oligodendroglia.

C – Vacuolization of myelin fibers with microcystic transformation of the white matter of the brain x200.

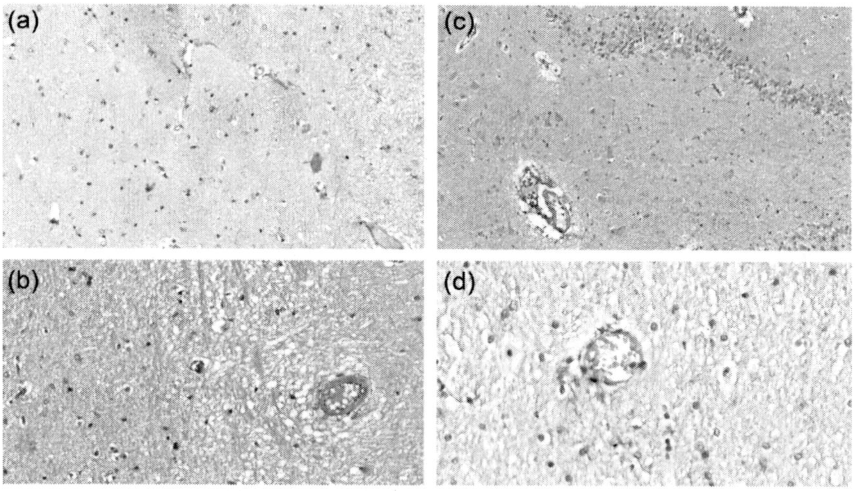

Figure 11.7 Immunohistochemical reactions with antibodies to Caspase-3 and CD20 x200.

A – Pronounced glial apoptosis in the brain stem. Caspase-3.

B – Weak glial apoptosis of the hippocampus. Caspase-3.

C – Moderate glial apoptosis of white matter in the edema zone. Caspase-3.

D – Perivascular B-cell infiltration. CD 200.

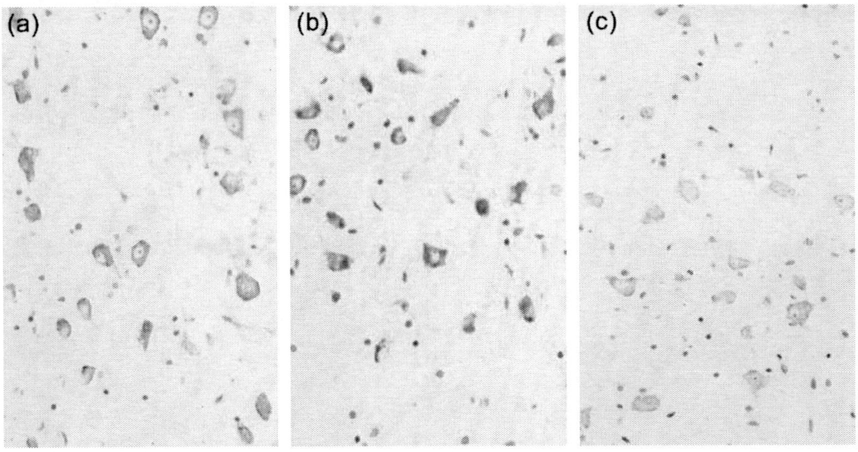

Figure 11.8 Necrobiotic changes of neurons in subcortical nuclei of cerebral hemispheres. Nissl staining x200.

A – Foci of neuronal prolapse. B – Karyolysis with wrinkled hyperchromic nucleus, karyorexis in combination with swelling of the neuron body. C – Hydropic changes with the formation of vacuoles and karyolysis, and karyorexis in combination with swelling of the neuron body.

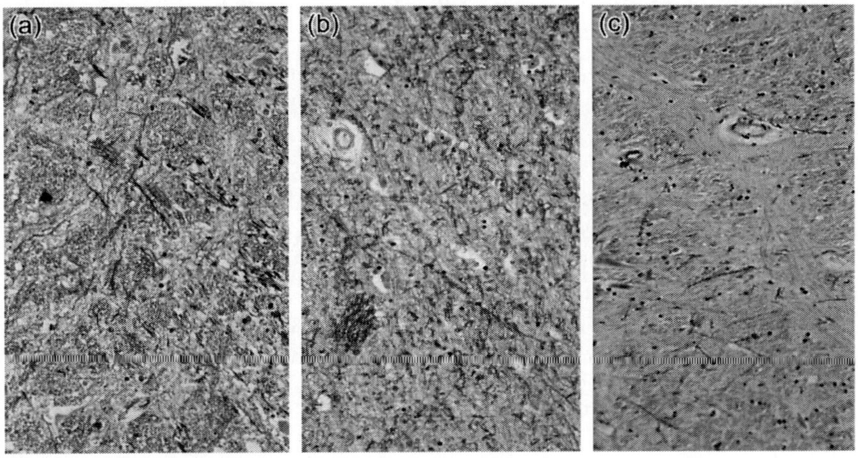

Figure 11.9 Necrotizing leukoencephalopathy. Spielmeyer staining.

A – Dystrophic changes with demyelination of fibers, their fragmentation x100.

B – Severe tissue rarefaction, formation of voids, fragmentation of myelin fibers x200.

C – Alternation and demyelination of myelin fiber with the formation of empty x200.

regulation of synaptic efficiency (Griesbach, and Hovda 2015; Gulyaeva N.V. 2017). As described above, in sepsis with the development of septic encephalopathy, there is a violation in blood circulation with a violation of the integrity of the vascular walls, the release of mediators, and cytokines, a deviation in the functional ability of each structure of the brain to perform its functions (Fairchild et al. 2011; Zakkar 2009; Unsinger 2010). As a result, compensatory and adaptive

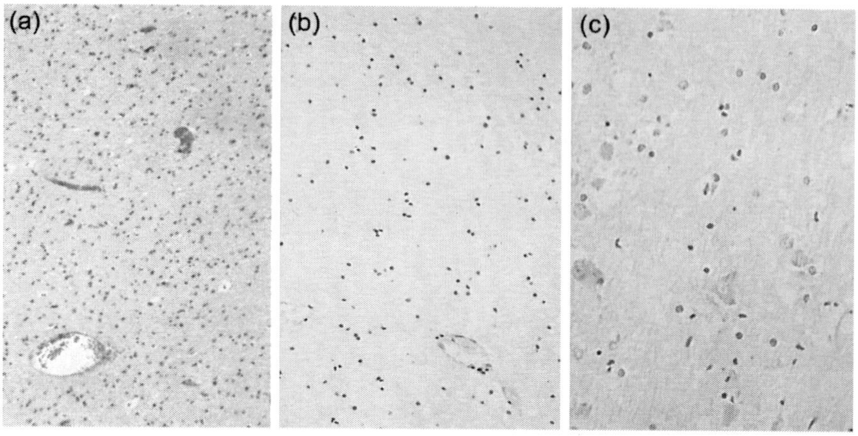

Figure 11.10 Glial reactions in white matter. Nissl staining x200.

A – Gliosis. B – Gliocytopenia. C – Gliocytopenia, necrobiotic changes of gliocytes, "shadow cells," and plasmorexis of cortical neurons.

processes are disrupted, which further leads to dystrophic and often irreversible consequences, excessive growth of astrocytic neuroglia with substitutive hyperplasia in response to death or damage to nervous tissue. In septic encephalopathy, the presence of opposite processes was noted, such as gliosis with an increase in the number of astrocytes, and gliocytopenia with loss of gliocytes in all parts of the brain (Moraes et al. 2021; Griesbach, and Hovda 2015; Winkler 2017).

Attention was drawn to the appearance of lipofuscinosis and its increase in cases with an increase in age-related changes. Inflammatory cell infiltration represented diffuse single-lying lymphocytes, in severe cases neutrophilic leukocytes were designated (**Fig. 11.7D**). The immunohistochemical studies are dominated by lymphoid cells, less often macrophages. There was a diffuse arrangement with a more crowded character in the perivascular zone (Qin et al. 2007; Rada et al. 1991; Unsinger 2010).

These changes were accompanied by clinical symptoms of circulatory insufficiency, which are characteristic of bacterial infections (Mal'ceva, and Bazilenko 2015; Matthay et al. 2012; Moraes et al. 2021; Xu, Yang, and Zhu 2020). It is worth noting that changes in vascular walls and a violation of the circulatory process are not the results of the action of microbiota on the vessel wall but are the reflection of the setting of vasomotor centers and the autonomic nervous system as a whole (Zhang, Sheng, and Yao 2014; Sonneville et al. 2015). Activation of bacterial flora by the type of autoinfection against the background of predisposing factors (decreased immunity, concomitant diseases) has great importance in thanatogenesis (Medvedev 2005; Tian et al. 2019). Such changes are most pronounced in septic encephalopathy. It should be noted that pathomorphological changes in the substance of the brain due to the altered reactivity of the body have an unexpressed picture, and are often distorted (Singer et al. 2016).

Morphological basis of insufficiency of the ANS in sepsis

The ANS, the endocrine system, and the circulatory system dependent on them are systems that integrate and ensure the functioning of the body as a whole. Long-term and numerous

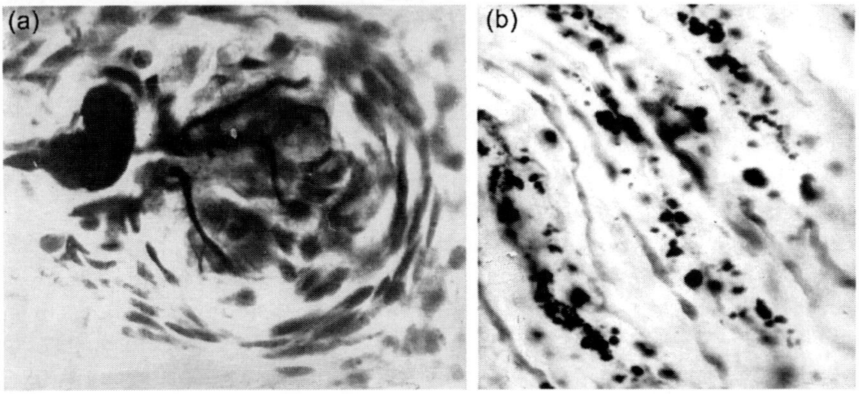

Figure 11.11 Afferent nerve fibers. Impregnation by Bilshovsky – Gross x400.

A – Neuroplasma surges, fields of sharp contractures, and ruptures of afferent nerve fibers forming glomerular receptors (3-day sepsis).

B – Complete destruction of the nerve plexus containing efferent and afferent nerve fibers in the lungs (9-day sepsis).

experimental studies on the plasticity of the nervous system in various injuries demonstrate the lack of specificity of changes in neurons (Purkayastha, Stokes, and Bell 2019; Xu, Yang, and Zhu 2020; Savvina, Petrova, and Zabrodskaya 2021).

Reactive-destructive changes in the structure of the neuron nucleus are manifested by invagination of the nuclear envelope, chromatin condensation, swelling of mitochondria and all cisternal structures (smooth and rough endoplasmic reticulum, Golgi apparatus, spike apparatus, changes in synaptic contacts, an increase in the number of active zones, the appearance of a large number of non-synaptic contacts, lysosomes, multivesicular bodies, etc.). These structural changes appear without any impact on the body and are a universal ultrastructural expression of the general adaptation syndrome, including sepsis (Plaschke, Do, and Uhle 2018).

Morphological changes appear earlier than functional ones and persist much longer. The organization of nerve cells into ensembles (modules) ensures the reliability and exceptional plasticity of the functional structures of the ANS (Kuchler et al. 2021)

Pathomorphological studies of the ANS, conducted on autopsy material, in any critical conditions, including sepsis, reveal severe dystrophic and destructive changes at all levels of the ANS (Medvedev 2005; Plaschke, Do, and Uhle 2018; Savvina, Petrova, and Zabrodskaya 2021).

Afferent department of visceral reflex arches

In the pathomorphological study of various structures of the afferent department (receptor apparatus and sensitive nerve fibers (dendrites), perceiving and conducting afferent impulses in the spinal (as a rule, Th2–Th4; L1–L4 were studied; S2–S3.) and similar cranial nerve ganglia (trigeminal, inferior node of the vagus nerve). It has been established that, regardless of the nature of the damaging causes, there are widespread and, as a rule, deep violations of the structure and, of course, the functions of the components of the afferent department, most of which should be qualified as irreversible (Medvedev 2005).

There is a partial or complete death of the sensitive nervous apparatus, the state of which largely determines both reactivity and plasticity in the implementation of an adaptive reaction. Changes were registered both from the glomerular and bush-shaped receptors. In the early stages of the disease, along the course of the adducting afferent nerve fiber forming the receptor, varicose thickenings, and "influx" of neuroplasma, which were five to six times larger than the diameter of the nerve fiber itself, are observed. Most often they are located in those areas where the fibers are dichotomically divided (Medvedev 2005; Savvina, Petrova, and Zabrodskaya 2021) **(Fig. 11.11)**.

Similar changes are found not only in the intramural plexuses but also in the trunk of the vagus nerve, which, as is known, carries, along with afferent, preganglionic fibers to intramural neurons. The same kind of destructive processes take place in the posterior roots of the spinal cord, where the axons of the neurons of the sensitive spinal ganglia pass, and in the sensitive ganglia themselves – the trophic centers of the sensory neurons.

Non-specific reactive changes are noted in them (marginal chromatolysis with preservation of the nucleus, central chromatolysis with preservation of the nucleus, central chromatolysis with "sintering" of lumps of Nissl substance along the periphery of neurons, hyperchromatosis of nuclei and cytoplasm of the cell in combination with edema and without it), as well as destructive irreversible phenomena were also represented by standard pictures (karyolysis with wrinkled hyperchromic nucleus, hydropic changes with the formation of vacuoles and karyolysis, karyorrhexis in combination with swelling of the neuron body) (Medvedev 2005) **(Fig. 11.12)**.

The total number of neurons involved in the reaction in the trigeminal ganglion can be almost 80%. Half of them detect reactive changes, and half of those who reacted died (41.4%). Approximately the same is the case in the spinal ganglia. Thus, the entire sensory tract, including its important components such as receptors, perikaryons of neurons, and intra- and extra-organ afferent nerve fibers, demonstrate a picture of a morphological catastrophe with an irreplaceable (if the patient had survived) loss of almost half of the sensitive cells (Xu, Yang, and Zhu 2020; Plaschke et al. 2021).

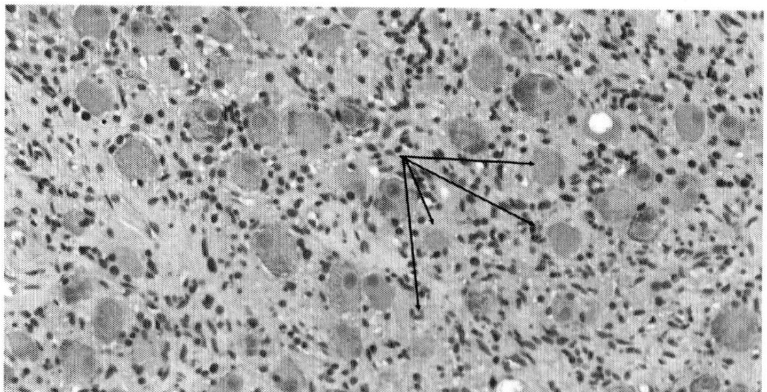

Figure 11.12 Nonspecific reactive changes in the central parts of the sympathetic and parasympathetic nervous system. Central and peripheral chromatolysis of neurons, acute cellular edema, and hyperchromatosis of nuclei and cytoplasm. Irreversible phenomena in neurons – karyocytolysis, karyolysis (arrows); lively glial reaction. H&E x200.

Central divisions of the autonomic nervous system

The central parts of the ANS are an associative (insertion) link of the visceral reflex arcs. The associative link of the sympathetic nervous system is represented by the nuclei of the lateral horns of the gray matter of the spinal cord in the thoracolumbar region. Ongoing studies of the spinal cord at the Th2–Th4, Th12, and L1–L2 levels, the insertion link of the parasympathetic nervous system at the mesencephalic (Yakubovich–Westphal-Edinger nucleus), and bulbar (autonomic vagus nerve nucleus) and sacral (S2–S3) levels also note widespread damage to mostly irreversible structures. Thus, there is partial or significant damage to the associative link, from which the efferent vegetative pathway begins.

Neurites (axons of associative neurons) leave the limits and reach the autonomic ganglia as part of peripheral nerves, where they end with synapses. Synaptic contacts are also established between associative neurons and axons of sensitive nerve cells. Thanks to synapses, all the links of the visceral reflex arcs are interconnected and, if necessary, can act as a whole. Significant changes are revealed in the synaptic apparatus of associative links (sympathetic and parasympathetic).

Normally synaptic endings look like delicate rings and loops, more rarely – buttons. Already in the early stages of the disease increases the affinity of synaptic rings to silver nitrate. They become argyrophilic. In the future, rings and loops thicken, their lumen is narrowed, the size increases, and they become spherical or bulbous shape, as a rule, hypertrophied. Argyrophilia and hypertrophy of synapses are the testimony of their reactive changes (**Fig. 11.13**).

However, destructive ones are revealed – fragmentation, granular-lumpy decay of presynaptic nerve fibers, and synaptic structures formed by them on associative neurons. The latter is more pronounced in long-term critical conditions of a patient with appropriate clinical symptoms. Reactive and destructive changes are detected among the associative neurons themselves.

Nonspecific reactive changes (central and peripheral chromatolysis, acute cellular swelling, process staining, and hyperchromatosis of nuclei and cytoplasm) are detected in the central parts of the sympathetic and parasympathetic nervous system. Irreversible destructive phenomena were standard (karyocytolysis, karyolysis). They probably represent different stages of neuronal death. There was a lively glial reaction (Qin et al. 2007).

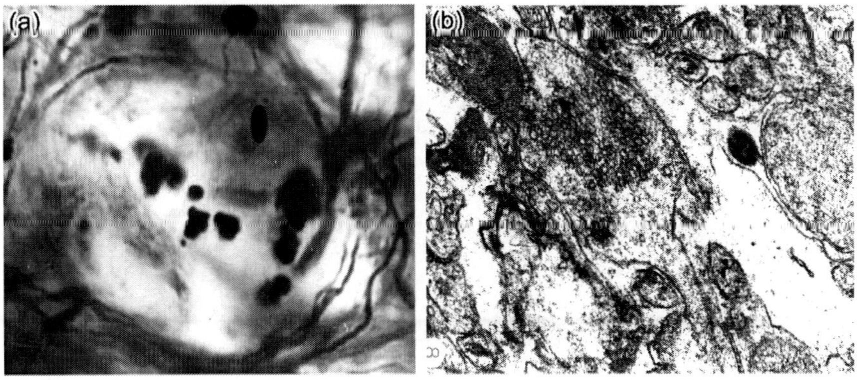

Figure 11.13 Sympathetic ganglion in 3-day sepsis.

A – Argyrophilia, hypertrophy, and deformation of synapses on neurons. Impregnation by Kahal x1000.

B – Destructive changes in the synaptic vesicle. Electronogram x1800.

Thus, the most critical, from a morphological point of view, the situation develops in the associative link of the sympathetic nervous system.

The death of neurons of nuclei in all parts of the hypothalamus (large-cell nucleus of the anterior hypothalamus, small-cell nuclei of the middle hypothalamus, nuclei, and pathways of the posterior) are also noted.

Efferent department of the visceral reflex arc

In the ANS, all effector neurons are located on the periphery. Most of them are located in the autonomic ganglia and synaptic contacts between associative and effector autonomic neurons are localized there. The efferent autonomic pathway is represented by the neurites of associative neurons (preganglionic fibers) and effector neurons and their neurites (postganglionic fibers). The latter reaches the innervated tissues, where they realize their impact.

When exposed to various damaging factors, including sepsis, extensive and deep structural, and, consequently, functional disorders of the main components of the autonomic ganglion, neurocytes are revealed. Qualifying them in a significant part as irreversible, we must take into account that not only the "management" of the special functions of some organs (glands, smooth muscles of internal organs and vessels, heart muscle, ciliary and pupillary muscles, etc.) is disrupted; however, the main thing is that the general adaptive and trophic function suffers (Matthay, Ware, and Zimmerman 2012).

Adhering to the structure of the visceral reflex arc, it is necessary to focus on preganglionic fibers that provide connections of associative neurons with effector ones. These connections are carried out by synapses that undergo reactive and destructive changes similar to those already described in the associative link.

In the sympathetic ganglia, a rather motley pattern of reactive changes is established: central and peripheral chromatolysis, total chromatolysis with preservation of the nucleus and nucleolus and "sintering" of chromatophilic substance along the edge of the neuron body, hyperchromatosis of the nucleus and perinuclear edema, wrinkling of nuclear material into a homogeneous structureless mass with total chromatolysis.

Quantitative analysis data show that the total number of neurocytes involved in the reaction with reversible and irreversible changes is greater in the sympathetic nodes. In the paravertebral nodes of the thoracic region, this indicator reaches 80–85.3%. In the same nodes, the highest percentage of dead neurons is observed (40–45.2%). The listed indicators are much lower in the parasympathetic nodes. In intramural, the percentage of neurocytes involved in the reaction and dead is almost half less and amounts to 59% and 20%, respectively (Medvedev 2005).

Finally, the last link of the visceral reflex arc is the postganglionic fibers, which originate in the autonomic ganglia and, as part of nerve trunks and bundles, penetrate all organs and tissues of the body, where they form effector nerve endings. Pronounced reactive and destructive changes of efferent nerve fibers and their terminals are observed in the composition of intra-organ nerve bundles. Both whole bundles of nerve fibers and efferent endings in tissues are subjected to destruction. Thus, the efferent part of the visceral reflex arches also detects gross dystrophic changes.

One of the indicators that correlate with the number of damaged and dead neurons is the time from the moment of the disease – the more the patient lived in critical condition, the more widespread the damage was (Matthay, Ware, and Zimmerman 2012).

The most vulnerable part of the visceral reflex arc – the efferent pathway – dies, of course, not because the irritation is above the threshold but due to more general influences – violations of water-electrolyte metabolism (hydration level, pH, osmolarity, etc.), the degree of oxygen starvation, intoxication. On the other hand, the death of neurons and their processes in some cases may be due to their overload, excessive functional stress, malfunctions in the rhythm of work, etc. (Mal'ceva, and Bazilenko 2015).

Some patients who have suffered severe critical conditions recover and return to life with a deeply disabled ANS. Following the raptures about the patient's recovery, a specialized system of medical and social rehabilitation should be built for those who leave the clinic with a disabled ANS, with a sharply narrowed range of adaptive reactions (Seymour et al. 2019; Savvina, Petrova, and Zabrodskaya 2021).

Death can occur (and it happens much more often than we assume) from the disintegration of the organism as a system, as a whole, with the relative safety of the components of the system (organs), with far from exhausted reserves (Anokhin 2008; Medvedev 2005; Czempik, Pluta, and Krzych 2020).

The ANS, the endocrine system, and the circulatory system dependent on them are systems that integrate and ensure the functioning of the body as a whole. The totality of dystrophic and necrobiotic changes detected in the ANS is the morphological equivalent of *vegetative distress syndrome* and ANS insufficiency (Medvedev 2005; Savvina, Petrova, and Zabrodskaya 2021).

The observed "collapse" of the ANS has as its consequence the disintegration of the organism as a whole, in its essence is a morphological manifestation of the *insufficiency* of the ANS (Medvedev 2005).

Conclusion

The studies reviewed above indicate that in the brain with sepsis, the same type of changes are observed, which are expressed in the defeat of the walls of the vessels of the microcirculatory bed, and the formation of microthrombi in vessels of small and medium diameter. There are also changes in the bodies of neurons and fibers with pronounced degenerative and dystrophic changes. There is pronounced swelling of the brain substance with the formation of microcystic areas, pronounced microglial reaction with proliferation and macrophage transformation into granular balls, and resorption of cerebral detritus without any specific signs. These changes are mainly the result of hypoxia and systemic inflammatory response to generalized infection and characterize septic encephalopathy. Ischemic lesions were found in areas of the brain sensitive to ischemia (hippocampus, basal ganglia, frontal cortex, dentate gyrus, olives of the medulla oblongata), but also in the sepsis-specific nuclei of the autonomic nervous system (amygdala, anterior and posterior hypothalamus, blue spot). In addition, pronounced neuronal apoptosis was detected in these areas. The defeat of the ANS with the development of vegetative distress syndrome with nonspecific reactions is included in the systemic response of the body in sepsis.

References

Aliev S.A., Aliev E.S., Gummatov A.F. 2020. "Sepsis: Old Dogs and the Evolution of Ideas." *Bulletin of the National Medical and Surgical Center Named After N. I. Pirogov* 15 (1): 132–136. https://doi.org/10.25881/BPNMSC.2020.32. (In Russ.).

Anokhin P.K. 2008. "Fundamental Issues of the General Theory of Functional Systems the General Theory of Functional Systems." 131 p. Moscow: Direct-Media. (In Russ.)

Barbosa-Silva M.C., Lima M.N., Battaglini D., Robba C., Pelosi P., Rocco P.R.M., Maron-Gutierrez T. 2021. "Infectious Disease-Associated Encephalopathies." *Critical Care Medicine* 25 (1): 236. https://doi.org/10.1186/s13054-021-03659-6.

Bodareva N.V., Zabrodskaya Y.M., Savvina I.A. 2021. "Pathomorphological Signs of Encephalopathy in Sepsis in Neurosurgical Patients." In *The Collection: Science and Innovation - Modern Concepts*, edited by Hysmatullin D.R., 71–78. Moscow: Infinity Publisher. (In Russ.)

Brinkhoff A., Zeng Y., Sieberichs A., Dolff S., Shilei X., Sun M., Engler H., Benson S., Korth J., Schedlowski M., Kribben A., Witzke O., Wilde B. 2019. "B-Cell Dynamics During Experimental Endotoxemia in Humans." *Bioscience Reports* 39 (5): BSR20182347. https://doi.org/10.1042/BSR20182347.

Burgaletto C., Munafò A., Di Benedetto G., De Francisci C., Caraci F., Di Mauro R., Bucolo C., Bernardini R., Cantarella G. 2020. "The Immune System on the TRAIL of Alzheimer's Disease." *Journal of Neuroinflammation* 17 (1): 298. https://doi.org/10.1186/s12974-020-01968-1.

Cai B. 2010. "Novel Insights for Systemic Inflammation in Sepsis and Hemorrhage." *Mediators of Inflammation* 10: 10. https://doi.org/10.1155/2010/642462.

Czempik P.F., Pluta M.P., Krzych Ł.J. 2020. "Sepsis-Associated Brain Dysfunction: A Review of Current Literature." *International Journal of Environmental Research and Public Health* 17 (16): 5852. https://doi.org/10.3390/ijerph17165852.

Fairchild K.D., Srinivasan V., Moorman J.R., Gaykema R.P., Goehler L.E. 2011. "Pathogen-Induced Heart Rate Changes Associated with Cholinergic Nervous System Activation." *American Journal of Physiology-Regulatory, Integrative and Comparative Physiology* 300: R330–R339. https://doi.org/10.1152/ajpregu.00487.2010.

Griesbach G.S., Hovda D.A. 2015. "Cellular and Molecular Neuronal Plasticity." *Handbook of Clinical Neurology* 128: 681–690. https://doi.org/10.1016/B978-0-444-63521-1.00042-X.

Gulyaeva N.V. 2017. "Molecular Mechanisms of Neuroplasticity: An Expanding Universe." *Biochemistry (Moscow)* 82(3): 237–242. https://doi.org/10.1134/S0006297917030014 (In Russ).

Kuchler J.C., Siqueira B.S., Ceglarek V.M., Chasko F.V., Moura I.C., Sczepanhak B.F., Vettorazzi J.F., Balbo S.L., Grassiolli S. 2021. "The Vagus Nerve and Spleen: Influence on White Adipose Mass and Histology of Obese and Non-obese Rats." *Frontiers in Physiology* 12: 672027. https://doi.org/10.3389/fphys.2021.672027.

Mal'ceva L.A., Bazilenko D.V. 2015. "The Role of Sepsis-Associated Encephalopathy in the Formation of Multiple Organ Failure Syndrome in Patients with Severe Sepsis and Septic Shock." *Journal of Intensive Care* 3: 11–15. (In Russ.)

Matthay M.A., Ware L.B, Zimmerman G.A. 2012. "The Acute Respiratory Distress Syndrome." *Journal of Clinical Investigation* 122: 2731–2740. https://doi.org/10.1172/JCI60331.

Mayr F.B., Yende S., Linde-Zwirble W.T., Peck-Palmer O.M., Barnato A.E., Weissfeld L.A., Angus D.C. 2010. "Infection Rate and Acute Organ Dysfunction Risk as Explanations for Racial Differences in Severe Sepsis." *Journal of the American Medical Association* 303: 2495–2503. https://doi.org/10.1001/jama.2010.851.

Medvedev Y.A. 2005. "Thanatological Analysis in Pathologo-anatomic Practice." Saint-Petersburg: Russian Polenov Scientific Research Neurosurgical Institute of Ministry of Health of Russia; 176. (In Russ.).

Medvedev Y.A., Rejnus K.B. 1989. "Hypothalamus in Neurosurgical Patients (Pathoanatomic and Clinical-Electrophysiological Correlations." *Archive of Pathology=Arkhiv patologii* 6: 37–43. (In Russ.)

Moraes C.A., Zaverucha-do-Valle C., Fleurance R., Sharshar T., Bozza F.A., d'Avila J.C. 2021. "Neuroinflammation in Sepsis: Molecular Pathways of Microglia Activation." *Pharmaceuticals (Basel)* 14 (5): 416. https://doi.org/10.3390/ph14050416.

Plaschke K., Do T.Q.M, Uhle F., Brenner T., Weigand M.A., Kopitz J. 2018. "Ablation of the Right Cardiac Vagus Nerve Reduces Acetylcholine Content without Changing the Inflammatory

Response during Endotoxemia." *International Journal of Molecular Sciences* 19 (2): 442. https://doi.org/10.3390/ijms1902044.
Purkayastha S., Stokes M., Bell K.R. 2019. "Autonomic Nervous System Dysfunction in Mild Traumatic Brain Injury: A Review of Related Pathophysiology and Symptoms." *Brain Injury* 33 (9): 1129–1136. PMID: 31216903. https://doi.org/10.1080/02699052.2019.1631488.
Qin L., Wu X., Block M.L., Liu Y., Breese G.R., Hong J.S., Knapp D.J., Crews F.T. 2007. "Systemic LPS Causes Chronic Neuroinflammation and Progressive Neurodegeneration." *Glia* 55 (5): 453–462. https://doi.org/10.1002/glia.20467.
Rada P., Mark G.P., Vitek M.P., Mangano R.M., Blume A.J., Beer B., Hoebel B.G. 1991. "Interleukin-1 Beta Decreases Acetylcholine Measured by Microdialysis in the Hippocampus of Freely Moving Rats." *Brain Research* 550: 287–290. https://doi.org/10.1016/0006-8993(91)91330-4.
Reale M., Costantini E. 2021. "Cholinergic Modulation of the Immune System in Neuroinflammatory Diseases." *Diseases* 9 (2): 29. https://doi.org/10.3390/diseases9020029.
Rello J., Leblebicioglu H. 2016. "Members of ESGCIP Sepsis and Septic Shock in Low-Income and Middle-Income Countries: Need for a Different Paradigm." *International Journal of Infectious Diseases* 48: 120–122. https://doi.org/10.1016/j.ijid.2016.04.017.
Rudnov V.A., Kulabuhov V.V. 2016. "Sepsis-3: Updated Key Provisions, Potential Problems and Further Practical Steps." *Vestnik anesteziologii i reanimatologii* 13 (4): 4–11. https://doi.org/10.21292/2078-5658-2016-13-4-4-11. (In Russ.).
Saharov V.I., Gulaj V.L., Ruslyakova I.A., Borzova Y.V. 2019. "Early Diagnosis of Sepsis in Elderly and Senile Patients with Comorbid Pathology." *Bulletin of the Bashkir State Medical University* 1 (2): 256–265. (In Russ).
Salomão R., Ferreira B.L., Salomão M.C., Santos S.S., Azevedo L.C.P., Brunialti M.K.C. 2019. "Sepsis: Evolving Concepts and Challenges." *Brazilian Journal of Medical and Biological Research* 52 (4): e8595. https://doi.org/10.1590/1414-431X20198595.
Savvina I.A., Petrova A.O., Zabrodskaya Y. M. 2021. "General Anesthesia and Autonomic Nervous System: Control and Management in Neurosurgery." *Autonomic Nervous System*. Ed. Intech Open; 24. https://doi.org/10.5772/intechopen.101829.
Savvina I.A., Zabrodskaya Y.M., Sebelev K.I., Petrova A.O., Bodareva N.V., Novikov V.Y., Rutkovskij R.V., Rasputina D.A. 2017. "Septic Encephalopathy: Pathophysiology, Pathomorphology, Clinical Syndromes, Therapeutic Tactics." *Neurosurgery and Neurology of Childhood* 4 (54): 20–33. https://doi.org/10.17116/hirurgia202207158. (In Russ.).
Serafim R., Gomes J.A., Salluh J. 2018. "A Comparison of the QuickSOFA and Systemic Inflammatory Response Syndrome Criteria for the Diagnosis of Sepsis and Prediction of Mortality: A Systematic Review and Meta-Analysis." *Chest* 153 (3): 646–655. https://doi.org/10.1016/j.chest.2017.12.015.
Serebryanaya N.B., Yakuceni P.P. 2020. "Platelets in the Development of Sepsis, Septic Shock and Multiple Organ Failure Syndrome." *Medical Immunology* 22 (6): 1085–1096. https://doi.org/10.15789/1563-0625-BPI-2090. (In Russ.).
Seymour C.W., Kennedy J.N., Wang S., Chang C.H., Elliott C.F., Xu Z., Berry S., Clermont G., Cooper G., Gomez H., Huang D.T., Kellum J.A., Mi Q., Opal S.M., Talisa V., van der Poll T., Visweswaran S., Vodovotz Y., Weiss J.C., Yealy D.M., Yende S., Angus D.C. 2019. "Derivation, Validation, and Potential Treatment Implications of Novel Clinical Phenotypes for Sepsis." *Journal of the American Medical Association* 321 (20): 2003–2017. https://doi.org/10.1001/jama.2019.5791.
Singer M., Deutschman C.S., Seymour C.W., Shankar-Hari M., Annane D., Bauer M. 2016. "The Third International Consensus Definitions for Sepsis and Septic Shock (Sepsis-3)." *Journal of the American Medical Association* 315: 801–810. https://doi.org/10.1001/jama.2016.0287.
Sonneville R., Verdonk F., Rauturier C., Klein I.F., Wolff M., Annane D. 2013. "Understanding Brain Dysfunction in Sepsis." *Annals of Intensive Care* 3 (1): 15. https://doi.org/10.1186/2110-5820-3-15.
Tian H.C., Zhou J.F., Weng L., Hu X.Y., Peng J.M., Wang C.Y., Jiang W., Du X.P., Xi X.M., An Y.Z., Duan M.L., Du B. 2019. "Epidemiology of Sepsis-3 in a Sub-District of Beijing: Secondary Analysis of a Population-Based Database." *Chinese Medical Journal* 132 (17): 2039–2045. https://doi.org/10.1097/CM9.0000000000000392.

Unsinger J. 2010. "IL-7 Promotes T Cell Viability, Trafficking, and Functionality and Improves Survival in Sepsis." *Journal of Immunology* 184: 3768–3779. https://doi.org/10.4049/jimmunol.0903151.

Varinthra P., Ganesan K., Huang S.P., Chompoopong S., Eurtivong C., Suresh P., Wen Z.H., Liu I.Y. 2021. "The 4-(Phenylsulfanyl) Butane-2-One Improves Impaired Fear Memory Retrieval and Reduces Excessive Inflammatory Response in Triple Transgenic Alzheimer's Disease Mice." *Frontiers in Aging Neuroscience* 13: 615079. https://doi.org/10.3389/fnagi.2021.615079.

Vincent J.L., Sakr Y., Sprung C.L. 2006. "Sepsis Occurrence in Acutely Ill Patients Investigators: Sepsis in European Intensive Care Units: Results of the SOAP Study." *Critical Care Medicine* 34: 344–353. https://doi.org/10.1097/01.ccm.0000194725.48928.3a.

Ward P.A. 2010. "The Harmful Role of C5a on Innate Immunity in Sepsis." *Journal of Innate Immunity* 2: 439–445. https://doi.org/10.1159/000317194.

Winkler M.S., Rissiek A., Priefler M., Schwedhelm E., Robbe L., Bauer A., Zahrte C., Zoellner C., Kluge S., Nierhaus A. 2017. "Human Leucocyte Antigen (HLA-DR) Gene Expression Is Reduced in Sepsis and Correlates with Impaired TNFα Response: A Diagnostic Tool for Immunosuppression?" *PLoS One* 12(8): e0182427. https://doi.org/10.1371/journal.pone.0182427.

Xu R., Yang C., Zhu B. 2020. "Research Progress of Delirium in Intensive Care Unit." *Zhonghua Wei Zhong Bing Ji Jiu Yi Xue* 32 (5): 636–640. https://doi.org/10.3760/cma.j.cn121430-20200204-00164.

Zakkar M. 2009. "Activation of Nrf2 in Endothelial Cells Protects Arteries from Exhibiting a Proinflammatory State." *Arteriosclerosis, Thrombosis, and Vascular Biology* 29: 1851–1857. https://doi.org/10.1161/ATVBAHA.109.193375.

Zhang Q.H., Sheng Z.Y., Yao Y.M. 2014. "Septic Encephalopathy: When Cytokines Interact with Acetylcholine in the Brain." *Military Medical Research* 1: 20. https://doi.org/10.1186/2054-9369-1-20.

Chapter 12

Molecular genetic aspects of diagnosis and clinical approaches of sepsis-associated encephalopathy

Irina A. Savvina[1,2*], MD., Ph.D., Kristina M. Bykova[1], MD, Eleonora T. Nazaralieva[3], MD., Ph.D.

[1] Department of Anesthesiology and Intensive Care, Almazov National Medical Research Centre of Ministry of Health Care of Russian Federation, Saint Petersburg, Russian Federation

[2] Department of Anesthesiology and Intensive Care named after V.L. Vanevskiy of the North-Western State Medical University named after Ilya I. Mechnikov of the Ministry of Health of Russian Federation, Saint Petersburg, Russian Federation

[3] Department of Pediatric Neurosurgery, Almazov National Medical Research Centre of Ministry of Health Care of Russian Federation, Saint Petersburg, Russian Federation

Abstract

Omics technologies based on the study of the human genome, proteome, and metabolome have opened up new possibilities for studying the pathophysiology of critical conditions, their diagnosis, and the development of modern targeted therapies for sepsis and sepsis-associated encephalopathy. In this chapter, the authors discuss strategies aimed at suppressing the neuroinflammatory cascade by targeting the nuclear protein HMGB1 using molecular inhibitors or inhibiting HMGB1 signaling pathways. They also examine the role of mtDNA and mitochondrial dysfunction in the pathophysiological cascades of SAE development, which will likely enable clinical trials soon using mitochondria-targeted therapeutic agents (e.g., mitochondrial antioxidants) that can prevent and/or treat delirium in sepsis. The authors present data on risk factors for SAE development, such as race/ethnicity, and the diagnostic role of microRNA in sepsis-associated encephalopathy.

Keywords: sepsis-associated encephalopathy, mitochondrial dysfunction, mtDNA, HMGB1 protein, microRNA.

* Corresponding author: Irina A. Savvina, Professor, MD., Ph.D.
e-mail address: irinasavvina@mail.ru

Editor: Irina A. Savvina, Natalia V. Beloborodova and Tatyana N. Trofimova
In: Sepsis-Associated Encephalopathy
ISBN: 979-8-89113-178-1

Introduction

Sepsis-associated encephalopathy (SAE) is the most common cause of encephalopathy in medical and surgical intensive care units. SAE is also associated with a higher risk of developing long-term cognitive impairments in sepsis survivors and an increased predisposition to neuropsychiatric disorders such as dementia, depression, anxiety, and post-traumatic stress disorder [1].

The results of experimental and clinical studies have shown that the inflammatory response in sepsis induces cellular and tissue stress characterized by increased production of reactive oxygen species (ROS), impaired oxygen delivery, oxygen extraction dysfunction, increased lactate production, and disrupted homeostasis regulation [2]. These events occur within the mitochondria, which regulate ROS production, oxygen metabolism, and nutrient metabolism. Mitochondrial dysfunction, such as impaired mitochondrial metabolism and mitochondrial biogenesis failure, has been associated with organ dysfunction in sepsis in numerous studies [3]. However, only a few have examined its impact on the brain, which is particularly vulnerable to metabolic and oxidative damage. Considering the evidence linking mitochondrial dysfunction to neurodegeneration [4], it could be expected that factors negatively affecting mitochondrial function during sepsis increase the risk of delirium.

High mobility group box 1 (HMGB1)

In preclinical studies, the role of high mobility group box 1 (HMGB1) alarmin in the complex pathogenesis of sepsis-associated encephalopathy (SAE) has been described. While limited data exist regarding the role of HMGB1 in neuroinflammation during sepsis, it is known to be involved in other neurological disorders (its translocation from the nucleus to the extracellular space triggers neuroinflammatory reactions and disrupts the blood-brain barrier). Suppression of the inflammatory cascade by targeting HMGB1 may serve as a complementary strategy to non-pharmacological therapy aimed at combating encephalopathy [5].

HMGB1 is a widely distributed nuclear protein that is highly conserved in mammals and belongs to the high-mobility group (HMG) protein family. It was initially identified as a chromatin-associated protein in the calf thymus and acquired its name due to its high electrophoretic mobility [6]. The nucleus of HMGB1 is involved in multiple important processes, such as DNA replication and repair, chromatin remodeling, transcription, and genome stabilization [7].

HMGB1 has been recognized as an important component in the inflammatory response during sepsis. It is released by immune cells and necrotic tissues and acts as a potent neuroinflammatory mediator [8]. When HMGB1 is present in the extracellular environment, it interacts with macrophage/monocyte receptors such as toll-like receptor 4 (TLR4) [9] and receptor for advanced glycation end products (RAGE) [10], leading to enhanced chemotaxis and activation of the NF-κB signaling pathway. This activates the gene expression and release of pro-inflammatory cytokines, including IL-6 and IL-1β. Strategies targeting HMGB1 using molecular inhibitors [11] or inhibiting HMGB1 signaling pathways [12] are effective in reducing mortality in experimental sepsis models and altering early cytokine profiles to patterns observed in survivors. In the brain, HMGB1 is expressed in all cell types, including microglia. Overexpression of extracellular HMGB1 has been observed in several neuroinflammatory conditions, including traumatic brain injury (TBI) [13], subarachnoid hemorrhage (SAH) [14], and neurodegenerative diseases [15]. Active translocation of HMGB1 from the nucleus to the extracellular space has been found to induce neuroinflammatory reactions and blood-brain barrier (BBB) damage. Furthermore, HMGB1 is capable of regulating the phenotypic polarization of M1/M2 microglia, leading to cortical damage [16], as well as alterations in the morphology and function of endothelial cells and pericytes in an experimental BBB model [17]. Therefore, HMGB1 has emerged as an extracellular target against a wide range of central nervous system (CNS) disorders, including sepsis-associated encephalopathy (SAE). Targeted therapy against HMGB1 has been shown to exert neuroprotective effects in CNS disorders, primarily by inhibiting its translocation and suppressing the immune response [13, 15].

Mitochondrial DNA haplogroups in sepsis

Genetic studies indicate that race can be a risk factor for the development of sepsis-associated encephalopathy (SAE). The research group of Samuels and Girard was the first to investigate the role of mitochondrial DNA (mtDNA) in the development of sepsis and SAE. After adjusting for age, they demonstrated a relative risk of 1.36 (95% CI: 1.13-1.64; p-value = 0.001) among individuals of European descent belonging to mtDNA haplogroup IWX compared to other haplogroups among Europeans, and a relative risk of 0.60 (95% CI: 0.38-0.94; p-value = 0.03) among African Americans belonging to mtDNA haplogroup L2 concerning the development of SAE [18]. These data suggest that certain ethnic groups are associated with a higher risk of developing SAE, while others appear to exhibit a protective factor.

Regarding HMGB1 levels, Chen et al. (2020) demonstrated a significantly elevated level in the cohort of Black individuals compared to the cohort of White individuals [19], which correlates with previous data on higher levels of pro-inflammatory markers such as hs-CRP and IL-6 in Black ethnic groups [20, 21]. Further research is needed to determine potential racial protective factors or risk factors for the development of SAE.

Unlike nuclear/chromosomal DNA, mtDNA does not undergo recombination and is exclusively inherited through the maternal lineage, leading to various maternal lineage-specific variations known as "haplogroups." MtDNA encodes 13 out of 90 oxidative phosphorylation proteins that control mitochondrial function [22, 23], and mtDNA haplogroups have been associated with neurodegenerative disorders such as Alzheimer's disease [24] and Parkinson's disease [25]. In sepsis, mtDNA haplogroups have been linked to mortality among Asian [26] and European [27] populations. These findings may be a result of haplogroup-associated alterations in oxidative phosphorylation or altered gene expression involved in inflammation, complement activation, and apoptosis, each of which has been associated with mtDNA variants determining haplogroup status [28].

Among Europeans, Baudouin et al. [29] found that haplogroup H is associated with improved survival in sepsis, while Lorente et al. [27] found that clade JT is a predictor of survival in septic patients. Alternatively, Jiménez-Sousa et al. [30] recently published a study of 507 European individuals with postoperative sepsis, in which the IWX clade was identified as a risk factor for mortality. Yan et al. [31] discovered that the Asian haplogroup R of mtDNA was a predictor of recovery from sepsis-associated encephalopathy, as diagnosed using the Glasgow Coma Scale.

If future studies confirm that mtDNA and mitochondrial dysfunction play a significant pathophysiological role in the development of sepsis-associated encephalopathy (SAE), clinical trials using mitochondria-targeted therapeutic agents (such as mitochondrial antioxidants) may be able to prevent and/or treat delirium during sepsis.

Furthermore, personalized management of sepsis patients based on haplogroups could be a promising direction, considering that the choice of antibiotics, thermoregulation management strategies, control of electrolyte balance and metabolites, nutritional strategies, selection of sedatives, and other aspects of intensive therapy may influence and/or be influenced by mitochondrial function. For instance, patients with the highest risk of mtDNA-associated delirium may have a higher likelihood of experiencing delirium due to benzodiazepines, which decrease cerebral metabolic rate by 20–30% and are associated with an increased risk of delirium in critical conditions in numerous observational [32, 33] and randomized studies [34]. Additionally, mtDNA haplogroups may potentially guide glucose [35] therapy and nutrition during sepsis in the future, considering that global cerebral metabolic rate dynamically decreases with glucose intake, and common medications may impede adaptive changes in carbon substrate transport that support the damaged brain.

The growing list of factors influencing cerebral metabolism and cognitive function during critical conditions suggests that new insights into the links between mtDNA haplogroups and sepsis-associated delirium are likely to shape future sepsis treatment trials and ultimately enable a personalized approach.

The diagnostic value of microRNAs in sepsis-associated encephalopathy

MicroRNAs have attracted attention for consideration in the context of sepsis-associated encephalopathy (SAE) as potential diagnostic and therapeutic targets for neurodegenerative diseases. They exist in various body fluids and are highly stable. Based on the specific characteristics of microRNAs as biomarkers for other neurodegenerative diseases, it is reasonable to conclude that microRNAs will be superior biomarkers for SAE [36].

They play an important role in various neurobiological processes, such as cell differentiation, proliferation, metabolism, regulation of the cell cycle, and apoptosis [37].

The high degree of microRNA differentiation indicates that a single microRNA can target multiple genes and regulate various biological pathways [38]. In pathological conditions such as neurodegenerative diseases, network patterns of gene regulation converge on different biological pathways to govern disease phenotypes [39].

Current evidence suggests that the blood-brain barrier (BBB) does not impede the passage of microRNAs between cerebrospinal fluid and blood [40]. MicroRNAs can enter the bloodstream from brain tissue through the BBB during various diseases, making them potential biomarkers for central nervous system (CNS) disorders [41].

Previous studies have shown that microRNAs, key gene regulators of various biological pathways, are closely associated with disease progression and play a crucial role in the onset and progression of neurodegenerative disorders, as well as in neuronal differentiation and synaptic plasticity [37, 42]. MicroRNAs have been extensively studied and can be used for the diagnosis of Alzheimer's disease, Parkinson's disease, multiple sclerosis, epilepsy, and other disorders [43, 44].

Studies have shown that levels of miR-370-3p increase in the brain and plasma during sepsis-associated encephalopathy (SAE), but not in uremic encephalopathy. Overexpression of miR-370-3p enhances susceptibility to apoptosis upon cytokine or lipopolysaccharide (LPS) activation. TNF-α induces apoptosis in PC-12 neurons by activating the expression of miR-370-3p in PC-12 neurons [45]. miR-370-3p is upregulated in SAE. YY1 may contribute to the polarization of M2 microglia by inhibiting the activity of the miR-130a-3p promoter, thereby improving SAE [46]. miR-25-3p is expressed at low levels in the brain cortex of mice with SAE, while microglia are hyperactivated. In vitro experiments have demonstrated that enhancing the expression of miR-25-3p can attenuate microglial activation in SAE by directly targeting Toll-like receptor 4 (TLR4) to inhibit the NLRP3/IL-1β/IL-18 axis, suggesting a protective role of miR-25-3p against SAE [47]. Although limited microRNAs have been studied in SAE, it is expected that certain microRNAs during sepsis may be associated with SAE, particularly those involved in inflammation.

In severe sepsis with thrombocytopenia, miR-130a is suppressed. The mechanism behind this involves the suppression of miR-130a leading to increased expression of IL-18, which worsens thrombocytopenia in severe sepsis [48]. In the study by Yao et al. (2015), miR-25 was found to be the most significantly altered RNA in sepsis, and decreased levels of miR-25 correlated with the severity of sepsis, SOFA scores, and CRP levels [49], which is consistent with the findings reported by Antonakos et al. (2022) [50].

Levels of miR-27a rapidly decrease in microglia after LPS stimulation, while overexpression of miR-27a significantly reduces the production of inflammatory cytokines such as IL-6, IL-1β, TNF-α, and NO. miR-27a directly inhibits the expression of TLR4 and IRAK4, key adaptor kinases in the TLR4/MyD88 signaling pathway [51]. The inhibitor of miR-210 can effectively suppress microglia-mediated neuroinflammation. miR-210 induces the activation of M1 microglia by targeting SIRT1, thereby reducing the deacetylation of the p65 NF-κB subunit and increasing NF-κB signaling activity [52]. Low levels of miR-210 exhibit neuroprotective effects in mice with hypoxic-ischemic encephalopathy [53]; however, its impact on SAE is yet to be studied.

Conclusion

Genetic studies indicate that race can be a risk factor for the development of SAE. It is well known that mitochondrial dysfunction underlies the pathophysiological events at the cellular level during critical conditions, including sepsis-associated encephalopathy. Recent experimental research findings are promising, suggesting that mitochondria-targeted therapeutic agents can alleviate the manifestations of SAE. Exploring the role of mtDNA and microRNAs in the development of critical conditions and sepsis opens up new possibilities for clinicians and enhances patients' chances of a favorable prognosis.

References

[1] Chung H-Y, Wickel J, Brunkhorst FM, et al. Sepsis-associated encephalopathy: From delirium to dementia? *J Clin Med* 2020; 9: 703. doi:10.3390/jcm9030703

[2] Andrades MÉ, Morina A, Spasić S, et al. Bench-to-bedside review: Sepsis - from the redox point of view. *Crit Care Lond Engl* 2011; 15: 230. doi:10.1186/cc10334

[3] Singer M. The role of mitochondrial dysfunction in sepsis-induced multi-organ failure. *Virulence* 2014; 5: 66–72. doi:10.4161/viru.26907

[4] Federico A, Cardaioli E, Da Pozzo P, et al. Mitochondria, oxidative stress, and neurodegeneration. *J Neurol Sci* 2012; 322: 254–262. doi:10.1016/j.jns.2012.05.030

[5] DeWulf B, Minsart L, Verdonk F, et al. High mobility group box 1 (HMGB1): Potential target in sepsis-associated encephalopathy. *Cells* 2023; 12: 1088. doi:10.3390/cells12071088

[6] Goodwin GH, Sanders C, Johns EW. A new group of chromatin-associated proteins with a high content of acidic and basic amino acids. *Eur J Biochem* 1973; 38: 14–19. doi:10.1111/j.1432-1033.1973.tb03026.x
[7] Agresti A, Bianchi ME. HMGB proteins and gene expression. *Curr Opin Genet Dev* 2003; 13: 170–178. doi:10.1016/S0959-437X(03)00023-6
[8] Diener KR, Al-Dasooqi N, Lousberg EL, et al. The multifunctional alarmin HMGB1 with roles in the pathophysiology of sepsis and cancer. *Immunol Cell Biol* 2013; 91: 443–450. doi:10.1038/icb.2013.25
[9] Yu M, Wang H, Ding A, et al. HMGB1 signals through toll-like receptor (TLR) 4 and TLR2. *Shock Augusta Ga* 2006; 26: 174–179. doi:10.1097/01.shk.0000225404.51320.82
[10] Sims GP, Rowe DC, Rietdijk ST, et al. HMGB1 and RAGE in inflammation and cancer. *Annu Rev Immunol* 2010; 28: 367–388. doi:10.1146/annurev.immunol.021908.132603
[11] Terrando N, Yang T, Wang X, et al. Systemic HMGB1 neutralization prevents postoperative neurocognitive dysfunction in aged rats. *Front Immunol* 2016; 7: 441. doi: 10.3389/fimmu.2016.00441
[12] Wei L, Zhang W, Li Y, et al. The SIRT1-HMGB1 axis: Therapeutic potential to ameliorate inflammatory responses and tumor occurrence. *Front Cell Dev Biol* 2022;10: 986511. doi: 10.3389/fcell.2022.986511
[13] Okuma Y, Liu K, Wake H, et al. Anti–high mobility group box-1 antibody therapy for traumatic brain injury. *Ann Neurol* 2012; 72: 373–384. doi:10.1002/ana.23602
[14] Sun Q, Wu W, Hu Y-C, et al. Early release of high-mobility group box 1 (HMGB1) from neurons in experimental subarachnoid hemorrhage in vivo and in vitro. *J Neuroinflammation* 2014; 11: 106. doi:10.1186/1742-2094-11-106
[15] Fujita K, Motoki K, Tagawa K, et al. HMGB1, a pathogenic molecule that induces neurite degeneration via TLR4-MARCKS, is a potential therapeutic target for Alzheimer's disease. *Sci Rep* 2016; 6: 31895. doi:10.1038/srep31895
[16] Sun Y, Hei M, Fang Z, et al. High-mobility group box 1 contributes to cerebral cortex injury in a neonatal hypoxic-ischemic rat model by regulating the phenotypic polarization of microglia. *Front Cell Neurosci* 2019; 13: 506. doi:10.3389/fncel.2019.00506
[17] Zhang J, Takahashi HK, Liu K, et al. Anti-high mobility group box-1 monoclonal antibody protects the blood-brain barrier from ischemia-induced disruption in rats. *Stroke* 2011; 42: 1420–1428. doi:10.1161/STROKEAHA.110.598334
[18] Samuels DC, Hulgan T, Fessel JP, et al. Mitochondrial DNA haplogroups and delirium during sepsis. *Crit Care Med* 2019; 47: 1065–1071. doi:10.1097/CCM.0000000000003810
[19] Chen L, Zhu H, Su S, et al. High-mobility group box-1 is associated with obesity, inflammation, and subclinical cardiovascular risk among young adults: A longitudinal cohort study. *Arterioscler Thromb Vasc Biol* 2020; 40: 2776–2784. doi:10.1161/ATVBAHA.120.314599
[20] Starzak DE, Semple SJ, Smith LL, et al. Differing cytokine responses by ethnic groups to a bout of exercise-induced muscle damage: A preliminary report. *J Sports Med Phys Fitness* 2016; 56: 665–677.
[21] Stepanikova I, Bateman LB, Oates GR. Systemic inflammation in midlife: Race, socioeconomic status, and perceived discrimination. *Am J Prev Med* 2017; 52: S63–S76. doi:10.1016/j.amepre.2016.09.026
[22] Gómez-Durán A, Pacheu-Grau D, Martínez-Romero I, et al. Oxidative phosphorylation differences between mitochondrial DNA haplogroups modify the risk of Leber's hereditary optic neuropathy. *Biochim Biophys Acta* 2012; 1822: 1216–1222. doi:10.1016/j.bbadis.2012.04.014
[23] Larsen S, Díez-Sánchez C, Rabøl R, et al. Increased intrinsic mitochondrial function in humans with mitochondrial haplogroup H. *Biochim Biophys Acta* 2014; 1837: 226–231. doi:10.1016/j.bbabio.2013.10.009
[24] Ridge PG, Maxwell TJ, Corcoran CD, et al. Mitochondrial genomic analysis of late-onset Alzheimer's disease reveals protective haplogroups H6A1A/H6A1B: The cache county study on memory in aging. *PloS One* 2012; 7: e45134. doi:10.1371/journal.pone.0045134
[25] Hudson G, Nalls M, Evans JR, et al. Two-stage association study and meta-analysis of mitochondrial DNA variants in Parkinson's disease. *Neurology* 2013; 80: 2042–2048. doi:10.1212/WNL.0b013e318294b434

[26] Yang Y, Shou Z, Zhang P, et al. Mitochondrial DNA haplogroup R predicts survival advantage in severe sepsis in the Han population. *Genet Med Off J Am Coll Med Genet* 2008; 10: 187–192. doi:10.1097/GIM.0b013e318163c343

[27] Lorente L, Iceta R, Martín MM, et al. Severe septic patients with mitochondrial DNA haplogroup JT show higher survival rates: A prospective, multicenter, observational study. *PloS One* 2013; 8: e73320. doi:10.1371/journal.pone.0073320

[28] Kenney MC, Chwa M, Atilano SR, et al. Inherited mitochondrial DNA variants can affect complement, inflammation and apoptosis pathways: insights into mitochondrial-nuclear interactions. *Hum Mol Genet* 2014; 23: 3537–3551. doi:10.1093/hmg/ddu065

[29] Baudouin SV, Saunders D, Tiangyou W, et al. Mitochondrial DNA and survival after sepsis: A prospective study. *Lancet Lond Engl* 2005; 366: 2118–2121. doi:10.1016/S0140-6736(05)67890-7

[30] Jiménez-Sousa MA, Tamayo E, Guzmán-Fulgencio M, et al. Mitochondrial DNA haplogroups are associated with severe sepsis and mortality in patients who underwent major surgery. *J Infect* 2015; 70: 20–29. doi:10.1016/j.jinf.2014.07.005

[31] Yang Y, Zhang P, Lv R, et al. Mitochondrial DNA haplogroup R in the Han population and recovery from septic encephalopathy. *Intensive Care Med* 2011; 37: 1613–1619. doi:10.1007/s00134-011-2319-9

[32] Pandharipande P, Shintani A, Peterson J, et al. Lorazepam is an independent risk factor for transitioning to delirium in intensive care unit patients. *Anesthesiology* 2006; 104: 21–26. doi:10.1097/00000542-200601000-00005

[33] Seymour CW, Pandharipande PP, Koestner T, et al. Diurnal sedative changes during intensive care: impact on liberation from mechanical ventilation and delirium. *Crit Care Med* 2012; 40: 2788–2796. doi:10.1097/CCM.0b013e31825b8ade

[34] Riker RR, Shehabi Y, Bokesch PM, et al. Dexmedetomidine vs midazolam for sedation of critically ill patients: A randomized trial. *JAMA* 2009; 301: 489–499. doi:10.1001/jama.2009.56

[35] Xu F, Liu P, Pascual JM, et al. Acute effect of glucose on cerebral blood flow, blood oxygenation, and oxidative metabolism. *Hum Brain Mapp* 2015; 36: 707–716. doi:10.1002/hbm.22658

[36] Yuechen Z, Shaosong X, Zhouxing Z, et al. A summary of the current diagnostic methods for, and exploration of the value of microRNAs as biomarkers in, sepsis-associated encephalopathy. *Front Neurosci* 2023; 17:1125888. doi: 10.3389/fnins.2023.1125888

[37] Nowakowski TJ, Rani N, Golkaram M, et al. Regulation of cell-type-specific transcriptomes by microRNA networks during human brain development. *Nat Neurosci* 2018; 21: 1784–1792. doi:10.1038/s41593-018-0265-3

[38] Valinezhad Orang A, Safaralizadeh R, Kazemzadeh-Bavili M. Mechanisms of miRNA-mediated gene regulation from common downregulation to mRNA-specific upregulation. *Int J Genomics* 2014; 2014: 970607. doi:10.1155/2014/970607

[39] Juźwik CA, S Drake S, Zhang Y, et al. microRNA dysregulation in neurodegenerative diseases: A systematic review. *Prog Neurobiol* 2019; 182: 101664. doi:10.1016/j.pneurobio.2019.101664

[40] Stoicea N, Du A, Lakis DC, et al. The MiRNA journey from theory to practice as a CNS biomarker. *Front Genet* 2016; 7: 11. doi:10.3389/fgene.2016.00011

[41] Dalkara T, Alarcon-Martinez L. Cerebral microvascular pericytes and neurogliovascular signaling in health and disease. *Brain Res* 2015; 1623: 3–17. doi:10.1016/j.brainres.2015.03.047

[42] Sohel MH. Extracellular/circulating MicroRNAs: Release mechanisms, functions and challenges. *Achieve Life Sci* 2016; 10: 175–186. doi:10.1016/j.als.2016.11.007

[43] Singh T, Yadav S. Role of microRNAs in neurodegeneration induced by environmental neurotoxicants and aging. *Ageing Res Rev* 2020; 60: 101068. doi:10.1016/j.arr.2020.101068

[44] Bazrgar M, Khodabakhsh P, Prudencio M, et al. The role of microRNA-34 family in Alzheimer's disease: A potential molecular link between neurodegeneration and metabolic disorders. *Pharmacol Res* 2021; 172: 105805. doi:10.1016/j.phrs.2021.105805

[45] Visitchanakun P, Tangtanatakul P, Trithiphen O, et al. Plasma miR-370-3P as a Biomarker of sepsis-associated encephalopathy, the transcriptomic profiling analysis of microrna-arrays from mouse brains. *Shock Augusta Ga* 2020; 54: 347–357. doi:10.1097/SHK.0000000000001473

[46] Peng L-S, Xu Y, Wang Q-S. YY1 promotes microglia M2 polarization through the MIR-130A-3P/TREM-2 axis to alleviate sepsis-associated encephalopathy. *Shock Augusta Ga* 2022; 58: 128–136. doi:10.1097/SHK.0000000000001914
[47] Luo X-Y, Ying J-H, Wang Q-S. miR-25-3p ameliorates SAE by targeting the TLR4/NLRP3 axis. *Metab Brain Dis* 2022; 37: 1803–1813. doi:10.1007/s11011-022-01017-1
[48] Cui Y-L, Wang B, Gao H-M, et al. Interleukin-18 and miR-130a in severe sepsis patients with thrombocytopenia. *Patient Prefer Adherence* 2016; 10: 313–319. doi:10.2147/PPA.S95588
[49] Yao L, Liu Z, Zhu J, et al. Clinical evaluation of circulating microRNA-25 level change in sepsis and its potential relationship with oxidative stress. *Int J Clin Exp Pathol* 2015; 8: 7675–7684.
[50] Antonakos N, Gilbert C, Théroude C, et al. Modes of action and diagnostic value of miRNAs in sepsis. *Front Immunol* 2022; 13: 951798. doi:10.3389/fimmu.2022.951798
[51] Lv Y-N, Ou-Yang A-J, Fu L-S. MicroRNA-27a negatively modulates the inflammatory response in lipopolysaccharide-stimulated microglia by targeting TLR4 and IRAK4. *Cell Mol Neurobiol* 2017; 37: 195–210. doi:10.1007/s10571-016-0361-4
[52] Li B, Dasgupta C, Huang L, et al. MiRNA-210 induces microglial activation and regulates microglia-mediated neuroinflammation in neonatal hypoxic-ischemic encephalopathy. *Cell Mol Immunol* 2020; 17: 976–991. doi:10.1038/s41423-019-0257-6
[53] Ma Q, Dasgupta C, Li Y, et al. Inhibition of microRNA-210 provides neuroprotection in hypoxic-ischemic brain injury in neonatal rats. *Neurobiol Dis* 2016; 89: 202–212. doi:10.1016/j.nbd.2016.02.011

Expert comments

Modern conception about the pathogenesis of sepsis-associated encephalopathy

The chapter "Modern conception about the pathogenesis of sepsis-associated encephalopathy" describes an important and interesting topic – a transient and reversible dysfunction of the brain that develops in a patient if there is a focus of infection as a source of sepsis outside the central nervous system, which leads to further cerebral damage due to different pathophysiological mechanisms in sepsis. The presented review covers the description of the basis pathogenetic links of the development of sepsis-associated encephalopathy (SAE) – diffuse neuroinflammation, ischemia, and neurotoxic processes.

The authors analyze a variety of mechanisms that may underlie damage to the blood–brain barrier (BBB), activation of microglia, neurotransmission imbalance, hypoperfusion, ischemic damage to neurons and violation of their trophy, astrogliosis, neuronal pyroptosis and apoptosis, secondary neuroanatomic changes in the brain in sepsis. Among these mechanisms, such as endothelial Injury and the role of endothelial factors such as impaired nitric oxide formation, endothelin-1 synthesis, mitochondrial dysfunction, and many others are noted. The authors describe the importance of two types of activated microglia phenotypes: pro-inflammatory phenotype M1 and anti-inflammatory M2, which is activated by anti-inflammatory cellular mediators, including IL-13 and IL-3, IL-10 and IL-17A, HMGB1 signaling pathways, and neurotrophic factors to repair brain tissue and neurons. In addition, the authors considered the role of mitochondrial cyclophilin D isomerase (CypD) in mitochondrial dysfunction and permeability, cellular apoptosis in SAE, oxidative stress cascade, family of transcription factors regulating cell migration, and other intracellular systems.

The literature list is sufficient, and modern sources are used. This chapter is quite voluminous and well-illustrated with original drawings. The present chapter describes the mechanisms of different cerebral structure damage and neuronal cell death in sepsis, including the hippocampus, which have been reviewed both on experimental material and the clinical studies. The chapter will be interesting because it describes all modern ideas about the mechanisms of the development of acute brain damage in sepsis and subsequent neurological and cognitive deficit.

Nikolay A. Belyakov, *D.Sc.Med., Professor,*
Academician of the Russian Academy of Sciences,
Honored Worker of Science,
Head of the Department of Socially Significant Infections and Phthisiopulmonology
Pavlov State University,
Saint Petersburg, Russia

Expert comments

Biomarkers of sepsis-associated encephalopathy

Sepsis is one of the most common complications in intensive care units leading to death. Critical factors causing severe septic shock include a systemic and intravascular inflammatory cascade in combination with impaired host immune response. Approximately one third of septic patients develop sepsis-associated encephalopathy (SAE). An early sign of SAE is impaired consciousness along with other manifestations including anxiety, depression, irritability, and cognitive decline. Neurological dysfunction can persist for several years in many sepsis survivors and seriously affect their quality of life. Important factors that can induce the development of SAE include neuroinflammation, blood–brain barrier destruction, metabolic disorders and neurovascular unit dysfunction. Early diagnosis and management of patients with SAE is essential to reduce disability and mortality.

There is an urgent need to develop biomarkers with high sensitivity and specificity to aid in early diagnosis and ultimately improve treatment outcomes for patients with SAE. The authors of the Chapter "Biomarkers of sepsis-associated encephalopathy" rightly noted, the evaluation of several biomarkers corresponding to one or another stage of the pathophysiological process may be more effective for the detection and monitoring of SAE. This chapter analyzes in detail the results of experimental and clinical studies of biomarkers, as known and the most promising. Individual groups of biomarkers are considered from the point of view of various stages of the pathophysiology of SAE. The authors summarized the data of the most significant works and presented them in the form of an original scheme. Further studies are needed to identify the correlation between neurophysiological parameters and individual groups of biomarkers.

In the future, the biomarkers of SAE will help develop comprehensive diagnostic algorithm that will allow clinicians to determine the degree of brain damage in septic patients and identify those who primarily need neurocognitive rehabilitation.

Zamyatin Mikhail Nikolaevich, *MD, PhD, Professor, Chief Specialist in Anesthesiology and Resuscitation of the N.I. Pirogov Scientific and Medical Surgical Center of the Ministry of Health of Russia, Moscow*

Expert comments

The role of microbiota and microbial metabolites in sepsis-associated encephalopathy

Along with the intensive study of sepsis, the number of studies of the mechanisms of sepsis-associated encephalopathy (SAE) development is growing all over the world, and new opportunities are being sought for the diagnosis, treatment and prediction of this severe complication of sepsis. The Chapter discusses the complex problem of the etiopathogenesis of SAE and the role of microbial factor, an attempt was made to consider the microbiota and its metabolites as active participants in encephalopathy developing during the septic process. This relatively new approach to the problem has become possible in recent years due to the improvement of microbiological methods, research has reached a new level of knowledge through the use of the metabolomic approach and technology based on chromatography-mass spectrometry.,

The authors of the chapter conducted a thorough search for published facts about bacteria, their structural components and their metabolites, confirming the connection with the development of encephalopathy. For an objective and comprehensive analysis, the authors used not only the latest data, publications for 2020–2023, but also paid tribute to fundamental research, referring to experiments conducted in the 80s of the last century. Systematization of data on microbial metabolites is certainly of great importance for future readers and for everyone who deals with the problem of sepsis-associated encephalopathy. The presented material will serve as a basis for the development of new methods of laboratory monitoring in septic patients, which will allow timely correction of metabolic disorders and reduce the frequency of such dangerous complications as SAE.

Pogorelskaya Lidiya V.,
PhD, DSMed, Professor,
Department of Infectious Diseases
Russian Academy of Continuing Professional
Education, Ministry of Health RF

Expert comments

Clinical assessment of sepsis-associated encephalopathy

The presented chapter is devoted to the topical issue of modern intensive care. Sepsis remains a widespread critical condition with a high mortality rate. One of the manifestations of sepsis is sepsis-associated encephalopathy (SAE), which also significantly aggravates the clinical course of the disease. These aspects determine the high importance of early diagnosis and adequate assessment of the severity of SAE, which is the subject of this manuscript.

The authors described approaches to the early diagnosis of SAE and the significance of differential diagnosis for primary and secondary CNS lesions of various origins. It was noted that SAE can be both an early manifestation of sepsis and an element of multiple organ failure. Approaches to neurological screening are described, including assessment by Confusion Assessment Methods for Intensive Care Unit (CAM-ICU), Intensive Care Delirium Screening Checklist (ICDSC), Full outline of UnResponsiveness score (FOUR) (these scales are also given in the appendices), and Glasgow Coma Scale (GCS). Much attention among the forms of SAE is given to delirium: direct and secondary etiological triggers, express diagnostic methods, like the Months of the Year Backwards (MOTYB), and the 4 A test (4AT), the importance of clinical neuromonitoring to diagnose concomitant neurological disorders are considered. The authors selected the methods for assessing the severity and prognosis in the development of multiple organ failure, including the SOFA and SAPS II scales. It is important to identify the clinical SAE phenotypes, including ischemic-hypoxic, metabolic, mixed, and unclassified, which makes it possible to understand the pathogenetic mechanisms of the patient's aggravation and also has prognostic significance. The mechanisms of development and the approach to the diagnosis of another significant complication, ICU-acquired weakness (ICUAW), are described. The possibilities of using the Medical Research Council Sum Score, Handgrip test, peroneal nerve test, and electroneuromyography in the diagnosis of this pathological condition are given. The authors detailed the patient's outcomes, in particular, prolonged cognitive impairment associated with SAE.

The considered approaches to the diagnosis and assessment of the severity of SAE and associated complications are modern and meet the requirements of clinical practice. The style of presentation is accessible and covers the most significant diagnostic techniques, the mentioned scales are given in the appendix section. The given author's schemes increase the visibility of the presentation of the material. The list of references includes 56 publications, at least half of which are in the last 5 years. Thus, this chapter will be useful for students, residents, postgraduates, and a wide range of practicing physicians.

Vadim I. Ershov, *Dr. Med. Sci., professor and chairman,*
Department of Anesthesiology and Intensive Care,
Director of University Scientific Clinical Center of Neurology,
Neuroreanimatology and Neurosurgery,
Orenburg Medical State University,
Orenburg, Russia

Expert comments

Neurophysiological assessment of sepsis-associated encephalopathy

The use of neurophysiological methods in severe brain injury has become a standard practice in intensive care units. The present chapter is devoted to their use in patients with sepsis-related encephalopathy characterized by diffuse brain damage.

The authors provide a detailed overview of the methodology and analysis of the results of electroencephalography and multimodal evoked potentials with a focus on their application in patients with sepsis-induced encephalopathy.

In addition to a detailed literature review, the results of our own scientific research are also presented.

The chapter is well illustrated with examples of long-term EEG monitoring in patients with sepsis-associated encephalopathy with varying severity of disease progression.

The section on multimodal evoked potentials includes images obtained from the study of visual, short-term somatosensory and auditory evoked potentials in the brainstem in both normal and sepsis brain damage.

The chapter devoted to neurophysiological research methods in sepsis-induced encephalopathy is important and useful for the reader of the monograph, as it is filled with scientific content.

M.V. Sinkin, *Doctor of Medical Sciences, Leading Researcher,*
Head of the Clinical Neurophysiology Group
Department of Emergency Neurosurgery,
N.V. Sklifosovsky Research Institute of Emergency Medicine,
Moscow, Russia

Expert comments

Neuroradiology of sepsis-associated encephalopathy

One of the most common neurological complications of sepsis is sepsis-associated encephalopathy (SAE), a diffuse cerebral dysfunction due to a systemic inflammatory response syndrome. The incidence of SAE in patients with sepsis is approximately 35–71% and is a risk factor for long-term disability and mortality, as well as the occurrence of long-term cognitive impairment. At the same time, the neuroimaging patterns of the SAE are poorly understood and require clarification and analysis. The foregoing substantiates the relevance of research conducted by a group of neuroradiologists headed by Professor T.N. Trofimova. The authors consider the leading neuroradiological patterns and give them a pathogenetic and pathophysiological assessment. Particular attention is paid to the combination of imaging findings. It is extremely important to discuss the differences and similarities in other sepsis-associated brain lesions. Thus, the topic of differentiation of sepsis-associated encephalopathy, sepsis-embolic encephalitis, and sepsis-metastatic encephalitis is very complex and controversial. The authors define the place of neuroimaging methods in the diagnostic algorithm, emphasizing the need to exclude other conditions that lead to brain dysfunction. The chapter is well illustrated whereby promoting a deeper understanding of the material presented. The presentation style chosen by the authors helps not only to state the current knowledge of neuroradiological semiotics but also outlines ways for further development of the topic of neuroimaging of sepsis-associated brain lesions.

Andrey Tulupov

MD, PhD, Professor, Member of the Russian Academy of Sciences.
Chief scientific secretary of The Siberian branch of the Russian Academy of Sciences.
Deputy Director, Chief researcher, Head of the Laboratory «MRT TECHNOLOGIES» of The Institute International Tomography Center of the Russian Academy of Sciences.
Professor at The Institute for the Medicine and Psychology of the Novosibirsk State University.

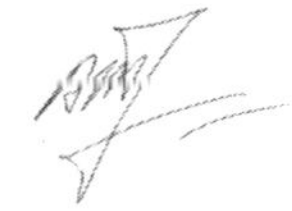

Expert comments

Positron emission tomography in sepsis-associated encephalopathy

Peer-reviewed chapter of the manuscript *Sepsis-Associated Encephalopathy: Clinical, Metabolomic, Neurophysiological and Neuroimaging Parallels* is devoted to the problem of diagnosing acute cerebral damage using positron emission tomography in patients with sepsis.

The possibility of early diagnosis of brain dysfunction is very significant due to high mortality and poor prognosis for the septic patient if brain damage progresses. Along with clinical and laboratory diagnosis of acute cerebral insufficiency, neuroimaging and the study of brain metabolism, neurotransmitter function, and cerebral perfusion are of particular importance. In this regard, the X-ray and PET technologies complement the data on sepsis-associated encephalopathy.

The chapter discusses the results of experimental and clinical studies of cerebral metabolism, perfusion, and neurotransmission in sepsis-associated encephalopathy using PET. The results of studies of Almazov National Medical Research Centre of patients with sepsis are also described.

Undoubtedly, the future in clinical medicine, including critical care medicine and sepsis, belongs to high-tech methods of hardware diagnostics. We will use a subtle tool for diagnosing cerebral dysfunction and complement the clinicians' understanding of the state of the patient's brain in the different stages of sepsis.

The chapter may be published in print.

Professor Luiza I. Korytova, *Ph.D.*,
Chief Researcher of the Department of Radiation and Combined Methods of Treatment,
Honored Worker of Science of Russian Federation,
Honorary Professor of
Russian Scientific Center for Radiology and Surgical Technologies
named after Academician A.M. Granova,
Saint Petersburg, Russia

Expert comments

Sepsis-associated encephalopathy as a component of multiple organ failure in ICU patients

The problem of multiple organ failure (MOF) in ICU patients is one of the most urgent and intractable problems of modern medicine. Despite advances in medical technology and intensive care, the morbidity and mortality of MOF in patients with sepsis remains unacceptably high. In most patients with sepsis, sepsis-associated encephalopathy (SAE) develops against the background of pre-existing organ dysfunction and homeostasis disorders, which makes the latter an integral component of the pathogenesis of SAE.

Because of the foregoing, this chapter will organically complement other chapters of the collective book on various aspects of pathophysiology, diagnosis, and treatment of SAE. The authors briefly described the general pathophysiology of MOF and SAE and emphasized the importance of differential diagnosis of acute encephalopathies in the ICU. In particular, the latest recommendations on the terminology and classification of acute encephalopathy, delirium, and coma are given. A distinctive feature of this chapter is a detailed theoretical analysis of the significance of dysfunction of remote organs, homeostasis disorders, and other extracerebral factors in the pathogenesis of SAE. In addition to hypoxia, disorders of macro- and microhemodynamics, fluid-electrolyte and metabolic disorders, and other manifestations of organ dysfunction, the authors also pay attention to more specific mechanisms of organ "cross-talk" that can exacerbate brain damage in sepsis. The potentially negative effects on the brain of several intensive care methods are also discussed in the chapter.

Thus, the presented chapter contains up-to-date information on the problem of SAE and will be of interest to both physicians and researchers interested in this area.

Aslan K. Shabanov,
M.D., Doctor of Medical Sciences,
Deputy Chief Physician for
Anesthesiology and Intensive Care in
Sklifosovsky Research Institute
of Emergency Medicine, Moscow, Russia

Expert comments

Features of sepsis-associated encephalopathy in children

The problem of effective treatment of sepsis in pediatric practice is significant due to the high mortality rate and the formation of delayed cognitive impairment in surviving patients. The damage to the central nervous system in sepsis determines the prognosis and severity of the course of the disease.

Undoubtedly, early diagnosis of sepsis-associated encephalopathy in the structure of multiple organ dysfunction in a child with sepsis will be a determining factor in the treatment strategy to prevent the development of acute cerebral dysfunction.

The authors of the chapter "Features of sepsis-associated encephalopathy in pediatric patients" describe the clinical picture of SAE in children with age characteristics. The stages of development of the child's brain from the moment of birth, the formation of neurotransmission, myelination, apoptosis, and the features of the functioning of the central nervous system in different periods of childhood, outlined in the chapter, are necessary for understanding what pathophysiological processes cause cognitive impairment in sepsis in children.

The authors brilliantly describe the methods of functional diagnostics used in pediatrics to verify cerebral dysfunction, bedside neuromonitoring methods, and laboratory diagnostic panels for confirming the diagnosis of SAE. The chapter is informative and good for reading for pediatric neurologists, pediatricians, neonatologists, intensivists, and medical students.

Yuri S. Alexandrovich, *Doctor of Medical Sciences, Professor,*
Honored Worker of Science,
Head of the Department of Anesthesiology, Resuscitation and
Emergency Pediatrics of AF and DPO,
Vice-Rector for Postgraduate,
Additional Professional
Education and Regional Health Development,
St. Petersburg State Pediatric Medical University,
Saint Petersburg, Russia

Expert comments

Therapeutic tactics in sepsis-associated encephalopathy: present and prospects

Sepsis is a common critical syndrome with a maximum mortality and complication rate. Sepsis-associated encephalopathy (SAE) is a leading sepsis syndrome with unclear pathophysiology and principles of therapy and diagnosis. These aspects determine the high importance of early diagnosis and adequate assessment of the severity of the patient's condition.

The article describes an approach to the diagnosis of encephalopathy and differentiation between sepsis and other causes of cerebral disorders. Approaches to neurological screening are described, including evaluation with the Intensive Care Unit Confusion Score (CAM-ICU), the Critical Care Delirium Screening Checklist (ICDSC), the Complete Immunity Rating Scale (FOUR) and Glasgow Coma Scale (GCS). Among the forms of SAE, much attention is paid to delirium: a description of the causes, the importance of clinical neuromonitoring for the diagnosis of concomitant diseases. The authors analyzed methods for assessing the severity and predicting the development of multiple organ failure, including the SOFA and SAPS II scales. Clinical and instrumental phenotypes of septic encephalopathy have been identified. The mechanisms of development and approaches to the diagnosis of another significant complication, acquired weakness in intensive care, are described. The style of presentation is accessible and covers the most significant diagnostic techniques, the indicated scales are given in the appendix section. The author's schemes increase the visibility of the presentation of the material. The chapter will be useful to ICU practitioners.

Head and Chair of the Department of ICU,
Scientific Research Institute for Complex Issues of
Cardiovascular Disease, Professor, MD., Ph. D.
Kemerovo
Russia

Evgeny Grigoryev

4 - July- 2023

Expert comments

Pathomorphology of sepsis-associated encephalopathy

Recently, in the problem of sepsis, the lesion of the nervous system has been isolated in a separate direction. The resulting septic encephalopathy most often determines the outcome of a septic condition. Pathomorphological changes of the brain in sepsis are presented in the literature in a very general and fragmentary way. The authors of the chapter present material not only on brain damage but also on structural changes in the autonomic nervous system, which gives a comprehensive idea of structural lesions in the nervous system. Due to the scarce literature data on the pathomorphology of the nervous system in sepsis, the text is accompanied by original photographs of micro-preparations. A red line through the whole narrative is the thought of the nonspecificity changes both in the brain and in the autonomic nervous system. A complex of reactive and destructive changes characterizes the insufficiency of the functions of the nervous system. This generalization on the pathomorphology of septic encephalopathy emphasizes the need for further systematic study of this issue, which opens up new prospects in understanding the mechanisms of development of this condition.

Olga Nikolaevna Gaikova, MD, Ph. D.,
Professor, Leading Researcher
Laboratory of Pathomorphology and Electron Microscopy
Golikov Institute of Toxicology,
St. Petersburg, Russia

Expert comments

Molecular genetic aspects of diagnosis and clinical approaches of sepsis-associated encephalopathy

The chapter *Molecular Genetic Aspects of Diagnosis and Clinical Approaches of Sepsis-Associated Encephalopathy* is devoted to the significant problem, concerning the management of critically ill patients in ICU using modern special tests and laboratory panels for diagnosis of acute cerebral damage in sepsis.

The chapter is written in a good manner with a literature review of modern molecular genetic methods of sepsis-associated encephalopathy diagnosis and clinical approaches to the treatment of acute cerebral insufficiency in the structure of multiple organ failure in sepsis.

The authors discuss strategies aimed at suppressing the neuroinflammatory cascade by targeting the nuclear protein HMGB1 using molecular inhibitors or inhibiting HMGB1 signaling pathways. They also examine the role of mtDNA and mitochondrial dysfunction in the pathophysiological cascades of SAE development, which will likely enable clinical trials soon using mitochondria-targeted therapeutic agents (e.g., mitochondrial antioxidants) that can prevent and/or treat delirium in sepsis. The authors present data on risk factors for SAE development, such as race/ethnicity, and the diagnostic role of microRNA in sepsis-associated encephalopathy.

Undoubtedly, this chapter will be useful to medical students, and doctors of various specialties, and can be published.

Professor Evgeny V. Grigoryev, MD., Ph.D.,
Head of the Department of ICU, Scientific Research Institute for Complex Issues of Cardiovascular Disease, Kemerovo, Russia

Biographical Sketches

Name: Polina Leonidovna Andropova

Affiliation: N.P. Behtereva Institute of the Human Brain of the Russian Academy of Sciences (IHB RAS)

Education: Federal State Budgetary Educational Institution of Higher Education «St. Petersburg State Pediatric Medical University» of the Ministry of Healthcare of the Russian Federation, qualification of a general practitioner (Specialist Degree in pediatrics). N.P. Behtereva Institute of the Human Brain of the Russian Academy of Sciences Radiology Residency and Postgraduate Medical Radiology course. ESOR Graz Tutorial (European School of Radiology).

Business Address: 197376, St.-Petersburg, Academician Pavlova street, 9.

Research and Professional Experience and Professional Appointments:

March 2020 – Today	St. Petersburg State Budgetary Institution of Healthcare "City Hospital of the Holy Martyr Elizabeth" – Radiologist of the CT department
Oct 2019 – Oct 2022	Postgraduate studies at the N. P. Bekhtereva Institute of the Human Brain of the Russian Academy of Sciences
Sep 2018 – Sep 2019	N. P. Bekhtereva Institute of the Human Brain of the Russian Academy of Sciences – Resident Doctor
Sep 2017 - Sep 2018	Saint-Petersburg State Research Institute of Phthisiopulmonology – Resident Doctor

My primary field of scientific interest is emergency neuroradiology, especially acute stroke, as well as the development of artificial intelligence and the introduction into the practice of a doctors.

Alongside with the research, I perform the duties of a clinical radiologist.

Publications from the Last 3 Years:

- Andropova P.L., Gavrilov P.V., Kazantseva I.P., Kochanova N.I., Narkevich A.N., Trofimova T.N. Interexpert agreement between emergency neuroradiologists with different levels of experience in the rating of aspects. *Radiology — Practice*. 2022. № 5 (95). C. 10–25. doi: http://dx.doi.org/10.52560/2713-0118-2022-5-10-25
- Andropova P.L., Gavrilov P.V., Savintseva Zh.I. ASPECTS: Interobserver agreement between radiologist. *Diagnostic Radiology and Radiotherapy*. 2022. Vol. 13, No. 1. P. 21–27, doi: http://dx.doi.org/10.22328/2079-5343-2022-13-1-21-27.
- Skvortsova T.Y., Savintceva Z.I., Zhavoronkova A.S., Gurchin A.F., Andropova P.L. Persistent nontumoral high-amino-acid uptake on brain [11C] methionine PET/CT in a

patient after combined glioma treatment. *Clinical Nuclear Medicine*. 2021. T. 46. № 7. C. E376–E377.

- Trofimova T.N., Andropova P.L., Savintseva J.I., Belyakov N.A. Radiology of the central nervous system of patients in the acute phase of COVID-19. *HIV Infection and Immunosuppressive Disorders*. 2021. Vol. 13, No. 2. P. 20–32, doi: http://dx.doi.org/10.22328/2077-9828-2021-13-2-20-32
- Andropova P.L., Gavrilov P.V., Savintseva Zh.I., Vovk A.V., Rybin E.V. Application of artificial intelligence systems in neuroradiology of acute ischemic stroke. *Diagnostic Radiology and Radiotherapy*. 2021. Vol. 12, No. 2. P. 30–36, http://dx.doi.org/10.22328/2079-5343-2021-12-2-30-36.
- Andropova P., Cheremisin D., Meldo A. A computer-aided diagnosis system in the diagnosis of multiple sclerosis. *Smart Innovation, Systems and Technologies*. 2021. T. 220. C. 277–284.
- Cheremisin D., Andropova P., Gavrilov P. Response to: BCG infection following immunotherapy for bladder cancer. *QJM: Quarterly Journal of Medicine*. 2020. T. 113. № 3. C. 232.
- Cheremisin D., Andropova P., Gavrilov P. A case of renal tuberculosis following BCG therapy for bladder cancer. *QJM: Quarterly Journal of Medicine*. 2019. T. 112. № 10. C. 797–798.

Name: Natalia V. Beloborodova

Affiliation: Federal Research and Clinical Center of Intensive Care Medicine and Rehabilitology, Negovsky Research Institute of General Reanimatology, Chief Scientific Officer, Head of the Laboratory of Metabolism in critical state

Education: Higher medical (Pirogov's 2st Moscow medical Institute, Faculty of Pediatrics, Moscow, Russia), degree of PhD since 1984, State Medical Academy of Postgraduate education, academic certification in clinical microbiology and chemotherapy, academic degree of Doctor of Medical Sciences since 1996, the title of Professor since 1998.

Natalia V. Beloborodova:

- Is Member of the European Academy of Natural Sciences since 2003 (Hannover, Germany)
- Is an expert of the Russian Science Foundation since 2017
- Have the title of Honored Worker of Sciences of the Russian Federation since 2021

Business Address: 25 build. 2 Petrovka str., Moscow107031, Russian Federation

Research interests: sepsis, infectious complications, biomarkers, antibiotic therapy, human microecology, microbiota, microbial biofilms, metabolomics, metabolic diagnostics, bacterial signaling molecules.

Research and Professional Experience:
Series of clinical and experimental studies on the role of microbial metabolites in normal and human pathologies were initiated. The results of the researches formed the basis for the concept of the integration of human metabolism and its microbiota (2012) and led to the discovery of signaling molecules involved in the mechanisms of sepsis, multiple organ failure and septic shock. New biomarkers have been developed for diagnostics, prognosis and monitoring of critical states and introduction into clinical practice.

Scientific and clinical studies of Beloborodova N.V. in the field of infections, antimicrobial therapy and dysbiosis are widely known in Russia.

Russian Honours:

- Diploma of Filatov in the field of pediatrics (1996);
- Prize of the Presidium of the Russian Academy of Medical Sciences in the field of fundamental medical research for the work "Development of the Fundamentals of Optimization of Antimicrobial Therapy" (2001);
- Diploma of the Pirogov Russian National Research Medical University for publishing textbooks and co-authoring textbooks on pediatric surgery and intensive care (2008);
- Medal and the Prize of Bakulev AN "For the success in solving the problem of infection in cardiosurgery" (2008).

Abroad Honours:

- Nominal Prize of Maria Koates "Best lecturer-scientist" at the "XVIII International Symposium on Gnotobiology" (2014);
- Medal of Robert Koch "For achievements in science" of the European Academy of Natural Sciences, Hannover, Germany (2013);
- Award at the "International Sepsis Forum-2014" for the best work «Tyrosine metabolism disorder and the potential capability of anaerobic microbiota to decrease the value of aromatic metabolites in critically ill patients», The Pasteur Institute, Paris, France.

The total number of scientific publications is more than 500, most of them in Russian. Below are some monographs and chapters from books from previous years:

1. MONOGRAPH "***SEPSIS. The metabolomic approach***". Beloborodova N.V. Publishing House Medical Information Agency (MIA), Moscow, 2018. – 272 p. ISBN 978-5-9986-0350-1
2. MONOGRAPH. ***Algorithms of antibacterial therapy in the era of antibiotic resistance***. Beloborodova N.V., Chernenkaya T.V., Bogdanov M.B. Moscow, Publisher: Medical Information Agency (MIA), 2019., – 360 p. ISBN 978-5-907098-26-8
3. Chapter in book «Sepsis». Ed. by Vijay Kumar. Published by InTech, Rijeka, Croatia, 2017 Print ISBN 978-953-51-3395-7. –158 p. DOI. 10.5772/65611 https://www.intechopen.com/books/sepsis. Chapter 1. Beloborodova N.V. «***Interaction of host-microbial metabolism in sepsis***» p. 3–19. DOI: 10.5772/68046
4. Chapter in Book InTechOpen «Metabolomics - New Insights into Biology and Medicine». 2019. Beloborodova N.V., Grechko A.V., Olenin A.Yu. Chapter «***Metabolomic Discovery of Microbiota Dysfunction as the Cause of Pathology***» DOI: 10.5772/intechopen.87176
5. Chapter in Book « Infectious process and Sepsis» Edit by V.Nery. Chapter 3. Chernevskaya E.A., Beloborodova N.V. «***Microbiota-oriented diagnostic and therapy in sepsis, utopia or necessity?***» 2019. DOI: 10.5772/intechopen.89187
6. MONOGRAPH. «***The role of microbial metabolites in mitochondrial dysfunction in sepsis***». Beloborodova N., Teplova V., Fedotcheva N. Publisher: LAP LAMBERT Academic Publishing, Saarbrucken, Germany, 2013. – 89 p. ISBN: 978-3-659-43111-1
7. MONOGRAPH. «***Infection in cardiac surgery***» L.A. Bokeria, N.V.Beloborodova. Moscow, Publishing house of the Scientific Research Center named after A.N.Bakulev, 2007. – 582 p. ISBN 978-5-7982-0206-5

8. MONOGRAPH ***«Sepsis in children»***. Yu.F.Isakov, N.V. Beloborodova. RAMS. Moscow. Publisher Mokeev, 2001. – 369 p. ISBN 5-93135-005-5
9. MONOGRAPH. ***«Surgical infection in newborns»***. T.V. Krasovskaya, N.V. Beloborodova, ,Moscow, Ed Medicine, 1993 – 224 p. ISBN 5-225-00810-0

Since 2010, the ORCID website contains 178 articles and 25 reviews in journals, authored by Beloborodova N. https://orcid.org/0000-0003-2328-1610

The ten most significant publications for the last 3 years (**2021-2023**):

1. **Beloborodova,** N.V. Serum aromatic microbial metabolites as biological markers in intensive care. In: Rajendram, R., Preedy, V.R., Patel, V.B. (eds) *Biomarkers in Trauma, Injury and Critical Care. Biomarkers in Disease: Methods, Discoveries and Applications.* Springer, Cham. **2023**. Chapter 13, P. 245–268.
   DOI:10.1007/978-3-031-07395-3_64
2. **Beloborodova** N., Pautova A., Grekova M., Yadgarov M., Grin O., Eremenko A., Babaev M. Microbiota metabolism failure as a risk factor for postoperative complications after aortic prosthetics // *Biomedicines*. – **2023**. – Vol. 11. – No. 5. – P. 1335.
3. Sorokina E., Pautova A., Fatuev O., Zakharchenko V., Onufrievich A., Grechko A., **Beloborodova** N., Chernevskaya E. Promising markers of inflammatory and microbiota disorders in patients with post-covid-19 syndrome // *Journal of Personalized Medicine*. – **2023**. – Vol. 13. – No. 6. – P. 971.
4. Pautova A.K., Meglei A.Yu., Chernevskaya E.A., Alexandrova I.A., **Beloborodova** N.V. 4-hydroxyphenyllactic acid in cerebrospinal fluid as a possible marker of post-neurosurgical meningitis: Retrospective study // *Journal of Personalized Medicine*. – **2022**. – Vol. 12. – No. 3. – P.399.
5. Pautova A.K., Samokhin A.S., **Beloborodova N.V.,** Revelsky A.I. Multivariate prognostic model for predicting the outcome of critically ill patients using the aromatic metabolites detected by gas chromatography-mass spectrometry // *Molecules*. – **2022**. – Vol. 27. – P. 4784.
6. Ivanova V., Chernevskaya E., Vasiluev P., Ivanov A., Tolstoganov I., Shafranskaya D., Ulyantsev V., Korobeynikov A., Razin S.V., **Beloborodova N.,** Ulianov S.V., Tyakht A. Hi-c metagenomics in the icu: Exploring clinically relevant features of gut microbiome in chronically critically ill patients // *Frontiers in microbiology*. – **2022**. – Vol. 12. – P. 770323.
7. Fedotcheva N., **Beloborodova N.** Influence of microbial metabolites and itaconic acid involved in bacterial inflammation on the activity of mitochondrial enzymes and the protective role of alkalization // *International Journal of Molecular Sciences*. – **2022.** – Vol. 23. – No. 16. – P. 9069.
8. Fedotcheva N., Olenin A., **Beloborodova N**. Influence of microbial metabolites on the nonspecific permeability of mitochondrial membranes under conditions of acidosis and loading with calcium and iron ions // *Biomedicines*. – **2021**. – Vol. 9. – No. 5. – P. 558. DOI:10.3390/biomedicines9050558
9. **Beloborodova** N., Grechko A. *"Dialogue" between the Human Microbiome and the Brain, Human Microbiome*, Natalia V. Beloborodova and Andrey V. Grechko, IntechOpen, **2021**. DOI: 10.5772/intechopen.94431. Available from: https://www.intechopen.com/chapters/73917
10. «Human Microbiome». **Beloborodova** N.V. and Grechko A.V., IntechOpen, **2021**. ISBN 978-1-78984-849-6. - 166 P.

Name: Natalya Valerievna Bodareva

Place of employment : Russian Research Neurosurgical Institute named after V.I. Polenov – branch of the Almazov National Medical Research Center of the Ministry of Health of Russia, Russian Federation

Education: St. Petersburg State Medical Academy named after Ilya I. Mechnikov, qualification pathologist. Internship, clinical residency, postgraduate study in pathological anatomy. Refresher course in pathological anatomy.

Legal address : 191014, Russian Federation, St. Petersburg, st. Mayakovsky, 12

Research and professional experience:
Highly qualified pathologist with more than 15 years of experience. Specialist in the field of pathomorphological diagnostics of oncological diseases and diseases of the nervous system.

We conduct scientific research in the field of diseases of the nervous system.

My scientific interests are related to the etiopathogenesis and pathomorphology of diseases in patients with neurosurgical pathology (brain aneurysms, cerebral infarctions), morphological assessment of the pathological process.

In 2013, he defended his Ph.D. thesis "Clinical-morphological and immunohistochemical features of the variants of the artificial bladder in different periods of functioning". It describes the adaptation of the urinary reservoir in new aggressive conditions, changes in the mucous membrane of the urinary reservoirs over a long period of time. Since 2014, I have been engaged in pathomorphological examination of the brain in sepsis in the field of neurosurgery.

In parallel with the research, he performed the duties of a clinical pathologist.

Professional appointments :
From 2007 to 2013 – internship, clinical postgraduate study, correspondence postgraduate study at the St. Petersburg Academy named after A.I. I.I. Mechnikov with a degree in pathological anatomy. For 15 years of his professional activity he has gone from an intern to a senior researcher.

Publications in the last 3 years:

1. Bodareva N.V., Zabrodskaya Yu.M., Savvina I.A. Pathomorphological signs of encephalopathy in sepsis in neurosurgical patients. In the collection: science and innovation - modern concepts. collection of scientific articles based on the results of the work of the International nauchnogo forum. Moscow, 2021. P. 71–78. ISBN 978-5-905695-44-5. (In Russ.)
2. Savvina I.A., Zabrodskaya Y.M., Sebelev K.I., Bodareva N.V., Lavrinenko N.V., Tkebuchava I.V. A method for predicting the development of infectious complications and sepsis in patients with severe traumatic brain injury. Patent number: RU 2743806 C1. Russia. 2021. Date of publication: 02/26/2021. (In Russ.)
3. Bodareva N.V., Zabrodskaya Y.M., Savvina I.A. To the question of septic encephalopathy: Clinical and morphological parallels. *Journal of Complementary Medicine Research.* 2021; 12(2): 52–60. doi: 10.5455/jcmr.2021.12.02.08
4. Bykova K.M., Savvina I.A., Bondareva N.V., Zabrodskaya Yu.M. Pathophysiological aspects and complex diagnostics of sepsis-associated encephalopathy: Prospects of etiopathogenetic therapy. *Journal of Anesthesiology and Resuscitation.* 2022; 4: 92–99. (In Russ.)

Name: Irina Vladimirovna Buyakova

Affiliation: Research Institute of General Resuscitation named after V.A. Negovsky Federal Scientific and Clinical Center of Resuscitation and Rehabilitation.

Education: N.I. Pirogov Russian State Medical University, Residency in neurology.
Postgraduate course in pathological physiology.

Business Address: 25, building 2, Petrovka Str., 107031 Moscow, RF.

Research and professional experience:
A highly qualified neurologist with more than 20 years of experience, as well as a research doctor. Specialist in the field of diseases of the nervous system from a practical and scientific point of view.

My research interests are related to the etiology, pathogenesis, and course of various diseases of the nervous system. I pay much attention to the study of the functioning of the microbiota in various diseases of the central nervous system.

In 2022, I defended my PhD thesis "Microbiota dysfunction in patients with severe brain damage", which describes a previously unexplored problema: changes in metabolism under the influence of altered microbiota in patients in a chronic critical condition. Microbial metabolites have been identified, which are important for predicting the course and outcome of the disease.

Along with research, I performed the duties of a neurologist.

Professional appointments:
2017-2020 - postgraduate studies at the Institute of Higher and Additional Professional Education of the Federal Scientific and Clinical Center of Intensive Care Medicines and Rehabilitation.

Since 2018, I have been a senior researcher at the Laboratory of Metabolism in Critical Conditions of the Research Institute of General Resuscitation named after V.A. Negovsky, Federal Scientific and Clinical Center of Intensive Care Medicines and Rehabilitation.

Publications for the last 3 years:

1. I. Buyakova. Host-microbiome interactions mediated by phenolic metabolites in chronically critically ill patients/ E. Chernevskaya, N. Klimenko, A. Pautova, I. Buyakova, A. Tyakht, N. Beloborodova // *Metabolites*. – 2021. – Vol. 11 – No. 2 – P. 1–16.
2. I. Buyakova. The connection of aromatic microbial metabolites, inflammatory and autoimmune biomarkers with clinical dynamics in severe diseases of the central nervous system / E. A. Chernevskaya, S. A. Zozulya, N. V. Beloborodova, T. P. Klyushnik, I. V. Buyakova // *Journal of Neurology and Psychiatry* named after S. S. Korsakov. – 2020. – No. 7 – C. 78–85.
3. I.V. Buyakova. Taxonomic changes in microbiota and serum biomarkers as a reflection of the severity of damage to the central nervous system / E. A. Chernevskaya, A.Yu. Megley, I.V. Buyakova, N.Y. Kovaleva, K.M. Gorshkov, V.E. Zakharchenko, N.V. Beloborodova // *Bulletin of RSMU*. – 2020. – No. 5 – P. 15–22.
4. I.V. Buyakova. Assessment of muscle tone in severe diseases of the central nervous system based on digital myotometry / H.V. Beloborodova, I.V. Buyakova // *Treatment and Prevention*. – 2020. – No. 10 – P. 55–63 (in Russ.).

5. Buyakova I.V. Microbiota dysfunction in patients with brain damage in a chronic critical condition / A.V. Grechko, I.V. Buyakova, N.V. Beloborodova // *Russian Neurological Journal*. – 2022. – Vol. 27 – No. 1 – P. 94–104.
6. I. Buyakova. Feasibility of quantitative assessment of mechanical properties of muscles in chronic critical ill patients / N. Beloborodova, M. Petrova, I. Buyakova, E. Chernevskaya // *Critical Care*. – 2020. – Vol. 24 – No. S1 – P. 4.
7. I. Buyakova. Features of the gut microbiota as a risk factor in chronically critically ill patients / E. Chernevskaya, N. Beloborodova, I. Buyakova, N. Klimenko, A. Tyakht, N. Kovaleva // *Shock*. –2020. – Vol. 53 – No. 1S – P. 75.
8. I.V. Buyakova. Assessment of muscle tone by MyotonPro apparatus in patients with severe central nervous system damage / N.V. Beloborodova, E.A. Chernevskaya, I.V. Buyakova. // *Materials of the XXII All-Russian Conference with International Participation "Life Support in Critical Conditions": Proceedings*. – 2020. – P. 19–20.
9. I.V. Buyakova. The experience of using a test system to assess the state of the intestinal microbiota by PCR in patients in a chronic critical condition / A.Yu. Megley, I.V. Buyakova, E.A. Chernevskaya // *X Anniversary International Scientific and Practical Conference "Molecular Diagnostics 2020": Proceedings*. – 2020. – P. 439–440.
10. I.V. Buyakova. The relationship neurospecific biomarkers and changes in the gut microbiota in critical conditions / A.Yu. Megley, I.V. Buyakova, E.A. Chernevskaya // *Materials of the Scientific and Practical Conference, the VI Russian Congress of Laboratory Medicine: A Collection of Abstracts*. – 2020. – P. 27 (in Russ.)

Name: Potemkina Elena Gennadevna

Affiliation: Russian Polenov Scienific Research Neurosurgical Institute – branch of the Almazov National Medical Research Centre of Ministry of Health Care of Russian Federation

Education: St. Petersburg State Pediatric Medical University

Business Address: 191014, 12 Mayakovskogo Str., Saint Petersburg, Russian Federation.

Research and Professional Experience: radiation diagnostics of cerebral vascular pathology

Professional Appointments: neurorentgenology

Honors: PhD

Publications from the Last 3 Years:

1. Potemkina E.G., Salomatina T.A., Andreev E.V., Abramov K.B., Bannikova V.D., Denygina N.O., Nezdorovina V.G., Zabrodskaya Yu.M., Samochernych K.A., Odintsova G.V. MR-morphometry use in epileptology:achievements and prospects. *Burdenko's Journal of Neurosurgery*. 2023. – Vol. 3. – P. 113–119. https://doi.org/10.17116/neiro202387031113
2. Savvina I.A., Zabrodskaya Yu.M., Rozhchenko L.V., Goroshchenko S.A., Potemkina E.G., Petrova A.O., Samochernykh K.A. Aneurysmal subarachnoid hemorrhage: From diagnosis to treatment. In: *Aneurysmal Subarachnoid Hemorrhage: From Diagnosis to Treatment*. Ed. by I.A. Savvina. New York: Nova Medicine α Health; 2022: 41–112 – ISBN:979-8-88697-298-6 (eBook)

3. Sidorin V.S., Zabrodskaya Yu.M., Sitovskaya D.A., Potemkina E.G., Panaskov A.V., Lyapakova M.O., Sokolova T.V. Isolated sarcoidosis of the brain. *Archive of Pathology.* 2022. – Vol. 84. – No. 4. – P. 56–61.
4. Kukanov K.K., Vorobyeva O.M., Zabrodskaya Yu.M., Potemkina E.G., Ushanov V.V., Tastanbekov M.M., Ivanova N.E. Intracranial meningiomas: Clinical-intrascopic and pathomorphological reasons of recurrence taking into account modern methods of treatment (literature review). *Siberian Oncological Journal.* 2022. – Vol. 21. – No. 4. – P. 110–123.
5. Zhukova T.V., Shanyko Yu.G., Beletskiy A.V., Nadzved M.K., Polyakova S.M., Guzov S.A., Shirinskiy A.A., Potemkina E.G., Sitovskaya D.A., Zrelov A.A., Ivanova N.E., Zabrodskaya Yu.M. Intraoperative diagnosis of peritumoral zone taking into account the glioma growth mechanisms. *Russian Neurosurgical Journal* named after Professor A.L. Polenov. 2022. – Vol. 14. – No. 1–2. – P. 46–49.
6. Kondratyeva E.A., Ivanova A.O., Yarmolinskaya M.I., Potemkina E.G. et al. Evaluation of structural variations in the pituitary gland, hormonal status and laboratory markers of the central nervous system functioning in patients with chronic disorders of consciousness. *Journal of Obstetrics and Women's Diseases.* 2021. – Vol. 70. – No. 5. – P. 23–36. DOI: 10.17816/JOWD77930.
7. Potemkina E.G. Treatment of patients with posthemorrhagic hydrocephalus / N.K. Samochernykh, K.B. Abramov, M.S. Nikolaenko [et al.] // *Russian Bulletin of Perinatology and Pediatrics.* 2021. – Vol. 66. – No. 5. – P. 97-104. DOI: 10.21508/1027-4065-2021-66-5-97-104.
8. Potemkina E.G. Comparative analysis of percutaneous endoscopic intralaminar discectomy and microdiscectomy in overweight patients / Yu. V. Belyakov, A.M. Meredzhi, A. Y. Orlov [et al.] // *The Russian Neurosurgical Journal* named after Professor A.L. Polenov. 2020. – Vol. 12. – No. 1. – P. 12–15.
9. Potemkina E.G. Primary multiple cerebral tumors of various histological structures (description of clinical cases) / N.E. Warriors, A.Y. Ulitin, P.V. Lavrovsky [et al.] // *The Russian Neurosurgical Journal* named after Professor A.L. Polenov. 2020. – Vol. 12. – No. 1. – P. 55–63.
10. Potemkina E.G. Comparative analysis of stereotactic and endoscopic methods of brain tumor biopsy (literature review) / K.K. Kukanov, A.A. Matrelov, K.A. Samochernykh [et al.] // *The Russian Neurosurgical Journal* named after Professor A.L. Polenov. – 2020. – Vol. 12. – No. 1. – P. 64–70.
11. Potemkina E.G. The frequency of infectious complications and features of the systemic inflammatory response in patients with prolonged impaired consciousness / N.V. Dryagina, E.A. Kondratieva, S.A. Kondratiev [et al.] // *Journal of Infectology.* 2020. – Vol. 12. – P. 21–28. DOI: 10.22625/2072-6732-2020-12-5-21-28.
12. Potemkina E.G. Pathomorphological manifestations of peritumorous inflammation in brain tumors / Yu. M. Zabrodskaya, T.V. Zhukova, A.F. Smeyanovich [et al.] // *Neurology and Neurosurgery. Eastern Europe.* 2020. – Vol. 10. – No. 3. – P. 392–399. DOI: 10.34883/PI.2020.10.3.034.
13. Potemkina E.G. Features of the atrophic process in progressive supranuclear paralysis according to magnetic resonance morphometry / E.V. Iskhakova, A.S. Lepekhina, Ya. B. Batozhargalova [et al.] // *Russian Electronic Journal of Radiation Diagnostics.* 2020. – Vol. 10. – No. 1. – P. 43–49. DOI 10.21569/2222-7415-2020-10-1-43-49.

Name: Andrey Viatcheslavovich Grechko

Affiliation: Federal Research and Clinical Center of Intensive Care Medicine and Rehabilitology, Director. Moscow, Russian Federation

Education: Higher medical (N.A. Semashko Moscow Medical Dental Institute), MD, PhD, DrSci, Professor, Corresponding member of the Russian academy of medical sciences.

Business Address: 107031, 25 Petrovka str., build. 2, Moscow, Russian Federation

Research and Professional Experience, professional Appointments:
In 2000 defended dissertation for the degree of Candidate of Medical Sciences. In 2004 defended dissertation for the degree of Doctor of Medical Sciences.

From 2000 to 2004 worked as a lecturer at the Department of Dermatology of the Moscow State Medical and Dental University. From 2004 to 2007 worked at the Ministry of Health and Social Development of the Russian Federation as the Head of the Structural Efficiency Improvement Department.

From 2007 to 2009 worked as the chief physician of polyclinic No. 2 of the Main Department of Internal Affairs in the city of Moscow. Since 2008 has been a professor at the I. M. Sechenov First Moscow State Medical University.

From 2009 to 2011 worked as a chief physician at the Central Clinical Hospital of the Ministry of Internal Affairs of the Russian Federation. From 2011 to 2012 held the position of Head of the Department of Medical Support of the Ministry of Internal Affairs of the Russian Federation. From 2013 to 2016 worked as the director of the Federal Scientific Treatment and Rehabilitation Center of the Russian Academy of Medical Sciences.

In 2015 A.V. Grechko was awarded the title of Professor of the Russian Academy of Sciences. Since 2016 A.V. Grechko has been the Director of the Federal Research and Clinical Center of Intensive Care Medicine and Rehabilitology.

A.V. Grechko is deputy editor-in-chief in the journals "Bulletin of the All-Russian Society of Specialists in Medical and Social Expertise, Rehabilitation and Rehabilitation Industry", "Medical and Social Expertise and Rehabilitation", member of the editorial board in the journals "Anesthesiology and Reanimatology", "General Reanimatology", "Physical and rehabilitation Medicine, medical Rehabilitation".

In November 2019 was elected a corresponding member of the Russian Academy of Sciences.

A.V. Grechko — created and headed a new scientific and clinical direction - early medical and social rehabilitation of critically ill patients with severe brain injuries; develops a new scientific direction in clinical medicine — the introduction of early rehabilitation in intensive care units; organizes testing of new methods of diagnosis, treatment and rehabilitation of patients with severe brain damage at different stages of the comatose and post-comatose period.

Honours:

- Medal of the Order of Merit for the Fatherland, II degree
- Honorary Worker of Science and High Technologies of the Russian Federation
- Medal "For contribution to the implementation of state policy in the field of scientific and technological development" (Ministry of Education and Science of Russia)

- Medal "For merits in management activities of the III degree"
- Badge "Excellent Health Worker"
- Badge of the Ministry of Emergency Situations of the Russian Federation "For the Commonwealth in the name of Salvation"
- Gratitude of the Chairman of the Federation Council of the Federal Assembly of the Russian Federation

Publications from the Last 3 Years:

A.V. Grechko is the author and co-author of 9 books and monographs, 13 patents for inventions, more than 250 scientific publications. The H-index according to the RSCI (Russian Science Citation Index) is 28, Scopus is 26, WoS is 17.
https://www.scopus.com/authid/detail.uri?authorId=57194278611

1. Human Microbiome, 2021. NV Beloborodova, AV Grechko. ISBN 978-1-78984-849-6
2. The effects of early postoperative neurocognitive disorders on clinically relevant outcomes: a meta-analysis. Likhvantsev VV, Landoni G, Berikashvili LB, Ermokhina NV, Yadgarov MY, Kotani Y, Kadantseva KK, Makarevich DM, **Grechko AV.** Korean J Anesthesiol. 2023 May 26. doi: 10.4097/kja.23126.
3. Morphologic Findings in the Cerebral Cortex in COVID-19: Association of Microglial Changes with Clinical and Demographic Variables. Babkina AS, Yadgarov MY, Lyubomudrov MA, Ostrova IV, Volkov AV, Kuzovlev AN, **Grechko AV**, Golubev AM. Biomedicines. 2023 May 9;11(5):1407. doi: 10.3390/biomedicines11051407.
4. Rapid Effects of BCI-Based Attention Training on Functional Brain Connectivity in Poststroke Patients: A Pilot Resting-State fMRI Study. Mayorova L, Kushnir A, Sorokina V, Pradhan P, Radutnaya M, Zhdanov V, Petrova M, **Grechko A.** Neurol Int. 2023 Mar 27;15(2):549-559. doi: 10.3390/neurolint15020033.
5. Mechanochemical Synergism of Reactive Oxygen Species Influences on RBC Membrane. Kozlova E, Sergunova V, Sherstyukova E, **Grechko A**, Lyapunova S, Inozemtsev V, Kozlov A, Gudkova O, Chernysh A. Int J Mol Sci. 2023 Mar 21;24(6):5952. doi: 10.3390/ijms24065952.
6. Bacteriophage Cocktails in the Post-COVID Rehabilitation. Zurabov FM, Chernevskaya EA, Beloborodova NV, Zurabov AY, Petrova MV, Yadgarov MY, Popova VM, Fatuev OE, Zakharchenko VE, Gurkova MM, Sorokina EA, Glazunov EA, Kochetova TA, Uskevich VV, Kuzovlev AN, **Grechko AV.** Viruses. 2022 Nov 23;14(12):2614. doi: 10.3390/v14122614.
7. Serum Levels of VEGF-A and Its Receptors in Patients in Different Phases of Hemorrhagic and Ischemic Strokes. Babkina AS, Yadgarov MY, Ostrova IV, Zakharchenko VE, Kuzovlev AN, **Grechko AV**, Lyubomudrov MA, Golubev AM. Curr Issues Mol Biol. 2022 Oct 14;44(10):4888-4901. doi: 10.3390/cimb44100332.
8. Detection of Preclinical Orthostatic Disorders in Young African and European Adults Using the Head-Up Tilt Test with a Standardized Hydrostatic Column Height: A Pilot Study. Dorogovtsev VN, Yankevich DS, Petrova MV, Torshin VI, Severin AE, Borisov IV, Podolskaya JA, **Grechko AV.** Biomedicines. 2022 Sep 1;10(9):2156. doi: 10.3390/biomedicines10092156.

9. Hypertension as a risk factor for atherosclerosis: Cardiovascular risk assessment. Poznyak AV, Sadykhov NK, Kartuesov AG, Borisov EE, Melnichenko AA, **Grechko AV**, Orekhov AN. Front Cardiovasc Med. 2022 Aug 22;9:959285. doi: 10.3389/fcvm.2022.959285
10. Effects of Metabolic Disorders in Immune Cells and Synoviocytes on the Development of Rheumatoid Arthritis. Blagov AV, **Grechko AV**, Nikiforov NG, Zhuravlev AD, Sadykhov NK, Orekhov AN. Metabolites. 2022 Jul 11;12(7):634. doi: 10.3390/metabo12070634.
11. Six-Month Quality of Life in COVID-19 Intensive Care Unit Survivors. Likhvantsev V, Landoni G, Perekhodov S, Chaus N, Kadantseva K, Ermokhina L, Baeva A, Yadgarov M, Berikashvili L, Kuzovlev A, **Grechko A.** J Cardiothorac Vasc Anesth. 2022 Jul;36(7):1949-1955. doi: 10.1053/j.jvca.2021.08.036.

Name: Gurskaya Viktoria Igorevna

Affiliation: Almazov National Medical Research Centre of Ministry of Health Care of Russian Federation

Education: Federal State Budgetary Educational Institution of Higher Education «Pacific State Medical University» of the Ministry of Healthcare of the Russian Federation

Business Address: 197341, 2 Accuratova Str., Saint Petersburg, Russian Federation.

Research and Professional Experience: anesthesiologic maintenance and intensive care of neurosurgical interventions for pediatric patients

In 2022, I defended my PhD thesis "Choice of anesthetic support method for neurosurgical operations and diagnostic procedures in children with craniosynostosis", which describes improving the safety profile of anesthesia monitoring based on the choice of anesthesia for reconstructive surgery in children of the first year of life with craniosynostosis.

Professional Appointments: anesthesiologist

Honors: no

Publications from the Last 3 Years:

1. Gurskaia VI, Ivanov VP, Novikov V Yu, Dryagina NV, Savvina IA. Systemic inflammatory response in infants with craniostenosis sedated with propofol. *Russian Journal of Pediatric Surgery, Anesthesia and Intensive Care.* 2021;11(3):297–306. https://doi.org/10.17816/psaic961
2. Gurskaya VI, Dryagina NV, Ivanov VP, Aleksandrovich Yu S, Khachatryan VA, Savvina IA. Effect of general anesthesia on systemic inflammatory response and neuronal damage in children with craniosynostosis in perioperative period. *Russian Journal of Anaesthesiology and Reanimatology = Anesteziologiya i Reanimatologiya.* 2021;1:39–45. (In Russ.). https://doi.org/10.17116/anaesthesiology202101139
3. Gurskaia VI. Effect of sevoflurane anesthesia on systemic inflammatory response in children with craniosynostosis undergoing MRI examination / N Dryagina, V Ivanov, I Savvina // *Abstract Book 17th World Congress of Anaesthesiologists.* – 2021. – P. 1221.

4. Gurskaia VI. Intraoperative evaluation of non-invasive hemoglobin in children with craniosynostosis / O Pulkina, V Ivanov, I Savvina // *Abstract Book 17th World Congress of Anaesthesiologists*. – 2021. – P. 1222.

Name: Sebelev Konstantin Ivanovich

Affiliation: Russian Polenov Scientific Research Neurosurgical Institute – branch of the Almazov National Medical Research Centre of Ministry of Health Care of Russian Federation, Russian Federation

Education : Leningrad First Medical Institute n.u. Academician I.P. Pavlov, qualification of a general practitioner. Residency in roentgenology. Postgraduate course in radiology.

Business Address : 191014, 12 Mayakovskogo Str., Saint Petersburg, Russian Federation

Research and Professional Experience:
Highly qualified radiologist with more than 40 years of experience. Specialist in the field of radiological diagnostic of nervous system (neurooncology, spine pathology, epilepsy).

I am also committed to conduct scientific research in this area.

My scientific interest is in MRI diagnostic of epileptogenic lesions such as cortical dysplasia, gray matter heterotopia, and hippocampal sclerosis.

In 1988, I defended my PhD thesis "Radiological studies in differentiation of spine and spinal cord pathology".

In 2011, I defended my doctoral dissertation on the topic "optimization of radiation diagnostic of degenerative diseases of the spine in the aspect of surgical treatment"

Professional Appointments :

1980-1982 - postgraduate studies at the Leningrad First Medical Institute, radiologist by profession.

1982-1987. Head of the Department of diagnostic radiology of the city Hospital № 3 (Leningrad).

Since 1989. Head of the Department of diagnostic radiology of the Polenov Scientific Neurosurgical Institute.

I am a Professor at the Department of Radiology and Medical Imagine of the Institute of Medical Education of the Almazov National Medical Research Centre.

Publications from the Last 3 Years:

Clinical structural and functional features of paroxismal syndrome in insular and temporal lobe tumors Khachatryan R. G., Bart V. A., Maslova L. N., Sebelev K. I., Tastanbekov M. M., Alekseeva T. M. Burdenko, s journal of neurosurgery, 2020, № 4, pp. 36-45

Clinical features of temporal lobe epilepsy with involvement of the insular lobe
Khachatryan R. G., Alekseeva T.M., Sebelev K. I., Khachatryan V. A.
S.S. Korsakov Journal of Neurology and Psychiatry 2021, vol.121, no. 6, pp. 7-12

The relationship of bioelectric activity and structural changes in the hippocampus at pharmacoresistant temporal lobe epilepsy
Astakhova E. A., Cherenkova S.E., Sebelev K.I., Marchenco E.V., Aleksandrov M.V.
Translational Medicine 2021, vol. 8, №2, pp. 6-12

Pharmacoresistant temporal epilepsy : the relationship of epileptiform activity and structural changes in the hippocampus
Cherenkova Y.D. ,Marchenko E.V., Aleksandrov M .V., Sebelev K.I., Arkhipova N.B., Chukhlovin A.A., Aleksandrov A.M.
Translation Medicine 2020, vol.7, № 6, pp. 46-54

Hippocampus role in predictive assessment of sepsis development in patients with head injury
Savvina I., Lavrinenko N., Zabrodskaya J., Sebelev K., Dolmatov D.
European Journal of Anesthesiology 2020, vol.37, pp.302-303 . Euroanesthesia 2020 . The European Anesthesiology Congress.

Name: Artem Nikolaevich Kuzovlev

Affiliation: Federal research and clinical center of intensive care medicine and rehabilitology, Head of the Negovsky research institute of general reanimatology

Education: Higher medical (I.M. Sechenov Moscow medical academy), anesthesia and intensive care medicine specialist, MD, PhD, DrSci.

Business Address: 107031, 25 Petrovka str., build. 2, Moscow, Russian Federation

Research and Professional Experience:

Currently – Federal research and clinical center of intensive care medicine and rehabilitology, Head of the V. A. Negovsky Research Institute of General Reanimatology. Investigation into new molecular biomarkers of ventilator-associated pneumonia, acute respiratory distress syndrome and sepsis, new modes of antibiotic therapy for ventilator-associated pneumonia.
Investigation into acute respiratory distress syndrome (ARDS)
2008 – 2010 – clinical investigation into the diagnosis of ARDS in nosocomial pneumonias (PhD)
2006 – 2007 – graduate scientific project dedicated to the role of ischemia and reperfusion in the ARDS pathogenesis.
2006 – experimental work in ventilator-induced lung injury.
2005 – apoptosis in ARDS, experimental work (TUNEL method)
2004 – 2005 – experimental work “Pulmonary microvasculature thrombosis and ARDS”
2004 – course paper “Acute Lung Injury – etiology and pathogenesis”
2007 – 2008 – Investigation into cardiopulmonary resuscitation. Experimental and clinical study. Institute for Experimental Medical Research, Ulleval Hospital, Oslo, Norway. Supervisor – Professor P.A. Steen

Professional Appointments:

2020 – currently - Federal research and clinical center of intensive care medicine and rehabilitology, Head of the V. A. Negovsky Research Institute of General Reanimatology;
2019 – 2020 – Federal research and clinical center of intensive care medicine and rehabilitology, Deputy Director for science;

2017 – 2019 - V. A. Negovsky Research Institute of General Reanimatology, Vice-Director for science.
2011 – currently – V. A. Negovsky Research Institute of General Reanimatology, Head of the Laboratory for clinical pathophysiology of critical states (part-time)
2009 – 2011 – V. A. Negovsky Research Institute of General Reanimatology, PhD fellowship (anesthesiology, "Diagnosis of acute respiratory distress syndrome in nosocomial pneumonia").
2007 – 2009 – V. A. Negovsky Research Institute of General Reanimatology, residence in anesthesiology.
2001 – 2007 - I.M. Sechenov Moscow Medical Academy (Faculty of training medical researchers and advisors).

Honours:

2017 – Prize of the Moscow Government to young scientists for 2016 (project "Increase of efficiency of diagnosis and treatment of infectious complications of critical states by modern technologies").
2014 – Presidential Scholarship for young researchers (for a period of 2015-2017).
2012 – Presidential Scholarship for young researchers (for a period of 2012-2014).

Some of the most significant publications in the last 3 years:

1. Salnikova LE, Khadzhieva MB, Kolobkov DS, Gracheva AS, **Kuzovlev AN**, Abilev SK. Cytokines Mapping for Tissue-Specific Expression, eQTLs and GWAS Traits. *Sci Rep.* 2020 Sep 7;10(1):14740. doi: 10.1038/s41598-020-71018-6
2. Khadzhieva MB, Kalinina EV, Larin SS, Sviridova DA, Gracheva AS, Chursinova JV, Stepanov VA, Redkin IV, Avdeikina LS, Rumyantsev AG, **Kuzovlev AN**, Salnikova LE. TREC/KREC Levels in Young COVID-19 Patients. *Diagnostics (Basel).* 2021 Aug 16;11(8):1486. doi: 10.3390/diagnostics11081486
3. Zurabov FM, Chernevskaya EA, Beloborodova NV, Zurabov AY, Petrova MV, Yadgarov MY, Popova VM, Fatuev OE, Zakharchenko VE, Gurkova MM, Sorokina EA, Glazunov EA, Kochetova TA, Uskevich VV, **Kuzovlev AN,** Grechko AV. Bacteriophage Cocktails in the Post-COVID Rehabilitation. *Viruses.* 2022 Nov 23;14(12):2614. doi: 10.3390/v14122614
4. Kashatnikova DA, Khadzhieva MB, Kolobkov DS, Belopolskaya OB, Smelaya TV, Gracheva AS, Kalinina EV, Larin SS, **Kuzovlev AN,** Salnikova LE. Pneumonia and Related Conditions in Critically Ill Patients-Insights from Basic and Experimental Studies. *Int J Mol Sci.* 2022 Aug 31;23(17):9896. doi: 10.3390/ijms23179896
5. Kolobkov DS, Sviridova DA, Abilev SK, **Kuzovlev AN,** Salnikova LE. Genes and Diseases: Insights from Transcriptomics Studies. *Genes (Basel).* 2022 Jun 28;13(7):1168. doi: 10.3390/genes13071168
6. Babkina AS, Ostrova IV, Yadgarov MY, **Kuzovlev AN**, Grechko AV, Volkov AV, Golubev AM. The Role of Von Willebrand Factor in the Pathogenesis of Pulmonary Vascular Thrombosis in COVID-19. *Viruses.* 2022 Jan 21;14(2):211. doi: 10.3390/v14020211
7. Babkina AS, Yadgarov MY, Ostrova IV, Zakharchenko VE, **Kuzovlev AN,** Grechko AV, Lyubomudrov MA, Golubev AM. Serum Levels of VEGF-A and Its Receptors in Patients

in Different Phases of Hemorrhagic and Ischemic Strokes. *Curr Issues Mol Biol*. 2022 Oct 14;44(10):4888-4901. doi: 10.3390/cimb44100332
8. Babkina AS, Yadgarov MY, Lyubomudrov MA, Ostrova IV, Volkov AV, **Kuzovlev** AN, Grechko AV, Golubev AM. Morphologic Findings in the Cerebral Cortex in COVID-19: Association of Microglial Changes with Clinical and Demographic Variables. *Biomedicines*. 2023 May 9;11(5):1407. doi: 10.3390/biomedicines11051407
9. Khadzhieva MB, Gracheva AS, Belopolskaya OB, Chursinova YV, Redkin IV, Pisarev MV, **Kuzovlev AN**. Serial Changes in Blood-Cell-Count-Derived and CRP-Derived Inflammatory Indices of COVID-19 Patients. *Diagnostics (Basel)*. 2023 Feb 16;13(4):746. doi: 10.3390/diagnostics13040746

Name: Konstantin Eduardovich Lebedev

Affiliation: Almazov National Medical Research Centre of Ministry of Health Care of Russian Federation, Russian Federation

Education: Leningrad Sanitary and Hygienic Medical Institute, qualification of a general practitioner. Residency in neurology. Postgraduate course in neurology.

Business Address: 197341, 2 Akkuratova street, Saint Petersburg, Russian Federation

Research and Professional Experience:
Highly qualified neurophysiologist with more than 30 years of experience. Specialist in the field of neurosurgical treatment of pharmacoresistent epilepsy.

I am also committed to conducting scientific research in this area.

My scientific interest is in the etiology, pathophysiology of epilepsy.

In 1996, I defended my PhD thesis "Functional state of the brain stem in patients with hydrocephalus.", which describes clinical symptoms of brainstem damage in hydrocephalus and assessment of the functional state by BAEP and EEG.

Alongside with the research I performed duties of a clinical neurophysiologist.

Professional Appointments:
1989-1991 - postgraduate studies at the Russian Polenov Scientific Research Neurosurgical Institute, neurologist.
In 1991, after my postgraduate study I got the position of a scientific research on a competitive basis. For 30 years of my professional activity, I have gone from an ordinary researcher to the senior research scientist.

Publications from the Last 3 Years:

1. Khachatryan V.A., Mamatkhanov M.R., Larionov S.N., Lebedev K.E. Reoperations in epilepsy surgery in children. *Questions of Neurosurgery*. N.N. Burdenko. – 2020. – Vol. 84, No. 5. PP. 21–27.
2. Lebedev K.E., Mamatkhanov M.R., Khachatryan V.A. Surgery for epilepsy in young children. *Russian Neurosurgical Journal*. A.L. Polenov. 2021. – Vol. 13. Specialist. Release. – P. 123.

3. Mamatkhanov M.R., Khachatryan V.A., Lebedev K.E. Analysis of the results of surgical treatment of epilepsy. *Russian Neurosurgical Journal.* A.L. Polenov. 2021. – Vol. 13. Specialist. Release. – PP. 124–125.
4. Mamatkhanov M.R., Khachatryan V.A., Lebedev K.E. Significance of structural changes in the brain in the development of epilepsy in children. *Russian Neurosurgical Journal.* A.L. Polenov. 2021. – Vol. 13. Specialist. Release. – P. 125.
5. Mamatkhanov M.R. Lebedev K.E. Khachatryan V.A. Epilepsy relapses and repeated operations in epilepsy surgery in children. V All-Russian congress on pediatric neurosurgery: Sat. theses, ed. Gorelysheva S.K. – M., 2021. – PP. 92–93.
6. Abramov K.B., Mamatkhanov M.R., Lebedev K.E., Samochernykh K.A., Khachatryan V.A., Ratnikov V.A. Personalized surgery for temporal lobe epilepsy in children. *Medical Bulletin of the North Caucasus.* – 2022. – Vol. 1, No. 2. – PP. 163–166.
7. Mamatkhanov M.R., Lebedev K.E., Kim A.V., Gerasimov A.P. Surgery for drug-resistant epilepsy in children. *Scientific and Practical Journal University Clinic.* Appendix (materials of the international medical forum of Donbass on December 15–16). – 2022. – Vol. 2. – P. 53.

Name: Bykova Kristina Mikhailovna

Affiliation: Almazov National Medical Research Centre of Ministry of Health Care of Russian Federation

Education: Voronezh State Medical University named after N. N. Burdenko (VSMU, Burdenko University)

Business Address: 197341, 2 Accuratova Str., Saint Petersburg, Russian Federation.

Research and Professional Experience: anesthesiologic maintenance of cardiosurgical interventions

Professional Appointments: anesthesiologist

Honors: no

Publications from the Last 3 Years:

1. Bykova K.M., Savvina I.A., Bodareva N.V., Zabrodskaya Yu.M. Pathophysiological aspects and complex diagnostics of sepsis-associated encephalopathy: Prospects for etiopathogenetic therapy (literature review) / *Anesthesiology and Resuscitation.* - 2022. - No. 4. – C. 92–98. (VAK, Scopus)
2. Bykova K.M., Savvina I.A., Rutkovsky R.V., Rodchenko A.M. The role of neuroinflammation in brain dysfunction in the perioperative period (literature review) / *Anesthesiology and Resuscitation.* - 2022. - No. 6. (VAK, Scopus)
3. Savvina I.A., Ryzhkova D.V., Bykova K.M., Lebedev K.E., Petrova A.O., Dryagina N.V., Potemkina E.G., Nazaralieva E.T. Diagnostics of central and autonomic nervous system dysfunction in patients with sepsis-associated encephalopathy /*Sepsis - New Perspectives*// Edit. by Dr. Lixing Huang, Dr. Youyu Zhang and Dr. Lingbin Sun. London: IntechOpen, 2022. https://www.intechopen.com/online-first/diagnostics-of-central-and-autonomic

-nervous-system-dysfunction-in-patients-with-sepsis-associated-e DOI: 10.5772/intechopen.108392 (ISBN 978-1-83768-236-2)
4. Bykova K.M., Savvina I.A. Assessment of neurological status in patients with septic encephalopathy / *17th All-Russian Conference with International Participation "The Problem of Infection in Critical Conditions"*. Moscow, 2022. - S. 22–23.
5. Savvina I.A., Bykova K.M. Monitoring dysfunction of the central and autonomic nervous system in patients with septic encephalopathy / *17th All-Russian Conference with International Participation "The Problem of Infection in Critical Conditions"*. Moscow, 2022. - S. 24–25.
6. Bykova K.M., Savvina I.A. Sepsis-associated encephalopathy: aspects of diagnosis and classification, treatment prospects / *Sat. abstract XX Congress of the Federation of Anesthesiologists and Resuscitators (FARR-2022)*. St. Petersburg, 2022 - email. edition. - P. 17–18.

Name: Eleonora T. Nazaralieva

Affiliation: Department of Paediatric Neurosurgery, Almazov National Medical Research Centre of Ministry of Health Care of Russian Federation, Saint Petersburg, Russian Federation;

Education: Kyrgyz State Medical Academy, Bishkek, Kyrgyzstan

Business Address: Department of Paediatric Neurosurgery, Almazov National Medical Research Centre of Ministry of Health Care of Russian Federation Akkuratova str. 2, 197341, Saint Petersburg, Russian Federation

Research and Professional Experience and Professional Appointments:

May 2021–Today	Department of Paediatric Neurosurgery, Almazov National Medical Research Centre of Ministry of Health Care of Russian Federation – Researcher, Neurosurgeon
Dec 2009–Sep 2018	National Hospital of Ministry of Health of Kyrgyz Republic, Bishkek, Kyrgyzstan - Neurosurgeon

Honours:

- Sep 2014: ASNS – scholarship for or the best achievements in the field of neurooncology among young scientists

Publications from the Last 3 Years:

Nazaralieva E.T., Gerasimov A.P., Nazaralieva Eln.T., Zabrodskaya Yu.M., Shevtsov M.A., Samochernych K.A. Modern approaches to predicting the course and outcomes of treatment of the most common malignant brain tumors in children (literature review). *Russian Neurosurgical Journal*. Professor A.L. Polenov. 2022. V. 14. No. 4. S. 122–132.

Nikolenko M.S., Samochernych N.K., Mamatchanov M.R., Gerasimov A.P., Nazaralieva E.T., Samochernych K.A. Evaluation of cerebrovascular infection in ventriculosinustransversostomy. *Russian Neurosurgical Journal*. Professor A.L. Polenov. 2022. V. 14. No. 4. S. 57–63

Nazaralieva E.T., Fedorov B.C., Zabrodskaya Yu.M., Kim A.V., Djanaliev B.R., Shevtsov M.A., Samochernych K.A. Heat shock proteins as diagnostic and prognostic markers in malignant tumors of the central nervous system. *Translational Medicine*. 2022. V. 9. No. 6. P. 29–39.

Nazaralieva E.T., Khachatryan W.A. Differential diagnosis and treatment tactics for subarachnoid hemorrhage in children / *Aneurysmal Subarachnoid Hemorrhage: From Diagnosis to Treatment* // Ed. by Irina Savvina. New York: Nova Science Publishers, 2022. P. 175-196.

Savvina I.A., Ryzhkova D.V., Bykova K.M., Lebedev K.E., Petrova A.O., Dryagina N.V., Potemkina E.G., Nazaralieva E.T. Diagnostics of central and autonomic nervous system dysfunction in patients with sepsis –associated encephalopathy/ *Sepsis - New Perspectives*//Ed.by Dr. Lixing Huang, Dr. Youyu Zhang and Dr. Lingbin Sun London: IntechOpen, 2022. DOI:10.5772/intechopen.108392 (ISBN 978-1-83768-236-2)

Atiskov Yu. A., Akshulakov S.K., Belkin A.A., Nazaralieva E.T., Riznich V.P., Safin Sh.M., Safin I.Sh., Gaydar B.V., Khachatryan W.A. Brain biomechanics: monitoring the biomechanical properties of the human craniospinal system. *Russian Journal of Biomechanics*. 2020. V. 24. No. 2. P. 111–124.

Atiskov Yu. A., Khachatryan W. A., Nazaralieva E. T., Malikov A.Ya., Riznich V. P. A craniospinal compliance monitor. *Biomedical Engineering*. 2021. V. 54. No. 6 (March). P. 380–383.

Nazaralieva E.T., Riznich V.P., Khachatryan W.A. New approaches to the diagnosis of intracranial hypertension. *Russian Neurosurgical Journal*. Professor A.L. Polenov. 2021. V. 13. No. S1. P. 156–157.

Nazaralieva E.T., Gerasimov A.P., Zabrodskaya Yu.M., Ivanova N.E., Shevtsov M.A., Khachatryan W.A. Some genetic markers of low-grade cerebral gliomas in children and their potential importance in the development of therapy. *Russian Neurosurgical Journal*. Professor A.L. Polenov. 2021. V. 13. No. 4. S. 103–110.

Nazaralieva E.T., Cherebillo V.Yu., Khachatryan W.A. Modern aspects of the study of pituitary adenomas and issues of epidemiology. *Modern Problems of Science and Education*. 2021. No. 4. P. 103.

Atiskov Yu.A., Akshulakov S.K., Belkin A.A., Kondratyev A.N., Larionov S.N., Nazaralieva E.T., Riznich V.P., Savvina I.A., SafinI Sh., Khachatryan W.A. Craniospinal compliance - new principles for monitoring intracranial pressure. *Anesthesiology and Resuscitation (Media Sphere)*. 2020. No. 6. P. 37–43.

Name: Petrova Anna Olegovna

Affiliation: Almazov National Medical Research Centre of Ministry of Health Care of Russian Federation

Education: The First Saint Petersburg Pavlov Medical State University

Business Address: 197341, 2 Accuratova Str., Saint Petersburg, Russian Federation.

Research and Professional Experience: anesthesiologic maintenance of neurosurgical interventions

In 2011, I defended my PhD thesis " Multimodal analgesia in pediatric neurosurgery", which describes the peculiarities of stress reactions in neurosurgery in paediatric patients and multimodal approach to maintenance of analgesia perioperatively in pediatric patients with intracranial hypertension, brain tumor, hydrocephalus.

Professional Appointments: anesthesiologist

Honors: no

Publications from the Last 3 Years:

1. Savvina I., Petrova A., Rutkovskiy R., Orechova E., Mertsalov S., Novikova A. Selective decontamination of the intestine in neurosurgical patients with subarachnoid haemorrhage in the acute period of cerebral aneurysm rupture/ *European Journal of Anaesthesiology*, June 2020. - Vol.37, e-Suppl.58. - P. 274–275. www.ejanaesthesiology.com
2. Petrov A., Ivanov A., Rozhchenko L., Petrova A., Bhogal P., Cimpoca A., Henkes H.J. Endovascular treatment of chronic subdural hematomas through embolization: A pilot study with a non-adhesive liquid embolic agent of minimal viscosity (squid). *Clin Med.* 2021 Sep 27;10(19):4436. doi: 10.3390/jcm10194436.
3. Savvina I.A., Petrova A.O. The Treatment of Acute Stroke. / In: *Ischemic Stroke*/ Edited by Pratap Sanchetee/ IntechOpen, London. - 2021. - P. 117. DOI: 10.5772/intechopen.86623
4. Savvina I.A., Zabrodskaya Y.M., Petrova A.O., Samochernykh K.A. Cerebral vasospasm: Mechanisms, pathomorphology, diagnostics, treatment / In: *Cerebrovascular Diseases*/ Edited by Patricia Bozzetto Ambrosi/ IntechOpen, London. - 2021. - P. 138. DOI: http://dx .doi.org/10.5772/intechopen.101229
5. Savvina I.A., Nutsalova H.S., Petrova A.O., Bykova K.M., Tkebuchava I.V. Replacement selenium therapy in acute cerebral damage. In: *Selenium and Human Health*. Book edited by: Dr. Volkan Gelen. IntechOpen, London. - P. 22. DOI: http://dx.doi.org/10.5772/intecho-pen.110505
6. Savvina I.A., Zabrodskaya Y.M., Petrova A.O., Rozhchenko L.V., Goroschenko S.A., Potemkina E.G., Samochernych K.A. Aneurysmal subarachnoid hemorrhage: From diagnosis to treatment/ *Aneurysmal Subarachnoid Hemorrhage: From Diagnosis to Treatment*/ Edited by Irina Savvina. - Nova Science Publishers, New York. - 2022. - P. 41–112.
7. Savvina I.A., Petrova A.O. Anesthetic management of cerebral aneurysm surgery/ *Aneurysmal Subarachnoid Hemorrhage: From Diagnosis to Treatment*/ Edited by Irina Savvina. - Nova Science Publishers, New York. - 2022. - P. 113–126.
8. Savvina I.A., Ryzhkova D.V., Bykova K.M., Lebedev K.E., Petrova A.O., Dryagina N.V., Potemkina E.G., Nazaralieva E.T. Diagnostics of central and autonomic nervous system dysfunction in patients with sepsis-associated encephalopathy/ *Sepsis - New Perspectives*/ Edited by Dr. Lixing Huang, Dr. Youyu Zhang and Dr. Lingbin Sun. London: Intech Open, 2022. https://www.intechopen.com/online-first/diagnostics-of-central-and-autonomic-nervous-system-dysfunction-in-patients-with-sepsis-associated-e DOI: 10.5772/intechopen.108392
9. Savvina I.A., Zabrodskaya Y.M., Petrova A.O., Samochernykh K.A. Cerebral vasospasm: Mechanisms, pathomorphology, diagnostics, treatment/ In: *Cerebrovascular Diseases — Elucidating Key Principles*/ Edited by Dr. Patricia Bozzetto Ambrosi/ IntechOpen, London. - 2022. - P. 138. *DOI:* http://dx.doi.org/10.5772/intechopen.101229
10. Savvina I.A., Zabrodskaya Y.M., Petrova A.O. General anesthesia and autonomic nervous system: Control and management in neurosurgery/ In: *Autonomic Nervous System – Special Interest Topics*/ Edited by Dr. Theodoros Aslanidis and M.Sc. Christos Nouris/ IntechOpen, London. - 2022. - P. 135. *DOI:* http://dx.doi.org/10.5772/intechopen.101829

Name: Irina Vasilievna Ostrova

Affiliation: Federal Research and Clinical Center of Intensive Care Medicine and Rehabilitology, V. A. Negovsky Research Institute of General Reanimatology, Moscow, Russia

Education: M.V. Lomonosov Moscow State University, Faculty of Biology, physiology.

Business Address: 107031, 25 bldg 2 Petrovka Str., Moscow, Russia

Research and Professional Experience:
I'm a qualified morphologist with more than 20 years of experience, leading researcher of Laboratory of cell pathology at critical states. My scientific interest is in the stress proteins and factors induced by ischemia-reperfusion, their relationships with dystrophic changes of brain neurons; the mechanisms of development of postischemic processes; morphological evaluation of the effectiveness of neuroprotective strategies.

In 2003, I successfully defended my PhD thesis on the topic "Postresuscitation changes in hippocampal pyramidal neurons: morphometric and immunocytochemical analysis" in the specialty "histology, cytology, cell biology". In 2009 I became a laureate of the Foundation for the Promotion of National Medicine. I'm a co-author of more than 100 publications in domestic and foreign journals. Also I have two patents for inventions.

Professional Appointments:

1993-1998 - M.V. Lomonosov Moscow State University
1997 - now (N.D) - V. A. Negovsky Research Institute of General Reanimatology
Since 2021, Leading researcher of Laboratory of cell pathology at critical states
of the V. A. Negovsky Research Institute of General Reanimatology

Honours:
2009 - I became a laureate of the Foundation for the Promotion of National Medicine.

Publications for the last 3 years:

1. Babkina AS, Golubev AM, Ostrova IV, Volkov AV, Kuzovlev AN. Brain morphological changes in COVID-19. *General Reanimatology.* 2021;17(3):4–15. https://doi.org/10.15360/1813-9779-2021-3-1-0
2. Babkina AS, Khadzhieva MB, Ostrova IV, Ryzhkov IA, Golubev AM. Global DNA methylation of brain neurons in acute poisoning with clozapine and its combination with alcohol: An experimental study. *Russian Open Medical Journal.* 2021; 10: e0306. DOI: 10.15275/rusomj.2021.0306
3. Ostrova IV, Kalabushev SN, Ryzhkov IA, Tsokolaeva ZI. A novel thromboplastin-based rat model of ischemic stroke. *Brain Science.* 2021;11:1475. https://doi.org/10.3390/brainsci11111475
4. Babkina AS, Khadzhieva MB, Ostrova IV, Ryzhkov IA, Golubev AM. Global DNA methylation of brain neurons in acute poisoning with clozapine and its combination with alcohol: An experimental study. *Russian Open Medical Journal.* 2021; 10: e0306. DOI: 10.15275/rusomj.2021.0306

5. Patent No. 2756427 Ostrov IV, Tsokolaeva ZI, Kalabushev SN, Ryzhkov IA, Babkina AS, Golubev AM. A method for modeling focal cerebral ischemic stroke. Received on 09/30/2021.
6. Chapter 2. Neuroprotection in the book: Biological markers of damage and regeneration of the central nervous system Babkina AS, Baeva AA, Bashirova AR, Blagonravov ML, Golubev AM, Grebenchikov OA, Grechko AV, Ershov AV, Zakharchenko VE, Kuzovlev AN, Muslimov BG, Ostrov IV, Perepelitsa SA, Petrova MV, Romanova OL, Saidov Sh.Kh., Silachev DN, Sundukov DV, Telipov IN, Usmanov E.Sh. and others. Edited by: Doctor of Medical Sciences, Professor, Honored Scientist of the Russian Federation A.M. Golubeva; Doctor of Medical Sciences, Professor, Corresponding Member of the Russian Academy of Sciences AV Grechko; Doctor of Medical Sciences. AN Kuzovlev; Doctor of Medical Sciences, Professor, Corresponding Member of the Russian Academy of Sciences V.V. Frost. Moscow, 2021. – P. 42–93.
7. Babkina AS, Ostrova IV, Yadgarov MY, Kuzovlev AN, Grechko AV, Volkov AV, Golubev AM. the Role of Von Willebrand factor in the pathogenesis of pulmonary vascular thrombosis in COVID-19. *Viruses*. 2022; 14(2): 211. DOI: 10.3390/v14020211
8. Ryzhkov I, Lapin K, Tsokolaeva Z, Kalabushev S, Ostrova I, Ershov A, Vladimir Dolgikh Microvascular and metabolic effects of a balanced electrolyte solution and heparinized autologous blood in hemorrhagic shock. *Archiv EuroMedica*. 2022; 12(3): e1. DOI: 10.35630/2022/12/3.10
9. Antonova VV, Silachev DN, Ryzhkov IA, Lapin KN, Kalabushev SN, Ostrova IV, Varnakova LA, Grebenchikov OA. Three-hour argon inhalation has no neuroprotective effect after open traumatic brain injury in rats. *Brain Science*. 2022; 12: 920. DOI: 10.3390/brainsci12070920

Name: Daria V. Ryzhkova

Affiliation: National Almazov Medical Research Centre

Education: Federal State Budgetary Educational Institution of the Highest Education "The First Saint Petersburg State Medical University named after Ivan P.Pavlov" of the Ministry of Health of the Russian Federation

Business Address: National Almazov Medical Research Centre, Saint-Petersburg, Akkuratova st.2

Research and Professional Experience and Professional Appointments:

1989-1995 – Diploma in Medicine
1995-1999 - Fellowship
1999-2003 – Postgraduate Student in Russian Research Centre of Radiology and Surgical Technology,
Since 2004 – PhD,
2003-2009 – Nuclear Medicine Doctor in PET center of Russian Research Centre of Radiology and Surgical Technology
2008– Doctor of Medical Sciences
2009-2015 – Head of the Scientific laboratory of Nuclear Cardiology

Since 2019 – Chief researcher of the Department of Nuclear Medicine and Theranostics National Almazov Medical Research Centre, Russia
Since 2020 – Head of the Department of Nuclear Medicine and Radiation Technologies with Clinic of the Institute of Medical Education, National Almazov Medical Research Centre, Russia

The scientific interest and educational activities are the radionuclide and hybrid imaging in cardiology, neurology and oncology; clinical trials of new positron-emitting radiopharmaceuticals for nuclear medicine.

Honours:

- 2008 – Doctor of Medical Sciences
- 2018 – Professor of the Russian Academy of Sciences
- 2021 - Honor healthcare specialist of the Russian Federation
- 2021 - Prize-winner of the award to the best doctors of Russia "Prizvanie"

Main publications from the Last 3 Years:

THE MYELOID SARCOMA TREATED BY VENETOCLAX WITH HYPOMETHYLATING AGENT FOLLOWED BY STEM CELL TRANSPLANTATION: RARE CASE REPORT	Print.	BMC Womens Health. 2021 May 1;21(1):184. doi: 10.1186/s12905-021-01328-y. PMID: 33933047; PMCID: PMC8088676.	IF=3,0 SJR 1,017	Shatilova A., Girshova L., Zaytsev D., Budaeva I., Mirolyubova Y., Ryzhkova D., Grozov R., Bogdanov K., Motorin D., Zammoeva D., Petukhov A., Nikulina T., Efremova S., Ivanov V., Alekseeva Y., Zaritskey A.
ONE-TISSUE COMPARTMENT MODEL FOR MYOCARDIAL PERFUSION QUANTIFICATION WITH N-13 AMMONIA PET PROVIDES MATCHING RESULTS: A CROSS-COMPARISON BETWEEN CARIMAS, FLOWQUANT, AND PMOD	Print.	J. Nucl. Cardiol. 29, 2543–2550 (2022). https://doi.org/10.1007/s12350-021-02741-4	IF=4,1 SJR 0,79	Nesterov S.V., Orozco L.E.J., Han C., Knuuti J.M., Sciagrà R., Settimo L., Prior J.O., Deshayes E., deKemp R.A., Ryzhkova D.V., Gwet K.L.
THE COINCIDENCE OF TWO RARE DISEASES WITH OPPOSITE METABOLIC PHENOTYPE: A CHILD WITH CONGENITAL HYPERINSULINISM AND BLOOM SYNDROME	Print.	Journal of Pediatric Endocrinology and Metabolism, vol. 35, no. 3, 2022, pp. 405-409. https://doi.org/10.1515/jpem-2021-0464	IF=1,42 SJR 0.502	Melikyan M.A., Gubaeva D.N., Nikitina I.L., Ryzhkova D.V., Mitrofanova L.B., Yukhacheva D., Pershin D.E., Shcherbina A.Yu., Vasilyev E., Proshchina A.E., Krivova Yu.S., Tyulpakov A.N.

(Continued)

(Continued)

DIFFERENTIAL MORPHOLOGICAL DIAGNOSIS OF VARIOUS FORMS OF CONGENITAL HYPERINSULINISM IN CHILDREN	Print.	Front Endocrinol (Lausanne). 2021 Aug 23;12:710947. doi: 10.3389/ fendo.2021.710947. PMID: 34497584; PMCID: PMC8419459.	IF=5,555	Mitrofanova L.B., Perminova A.A., Ryzhkova D.V., Sukhotskaya A.A., Bairov V.G., Nikitina I.L.
Dual-tracer PET/CT imaging to determine tumor heterogeneity in a patient with metastatic ACTH-secreting neuroendocrine neoplasm: A case report and literature review	Print.	Front Endocrinol (Lausanne). 2022 Sep 5;13:958442. doi: 10.3389/ fendo.2022.958442. PMID: 36133304; PMCID: PMC9483167.	IF=6.055	Ryzhkova, D., Mitrofanova, L., Tsoy, U., Grineva, E., Schlyakhto, E.
Case Report: Primary Leptomeningeal Medulloblastoma in a Child: Clinical Case Report and Literature Review	Print.	Front Pediatr. 2022 Jul 11;10:925340. doi: 10.3389/ fped.2022.925340. PMID: 35899134; PMCID: PMC9309486.	IF=3.569	Morgacheva D, Daks A, Smirnova A, Kim A, Ryzhkova D, Mitrofanova L, Staliarova A, Omelina E, Pindyurin A, Fedorova O, Shuvalov O, Petukhov A and Dinikina Y
Myocardial perfusion quantification with Rb-82 PET: good interobserver agreement of Carimas software on global, regional, and segmental levels	Print.	Ann Nucl Med. 2022 Jun;36(6):507-514. doi: 10.1007/ s12149-022-01729-5. Epub 2022 Feb 22. PMID: 35192160; PMCID: PMC9132838.	IF=2.258	Nesterov S.V., Juarez-Orozco L.E., Malaspina S., Han C., Knuuti J.M., Deshayes E., Prior J.O., deKemp R.A., Sciagrà R., Settimo L., Ryzhkova D.V., Kostina I.S., Gwet K.L
Prediction of Aortic Stenosis Progression by 18F-FDG and 18F-NaF PET/CT in Different Aortic Valve Phenotypes	Print.	Front Pharmacol. 2022 May 24;13:909975. doi: 10.3389/ fphar.2022.909975. PMID: 35685632; PMCID: PMC9171046.	IF=5.988	Murtazalieva P, Ryzhkova D, Malev E, Zhiduleva E and Moiseeva O
Preclinical Characterisation of PSMA/GRPR-Targeting Heterodimer [68Ga]Ga-BQ7812 for PET Diagnostic Imaging of Prostate Cancer: A Step towards Clinical Translation	Print.	Cancers (Basel). 2023 Jan 10;15(2):442. doi: 10.3390/ cancers15020442. PMID: 36672390; PMCID: PMC9856709.	IF=5.6	Lundmark F, Abouzayed A, Rinne SS, Timofeev V, Sipkina N, Naan M, Kirichenko A, Vasyutina M, Ryzhkova D, Tolmachev V, Rosenström U, Orlova A.

Name: Anton Vladimirovich Ryzhkov

Affiliation: Federal State Budgetary Institution «V. A. Almazov National Medical Research Center» of the Ministry of Health of the Russian Federation (V. A. Almazov NMRC).

Education: The Yaroslav-the-Wise Novgorod State University.Residency in radiology. Postgraduate course in radiology.

Business Address: 197341, 2 Akkuratova str., Saint Petersburg, the Russian Federation.

Research and Professional Experience:
A highly qualified radiologist with more than 15 years of experience, skilled in all modern methods of radiation diagnostics, such as traditional X-ray researching, computer tomography and MRI. The main areas of work are ~~is~~ MR cardioimaging and neuroimaging. I see my further scientific development in these areas.

My research interests are related to MRI of the heart, in particular way the study of another possibility of MRI, such as the assessment of pulmonary artery distensibility of patients with pulmonary hypertension using the method of MRI.

Professional Appointments:
In 2008 I completed advanced training in scientific research planning in the North-Western State Medical University of I.I. Mechnikov.

Since March, 2009 to present I have been a radiologist at the Department of Magnetic Resonance of the Federal State Budgetary Institution "V. A. Almazov National Medical Research Center" of the Ministry of Health of the Russian Federation (V. A. Almazov NMRC).

Since September, 2015 to present I am a Head of the Department of Magnetic Resonance Imaging of the Federal State Budgetary Institution "V. A. Almazov National Medical Research Center" of the Ministry of Health of the Russian Federation (V. A. Almazov NMRC). Since 2019 I was qualified as a highest category radiologist.

Since 2022 I have been a researcher at the Department of Pathology of the Institute of Medical Education of the Almazov National Medical Research Center.

Publications over the past 3 years

1. Clinical Application of T1-Myocardial Mapping: Review of Literature and First Experience of Clinical Application. Baev, M.S., Ryzhkov, A.V., Gavrilova, E.A., Trufanov, G.E. Sibirskij. Zurnal Kliniceskoj I Eksperimental'noj Mediciny, 2022, 37(1), Pp. 17–26.
2. Simple Predictors for Cardiac Fibrosis in Patients with Type 2 Diabetes Mellitus: The Role of Circulating Biomarkers and Pulse Wave Velocity.
   Luneva E.B., Vasileva A.A., Karelkina E.V., Boyarinova M.A., Mikhaylov E.N., Ryzhkov A.V., Babenko A.Y., Konradi A.O., Moiseeva O.M. *Journal of Clinical Medicine.* 2022. T. 11. № 10. C. 2843.
3. A Comprehensive Approach to Predicting the Outcomes of Transsphenoidal Endoscopic Adenomectomy in Patients with Cushing's Disease. Kuritsyna N.V., Tsoy U.A., Cherebillo V.Y., Paltsev A.A., Ryzhkov A.V., Ryazanov P.A., Ryzhkov V.K., Grineva E.N. *Journal of Personalized Medicine.* 2022. T. 12. № 5.
4. A Case of a Rare Form of Arrhythmogenic Cardiomyopathy in a 5-Year-Old. Fetisova S.G., Sivushchina E.S., Kofeynikova O.A., Vershinina T.L., Sokolnikova P.S., Kostareva A.A.,

Ryzhkov A.V., Vasichkina E.S. *Russian Journal of Personalized Medicine*. 2022. V. 2. No. 2. p. 104–112.

5. Features of the Diagnosis of Multiple Organ Disorders Associated with Covid-19 in a Child of Primary School Age. Fetisova S.G., Starshinova A.Ya., Kofeynikova O.A., Starshinova A.A., Sheyanova E.S., Vershinina T.L., Ryzhkov A.V., Skripnik A.Yu., Pervunina T .M., *Vasichkina. Journal of Infectology*. 2022. V. 14. No. 5. p. 90–100.

Name: Ivan A. Ryzhkov

Affiliation: Federal Research and Clinical Center of Intensive Care Medicine and Rehabilitology, Moscow, Russian Federation

Education: Medical Faculty of First Moscow State Medical University (Sechenov University) (Russia). Residency in Anesthesiology and Intensive Care Medicine.

Business Address: 25/2 Petrovka street, Moscow, 107031, Russian Federation

Research and Professional Experience:
My research interests are cardiac arrest and resuscitation, cardiovascular pathophysiology, microcirculatory disorders in hemorrhagic shock, laser methods for studying microcirculation (LDF, LSCI), neuroprotection, laboratory animal anesthesia and pharmacology of anesthetics.

In 2020 I received my Ph.D. in Pathophysiology and Critical Care Medicine. Thesis title: «Microcirculation disorders in the skin and brain in acute blood loss and their correction».

I am an instructor in European Resuscitation Council (Basic Life Support and Advanced Life Support courses).

As an intensive care specialist, I am involved in the management of surgical and medical patients with postoperative complications, sepsis, multiple organ failure and other critical illnesses.

Professional Appointments:

2018 – Present - Senior Researcher and Head of the Laboratory of Experimental Research in V. A. Negovsky Research Institute of General Reanimatology of Federal Research and Clinical Center of Intensive Care Medicine and Rehabilitology, Moscow, Russian Federation

2013 – Present - Anesthesiologist and Intensive Care Physician in the Department of Anesthesiology and Intensive Care Medicine in N.I. Pirogov National Medical and Surgical Center, Moscow, Russian Federation

2010 – 2013 - Intensive Care Physician in the ICU of Clinical Hospital No. 1 of Department of Presidential Affairs, Moscow, Russian Federation

Publications from the Last 3 Years:

1. Babkina A.S., Sundukov D.V., Golubev A.M., **Ryzhkov I.A.**, Tsokolaeva Z.I., Zarzhetsky YuV. Determination of the fluorescence intensity of coenzymes NADH and FAD in the skeletal muscle of the rat depending on the post-mortem interval. *Forensic Medical Expertise = Sudebno-meditsinskaya ekspertiza*. 2020;63(1):31–35. https://doi.org/10.17116/sudmed20206301131

2. Goloubev A., Babkina A., Khadzhieva M., Rhyzhkov I., Kuzovlev A., Bashirova A., Sundukov D. Epigenetic and morphological aspects of brain damage in acute exposure to clozapine combined with ethanol (experimental study). *Critical Care*. 2020; 24(S1):291.
3. **Ryzhkov I.A.,** Babkina A.S., Tsokolaeva Z.I., Kalabushev S.N., Antonova V.V., Sergeeva M.V., Ershov A.V. Morphology and Function of Myocardium and Skin Microcirculation 24 Hours after Clozapine Poisoning. *General Reanimatology*. 2020;16(5):56–64. https://doi.org/10.15360/1813-9779-2020-5-56-64
4. Kuzovlev A.N., Shpichko A.I., **Ryzhkov I.A.**, Grebenchikov O.A., Shabanov A.K., Khusainov S.Z., Tsokolaeva Z.I., Lobanov A.V. Effect of Xenon on the Phosphorylation of Glycogen Synthase Kinase 3β and Antioxidant Enzymes in Rat Brain. *Russian Sklifosovsky Journal "Emergency Medical Care"*. 2020;9(4):564–572. (In Russ.) https://doi.org/10.23934/2223-9022-2020-9-4-564-572
5. Filev A.D., Silachev D.N., **Ryzhkov I.A.**, Lapin K.N., Babkina A.S., Grebenchikov O.A., Pisarev V.M. Effect of Xenon Treatment on Gene Expression in Brain Tissue after Traumatic Brain Injury in Rats. *Brain Sciences*. 2021; 11(7):889. https://doi.org/10.3390/brainsci11070889
6. Babkina A.S., Khadzhieva M.B., Ostrova I.V., **Ryzhkov I.A.**, Golubev A.M. Global DNA methylation of brain neurons in acute poisoning with clozapine and its combination with alcohol: An experimental study. *Russian Open Medical Journal*. 2021; 10:e0306. DOI: 10.15275/rusomj.2021.0306
7. Lapin K.N., **Ryzhkov I.A.**, Maltseva V.A., Udut E.V. Vascular catheterization in small laboratory animals in biomedical research: Technological aspects of the method (review article). *Bulletin of Siberian Medicine*. 2021; 20 (3):168–181. https://doi.org/10.20538/1682-0363-2021-2-168-181
8. Ostrova I.V., Kalabushev S.N., **Ryzhkov I.A.**, Tsokolaeva Z.I. A novel thromboplastin-based rat model of ischemic stroke. *Brain Sciences*. 2021; 11(11):1475. https://doi.org/10.3390/brainsci11111475
9. **Ryzhkov I.**, Lapin K., Tsokolaeva Z., Kalabushev S., Ostrova I., Ershov A., Dolgikh V. Microvascular and metabolic effects of a balanced electrolyte solution and heparinized autologous blood in hemorrhagic shock. *Archiv EuroMedica*. 2022; 12(3):e1. DOI 10.35630/2199-885X/2022/12/3.10
10. Antonova V.V., Silachev D.N., **Ryzhkov I.A.**, Lapin K.N., Kalabushev S.N., Ostrova I.V., Varnakova L.A., Grebenchikov O.A. Three-hour argon inhalation has no neuroprotective effect after open traumatic brain injury in rats. *Brain Sciences*. 2022; 12(7):920. https://doi.org/10.3390/brainsci12070920

Name: Irina Alexandrovna Savvina

Affiliation: Almazov National Medical Research Centre of Ministry of Health Care of Russian Federation

Education:
The First Saint Petersburg Pavlov Medical State University, Saint Petersburg. Residency in Anesthesiology and Intensive Care.

Postgraduate course in Anesthesiology and Intensive Care.

Business Address: 197341, 2 Akkuratova str., Saint Petersburg, Russian Federation

Research and Professional Experience:
Highly qualified anesthesiologist with 35 years of experience. Specialist in the field of Neuroanesthesiology and NeuroIntensive Care.

I am also committed to conducting scientific research in this area.

My scientific interest is in the study of septic encephalopathy, molecular genetic aspects of general anesthesia and systemic inflammation response during general anesthesia in neurosurgery including pediatric neurosurgery, personified premedication in neurosurgical patients.

In 1994, I defended my PhD thesis "Opioid anesthesia in pediatric neurosurgery", which describes the peculiarities of opioid anesthesia in pediatric patients with intracranial hypertension, intracranial pressure dynamics during induction of anesthesia in neurosurgical patients with brain tumor, hydrocephalus.

In 2000, I defended my doctoral dissertation on the topic " Anesthesia management system of neurosurgical operations and diagnostic proceeders in pediatric patients", which presents the structure of general anesthesia and choice of anesthetic agents according to the anesthetic influence on the stress-limiting antinociceptive neuroregulatory systems of the brain.

In 2001 I received the degree of Doctor of Medical Sciences.

Alongside with the research I performed duties of a clinical anesthesiologist.

Professional Appointments:

1987-1988 - postgraduate study at the First Saint Petersburg Pavlov Medical State University, anesthesiologist by profession.

In 1988, after my postgraduate study I got the position of a scientific researcher on a competitive basis of the Russian Polenov Scientific Research Neurosurgical Institute. For 30 years of my professional activity, I have gone from the junior researcher to the Chief Researcher.

2008-2010 - Head of the Research Department of Anesthesiology and Intensive Care of the Research Institute of Children's Infections, Saint Petersburg, Russian Federation

From 2001 to the present time – Professor of the Vladimir L. Vanevskii Department of Anaesthesiology and Reanimatology of the North-Western State Medical University named after Ilya I. Mechnikov of Ministry of Health Care of Russian Federation, Saint Petersburg, Russian Federation

Honors: I am awarded the medal " To the 300th anniversary of St. Petersburg", the medal " For contribution to the development of science named after the Nobel laureate Ivan P. Pavlov", the medal " Personality of St. Petersburg".

Publications from the Last 3 Years:

1. Gurskaia V.I., Dryagina N.V., Ivanov V.P., Savvina I.A. General inhalation sevoflurane anesthesia effect on the inflammatory and brain damage biomarkers blood serum levels in the paediatric patients with craniosynostosis during MRI invetigation: A cohort study. *Science Education Practice: Materials of the International University Science Forum (Canada, Toronto)*, April 22, 2020. - Infinity Publishing. - P. 119–124. DOI: 10.34660/INF.2020.1.61638 URL http://naupers.ru/wp-content/uploads/2020/04/Canada-April-22-Part-2.pdf#page=119

2. Savvina I., Orechova E., Gulyaev D. Personify premedication in the structure of general anaesthesia in neurosurgical patients with intracranial neoplasm. *European Journal of Anaesthesiology.* - 2020. - Vol. 37. – No. suppl. 58. - P. 182–183. www.ejanaesthesiology .com
3. Savvina I.A., Lavrinenko N.V., Zabrodskaya Yu. M., Sebelev K. I., Dolmatov V. Hippocampus role in predictive assessment of sepsis development in patients with severe traumatic brain injury. *European Journal of Anaesthesiology.* - 2020. - Vol. 37. - No. suppl. 58. - P. 302–303. www.ejanaesthesiology.com
4. Savvina I., Petrova A., Rutkovskiy R., Orechova E., Mertsalov S., Novikova A. Selective decontamination of the intestine in neurosurgical patients with subarachnoid haemorrhage in the acute period of cerebral aneurysm rupture. *European Journal of Anaesthesiology.* - June 2020. -Vol. 37. – No. suppl. 58. – P. 274–275. www.ejanaesthesiology.com
5. Savvina I.A., Alexandrovich Yu. S., Lekmanov A.U., Semenova Zh. B., Khachatryan V.A. Management of pediatric severe traumatic brain injury: What are news? *EC Anaesthesia.* - 2020. - Vol. 6. - No. 10. - P. 1–14. https://www.ecronicon.com/anaesthesia.php
6. Atiskov Yu.A., Akshulakov S.K., Belkin A.A., Kondratiev A.N., Larionov S.N., Nazaralieva E.T., Riznich V.P., Savvina I.A., Safin I.S.h., Khachatryan V.A. Craniospinal compliance — New principles for intracranial pressure monitoring. *Russian Journal of Anaesthesiology and Reanimatology.* - 2020. Vol. 6. - P. 37–43. https://doi.org/10.17116/ana esthesiology202006137
7. Bodareva N.V., Zabrodskaya Yu.M., Savvina I.A. Pathomorphological signs of encephalopathy in sepsis in neurosurgical patients. In the collection: Science and innovation - modern concepts. Collection of scientific articles based on the results of the work of the International nauchnogo forum. Moscow, 2021. P. 71–78. ISBN 978-5-905695-44-5. (In Russ.)
8. Savvina I.A., Zabrodskaya Y.M., Sebelev K.I., Bodareva N.V., Lavrinenko N.V., Tkebuchava I.V. A method for predicting the development of infectious complications and sepsis in patients with severe traumatic brain injury. Patent number: RU 2743806 C1. Russia. 2021. Date of publication: 02/26/2021. (In Russ)
9. Bodareva N.V., Zabrodskaya Y.M., Savvina I.A. To the question of septic encephalopathy: Clinical and morphological parallels. *Journal of Complementary Medicine Research.* - 2021. - 12. - No. 2. - P. 52–60 doi: 10.5455/jcmr.2021.12.02.08
10. Bykova K.M., Savvina I.A., Bondareva N.V., Zabrodskaya Yu.M. Pathophysiological aspects and complex diagnostics of sepsis-associated encephalopathy: Prospects of Etiopathogenetic Therapy. *Journal of Anesthesiology and Resuscitation.* 2022. - Vol. 4. - P. 92–99 (In Russ.)
11. Savvina I.A., Kondratieva E.A., Grekhov E.V., Morozov K.A., Biktasheva L.Z., Gurskaya V.I., Stepanova K.V., Novikov V.Yu., Kim A.V., Lebedev K.E., Sereda E.O., Ryzhkov A.V., Efimtsev A.Yu., Trufanov G.E., Ryzhkova D.V., Pervunina T.M., Khachatryan V.A., Shlyakhto E.V. Consciousness recovery in a child with hypoxic brain damage after surgical treatment of congenital heart disease. *Russian Journal of Anaesthesiology and Reanimatology.* 2021. - Vol. - 1. - P. 81–90. https://doi.org/10.17116/anaesthesiology 202101181
12. Gurskaya V.I., Dryagina N.V., Ivanov V.P., Aleksandrovich Yu.S., Khachatryan V.A., Savvina I.A. Effect of general anesthesia on systemic inflammatory response and neuronal damage in children with craniosynostosis in perioperative period. *Russian Journal*

of Anaesthesiology and Reanimatology. 2021. - Vol. 1. - P. 39–45. https://doi.org/10.17116/anaesthesiology202101139

13. Gurskaya V.I., Ivanov V.P., Novikov V.Yu., Dryagina N.V., Savvina I.A. Systemic inflammatory response in infants with craniostenosis sedated with propofol. *Russian Journal of Pediatric Surgery, Anesthesia and Intensive Care*. 2021. - Vol. 11. - No. 3. - P. 297–306. DOI: https://doi.org/10.17816/psaic961
14. **Savvina I.A.**, Petrova A.O. The treatment of acute stroke. / In: Ischemic Stroke/ Edited by Pratap Sanchetee/ IntechOpen, London.-2021.- 117 P. DOI: 10.5772/intechopen.86623 ISBN: 978-1-83962-395-0
15. *Aneurysmal Subarachnoid Hemorrhage: From Diagnosis to Treatment* / Ed. by **Irina Savvina**. - Nova Science Publishers, New York. - 2022. - 266 P. ISBN 9798886972511 (hard cover); ISBN 9798886972986 (eBook) DOI: 10.52305/dngf4073
16. **Savvina I.A.**, Zabrodskaya Y.M., Petrova A.O., Rozhchenko L.V., Goroschenko S.A., Potemkina E.G., Samochernych K.A. Aneurysmal subarachnoid hemorrhage: From diagnosis to treatment / *Aneurysmal Subarachnoid Hemorrhage: From Diagnosis to Treatment* // Ed. by Irina Savvina. - Nova Science Publishers, New York. - 2022. - P. 41–112. ISBN 9798886972511 (hard cover); ISBN 9798886972986 (eBook)
17. **Savvina I.A.,** Petrova A.O. Anesthetic management of cerebral aneurysm surgery / *Aneurysmal Subarachnoid Hemorrhage: From Diagnosis to Treatment* // Ed. by Irina Savvina. - Nova Science Publishers, New York. - 2022. - P. 113–126. ISBN 9798886972511 (hard cover); ISBN 9798886972986 (eBook)
18. **Savvina I.A.** Preface/ *Aneurysmal Subarachnoid Hemorrhage: From Diagnosis to Treatment* // Ed. by Irina Savvina. Nova Science Publishers, New York. - 2022. – ix–x. ISBN 9798886972511 (hard cover); ISBN 9798886972986 (eBook)
19. **Savvina I.A.,** Ryzhkova D.V., Bykova K.M., Lebedev K.E., Petrova A.O., Dryagina N.V., Potemkina E.G., Nazaralieva E.T. Diagnostics of central and autonomic nervous system dysfunction in patients with sepsis-associated encephalopathy / *Sepsis - New Perspectives* // Edit. By Dr. Lixing Huang, Dr. Youyu Zhang and Dr. Lingbin Sun. London: IntechOpen, 2022. DOI: 10.5772/intechopen.108392 (ISBN 978-1-83768-236-2)
20. Bykova K.M., Savvina I.A., Bodareva N.V., Zabrodskaya Yu.M. Pathophysiological aspects and complex diagnosis of sepsis-associated encephalopathy: Perspectives of etiopathogenetic therapy. *Russian Journal of Anaesthesiology and Reanimatology*. 2022. - Vol. 4. - P. 92–98.
21. Bykova K.M., Savvina I.A., Rutkovskiy R.V., Rodchenko A.M. The role of neuroinflammation in the dysfunction of the brain in the perioperative period. *Russian Journal of Anaesthesiology and Reanimatology*. 2022. - Vol. 6. - P. 99–106.
22. *Zabolotskikh I.B., Belkin A.A., Butrov A.V., Gorbachev V.I., Golubtsov V.V., Ershov V.I., Kondratyev A.N., Kuzovlev A.N., Lebedinskiy K.M., Lubnin A.Yu., Magomedov M.A., Ovechkin A.M., Savvina I.A., Shadrin R.V., Shifman E.M. Schegolev A.V. Perioperative management of patients with neuromuscular diseases. Russian Journal of Anaesthesiology and Reanimatology*. 2022. - Vol. 6. - P. 6–28.
23. Semenova Zh.B., Melnikov A.V., Mesxheryakov S.A., Ahadov T.A., Savvina I.A., Lekmanov A.U., Valiullina S.A., Ponina I.V., Gorelyishev S.K., Khachatryan W.A. Clinical recommendations of ministry of health care of Russian federation. *Pediatric Traumatic Brain Injury*. 2022. - P. 93. https://apicr.minzdrav.gov.ru

24. Savvina I.A. *Intensive Care of the Stroke*. Saint Petersburg: Publishing house of the North-West State Medical University named after Ilya I. Mechnikov, 2022. - P. 44.
25. Bairova T.V., Savvina I.A. *Selected Issues of Intensive Care in Pediatrics*. Saint Petersburg: Publishing house of the North-West State Medical University named after Ilya I. Mechnikov, 2022. - P. 92.
26. Savvina I.A., Zabrodskaya Y.M., Petrova A.O., Samochernykh K.A. Cerebral vasospasm: Mechanisms, pathomorphology, diagnostics, treatment / In: *Cerebrovascular Diseases — Elucidating Key Principles* / Edited by Dr. Patricia Bozzetto Ambrosi// IntechOpen, London. - 2022. - P. 138. *DOI:* http://dx.doi.org/10.5772/intechopen.101229
27. Savvina I.A., Zabrodskaya Y.M., Petrova A.O. General anesthesia and autonomic nervous system: Control and management in neurosurgery / In: *Autonomic Nervous System – Special Interest Topics* / Edited by Dr. Theodoros Aslanidis and M.Sc. Christos Nouris // IntechOpen, London. - 2022. - P. 135. *DOI:* http://dx.doi.org/10.5772/intechopen.101829
28. Sinbukhova E.V., Protsenko D.N., Lubnin A.Yu., Savvina I.A., Tyurin I.N. Happiness of anesthesiology and intensive care staff in the context of life satisfaction and burnout. *Russian Journal of Anaesthesiology and Reanimatology*. 2022. - Vol. - 1. - P. 76–83. DOI: 10.17116/anaesthesiology202201176. https://istina.msu.ru/publications/article/435003068/
29. Savvina I.A., Nutsalova H.S., Petrova A.O., Bykova K.M. and Tkebuchava I.V. Replacement selenium therapy in acute cerebral damage. In: *Selenium and Human Health*. Book edited by: Dr. Volkan Gelen. IntechOpen, London. - P. 22. (ISBN 978-1-83768-911-8) DOI: http://dx.doi.org/10.5772/intechopen.110505
30. Petrova T.A., Kondratyev S.A., Kostareva A.A., Rutkovskiy R.V., Savvina I.A., Kondratyeva E.A. miR-21, miR-93, miR-191, miR-let-7b, and miR-499 expression level in plasma and cerebrospinal fluid in patients with prolonged disorders of consciousness. *Neurology International*. 2023. - Vol. 15. - P. 40–54. https://doi.org/10.3390/neurolint15010004

website: irinasavvina.com

Name: Rustam Sabirovich Talybov

Affiliation: Regional Clinical Hospital №2, Russian Federation

Education: Tyumen Medical Academy (Tyumen Medical University), qualification of a general practitioner. Residency in radiology. Postgraduate course in radiology.

Business Address: 625039, 75 Melnikaite Str., Tyumen, Russian Federation

Research and Professional Experience:
Highly qualified radiologist with more than 10 years of experience. Specialist in the field of neuroradiology. I am also committed to conducting scientific research in this area.

My scientific interest is in the vizualisation and differential diagnosis of brain tumors, intraoperative neuronavigation and neurovizualisation malignant glial tumors.

In 2021 entered to postgraduate studies at the research institute of the human brain (NP Bechtereva Institute of the Human Brain) for the degree of Candidate of Medical Sciences on the topic «Intraoperative CT perfusion in diffuse high-grade gliomas» , which presents use intraoperative CT perfusion in the evaluation high-grade gliomas surgery . Alongside with the research I performe duties of head of radiologist department. For 10 years of my professional activity, I have gone from an ordinary radiologist to the head of department. Since 2015, Head of the radiology department of the Regional Clinical Hospital .

Professional Appointments:
2012-2013 - clinical internship at the Tyumen Medical Academy radiologist by profession. In 2013, after my postintership study I got the position of a radiologist.

Honours:.

- 2016: Health department award– award for contribution to the development of health care.
- 2021: City government award - award for highest level results in medicine.

Publications from the Last 3 Years:

1. Surgical treatment of patients with primary and metastatic spinal tumor with use of the O-Arm intraoperative portable computed tomography scanner. A. A. Sufianov, V. I. Manashchuk, D. N. Nabiev, R. S. Talybov et al. *Russian Journal of Neurosurgery*, 2019, 21 (4), p. 39–49.
2. The use of intraoperative ultrasound in patients with focal cortical dysplasia: Preliminary observations. A. A. Sufianov, S. V. Mirhaydarov, Yu. A. Yakimov, R. S. Talybov et al. *Epilepsy and Paroxysmal Conditions*, 2020, 11 (4), p. 335–347.
3. Circulating miRNAs as diagnostic and prognostic biomarkers in high-grade gliomas. J. Wu, A. Al-Zahrani, O. Beylerli, R. Talybov et al. *Frontiers in Oncology*, 2022, 12, p. 12–12.
4. Multiparametric MR imaging features of primary CNS lymphomas. R. Talybov, T. Trofimova, V. Mochalov et al. *Frontiers in Surgery*, 2022, 18, p. 9–9.
5. Differencial diagnosis of primary central nervous system lymphomas based on multiparametric MRT mapping. R. Talybov, T. Trofimova. *Diagnostic Radiology and Radiotherapy*, 2022, 13(2), p. 36–49.
6. Reliability of diffusion-weighted imaging and perfusion parameters in the differential diagnosis of intracranial meningiomas and solitary dural metastasis: A single-center study. R. Talybov, T. Trofimova et al. *Diagnostic Radiology and Radiotherapy*, 2023, 14(2), p. 28–43.

Name: Tatiana N. Trofimova

Affiliation: The Human Brain State Institute named after Natalya P. Bekhtereva of Russian Academy of Science

Education: Federal State Budgetary Educational Institution of the Highest Education "The First Saint Petersburg State Medical University named after Ivan P.Pavlov" of the Ministry of Health of the Russian Federation

Business Address: The Human Brain State Institute named after Natalya P.Bekhtereva of Russian Academy of Science Saint-Petersburg, Acad. Pavlov st.9

Research and Professional Experience and Professional Appointments:

Sept 2009 - Today The Human Brain State Institute named after Natalya P.Bekhtereva of Russian Academy of Science Neuroimaging Laboratory, Chief researcher

Oct 1995 - Oct 2008 Medical Academy of Postgraduated Studies, Deputy Director, Head of the Radiological department

Honours:

- 1999 – Doctor of Medical Sciences
- 2001 – professor
- 2009 – Vice-President of the Saint-Petersburg Radiological Society
- 2011 – Laureate of the Government of the Russian Federation Award
- 2013 – Chief Medical Radiology Specialist of Saint Petersburg
- 2015 – Honor healthcare specialist of the Russian Federation
- 2015 – Member of the Public Chamber of Saint-Petersburg
- 2017 – Chief Medical Radiology Specialist of the Ministry of Health of the Russian Federation for the North-Western Federal District
- 2019 – Chairman of the Commission on Healthcare and Public Health of the Public Chamber of Saint-Petersburg
- 2022 - Laureate of the Saint-Petersburg Government Award
- 2022 – Corresponding member of the Russian Academy of Sciences

Main publications from the Last 3 Years:

Human biocenosis and hospital environment	Print.	Saint-Petersburg.: Baltic Medical Educational Center, 2023.-424 p.		N.A.Belyakov S.F.Bagnenko, T.N.Trofimova et. al.
Multiparametric MR Imaging Features of Primary CNS Lymphomas	Print.	Frontiers in Surgery 887249 April 2022, Vol. 9, article 887249 doi: 10.3389/fsurg.2022.		R. Talybov, O. Beylerli, T. Trofimova, Y. Guang et al.
Prevalence and outcomes of pregnancies in women with HIV over a 20-year period	Print.	AIDS. – 2021. – Vol.35. – №12. – P. 2025–2033.	9	J.D. Kowalska A. Pelchen-Matthews A. Mocroft L. Ryom D. Raben M.H. Losso et al
Neuroradiology in the acute phase of coronavirus infection - COVID-19	Print.	HIV-infection and immunosupressions. – 2021. – Vol.13. – №2. – P. 20–32.	13	P.L.Andropova Zh.I.Savintseva N.A.Belyakov
The dynamics of the COVID-19 pandemia and the formation of the post-COVID period in Russia	Print.	HIV-infection and immunosupressions. – 2021. – Vol.13. – №2. – P. 7–19.	13	N.A.Belyakov O.E.Simakina V.V.Rassohin S.L.Serebryakova

(Continued)

(Continued)

Comparison of radiotracers of the amino acid class L-[methyl-11C]methionine and O-2-[18F] fluoroethyl-L-tyrosine in the diagnosis of glial brain tumors by PET/CT	Print.	Diagnostic Radiology and Radiotherapy. – 2021.–№1(12). – P. 49–58.	10	T.U.Skvortsova Zh.I.Savintseva D.V.Zahs R.V.Tyurin A.F.Gurchin A.I.Holyavin
Comparison of combined positron emission and computed tomography with 11C-methionine and the KI-67 proliferation index in assessing the aggressiveness of cerebral gliomas	Print.	Radiology – practice. – 2021. – №4(88). – P. 34–48.	15	T.U.Skvortsova Zh.I.Savintseva D.V.Zahs A.F.Gurchin A.I.Holyavin Yu.M.Zabrodskaya
The prognostic power of MRI criteria in the diagnosis of immunity restoration syndrome in HIV-infected patients on the example of comparison of classification by the method of decision trees and ROC analysis	Print.	Diagnostic Radiology and Radiotherapy. – 2021. –№3(12). – P. 16–25.	10	E.G.Bakulina G.V.Katayeva
Healthcare delivery for HIV-positive people with tuberculosis in Europe	Print.	HIV medicine. –2021. – №22(4) . – P. 283-293.	11	A.K. Bentzon J.D. Lundgren D. Podlekareva O. Kirk A. Panteleev V. Mitsura E. Borodulina A. Skrahina E. Denisova et al.
The influence antiretroviral therapy on brain imaging in HIV infection	Print.	ECR 2020 Book of Abstracts. Insights Imaging. – 2020. –Vol.11:34. – P. 1–6	5	E.G.Bakulina
Personalized HIV medicine (monograph)	Print.	Saint-Petersburg.: Baltic Medical Educational Center, 2020. – 326 p.: ill.	326	N.A.Belyakov V.V.Rassohin A.E.Kolbin N.G.Neznanov A.A.Totolyan et. al.
Psychoemotional state and cognitive functions in HIV-infected patients and functional state of brain structures (according to positron emission tomography and magnetic resonance spectroscopy)	Print.	Clinical and special psychology. – 2020.– Vol.9.– № 1.– P. 78–103.	25	G.V.Katayeva Yu.G.Homenko I.A.Kotomin A.A.Bogdan E.A.Gromova A.V.Kosyh V.V.Rassohin N.A.Belyakov

(Continued)

(Continued)

HIV infection and comorbid conditions (educational manual)	Print.	Saint-Petersburg.: Baltic Medical Educational Center, 2020. –680 p. ill.	680	V.V.Rassohin N.A.Belyakov M.R.Bobkova E.V.Boyeva V.E.Zholobov A.Yu.Kovelenov A.S.Kolbin O.N.Leonova 3Z.A.Lisitsina N.G.Neznanov A.M.Panteleyev A.V.Samarina N.V.Sizova E.V.Stepanova N.B.Khalezova
Radiology of cerebral gliomas: diagnosis and monitoring / Edited by Trofimova T.N. (monograph)	Print.	Saint-Petersburg: LLC "Foliant Publishing House». –2020. – 564 p.	564	T.U.Skvortsova Zh.I.Savintseva M.A.Zhuravleva

Name: Khachatryan William A.

Affiliation: Department of Paediatric Neurosurgery, Almazov National Medical Research Centre of Ministry of Health Care of Russian Federation, Saint Petersburg, Russian Federation;

Education: Yerevan Medical Institute, Yerevan, Armenia

Business Address: Department of Paediatric Neurosurgery, Almazov National Medical Research Centre of Ministry of Health Care of Russian Federation Akkuratova str. 197341, Saint Petersburg, Russian Federation

Research and Professional Experience and Professional Appointments:
May 1980 - Today Department of Paediatric Neurosurgery, Almazov National
Medical Research Centre of Ministry of Health Care of
Russian Federation – Head of the Research
Laboratory of Pediatric Neurosurgery

Honours:
2014 - Honorary Professor of the Center for Neurosurgery, Nur-Sultan, Kazakhstan
2007- Awarded the title of Academician of the Academy of Medical and Technical Sciences of the Russian Federation.
2002 - Editor-in-chief of the scientific and practical journal "Neurosurgery and neurology of childhood"
1998 - Awarded the title of professor.

Publications from the Last 3 Years:

Nizolin D.V., Fedorov E.V., Kim A.V., Mitrofanova L.B., Khachatryan W.A. Combination of tumors of different histogenesis in pediatric neurosurgery. *Questions of Neurosurgery*. N.N. Burdenko. 2021. V. 85. No. 2. S. 80–90.

Volkodav O.V., Khachatryan W.A. Methods for improving the effectiveness of hydrocephalus treatment in neonatal practice. *Russian Bulletin of Perinatology and Pediatrics*. 2021. V. 66. No. 4. S. 141–147.

Mamatkhanov M.R., Khachatryan W.A., Lebedev K.E. Analysis of the results of surgical treatment of epilepsy. *Russian Neurosurgical Journal*. Professor A.L. Polenov. 2021. Vol. 13. No. S1. pp. 124–125.

Kim A.V., Fedorov E.V., Khachatryan W.A. Recurrence of neuroepithelial brain tumors in children. *Russian Neurosurgical Journal*. Professor A.L. Polenov. 2021. Vol. 13. No. S1. S. 123.

Atiskov Yu. A., Akshulakov S.K., Belkin A.A., Nazaralieva E.T., Riznich V.P., Safin Sh.M., Safin I.Sh., Gaydar B.V., Khachatryan W.A. Brain biomechanics: Monitoring the biomechanical properties of the human craniospinal system. *Russian Journal of Biomechanics*. 2020. Vol. 24. No. 2. pp. 111–124.

Atiskov Yu. A., Khachatryan W.A., Nazaralieva E.T., Malikov A.Ya., Riznich V.P. A Craniospinal compliance monitor. *Biomedical Engineering*. 2021. Vol. 54. No. 6 (March). pp. 380–383.

Nazaralieva E.T., Riznich V.P., Khachatryan W.A. New approaches to the diagnosis of intracranial hypertension. *Russian Neurosurgical Journal*. Professor A.L. Polenov. 2021. Vol. 13. No. S1. pp. 156–157.

Nazaralieva E.T., Gerasimov A.P., Zabrodskaya Yu.M., Ivanova N.E., Shevtsov M.A., Khachatryan W.A. Some genetic markers of low-grade cerebral gliomas in children and their potential importance in the development of therapy. *Russian Neurosurgical Journal*. Professor A.L. Polenov. 2021. V. 13. No. 4. S. 103–110.

Nazaralieva E.T., Cherebillo V.Yu., Khachatryan W.A. Modern aspects of the study of pituitary adenomas and issues of epidemiology. *Modern Problems of Science and Education*. 2021. No. 4. P. 103.

Atiskov Yu.A., Akshulakov S.K., Belkin A.A., Kondratyev A.N., Larionov S.N., Nazaralieva E.T., Riznich V.P., Savvina I.A., Safin I. Sh., Khachatryan W.A. Craniospinal compliance - New principles for monitoring intracranial pressure. *Anesthesiology and Resuscitation (Media Sphere)*. 2020. No. 6. P. 37–43.

Nazaralieva E.T., Khachatryan W.A. Differential diagnosis and treatment tactics for subarachnoid hemorrhage in children / *Aneurysmal Subarachnoid Hemorrhage: From Diagnosis to Treatment* // Ed. by Irina Savvina. New York: Nova Science Publishers, 2022. P. 175–196.

Name: Yulia Mikhailovna Zabrodskaya

Affiliation: Russian Polenov Scientific Research Neurosurgical Institute – branch of the Almazov National Medical Research Centre of Ministry of Health Care of Russian Federation, Russian Federation

Education:Leningrad Sanitary and Hygienic Medical Institute, qualification of a general practitioner. Residency in pathological anatomy. Postgraduate course in pathological anatomy.

Business Address:191014, 12 Mayakovskogo Str., Saint Petersburg, Russian Federation

Research and Professional Experience:
Highly qualified pathologist with more than 25 years of experience. Specialist in the field of pathomorphological diagnostics of diseases of the nervous system and neurooncology.

I am also committed to conducting scientific research in this area.

My scientific interest is in the etiology of brain aneurysm, brain pathology in critical conditional and sepsis, wound process, pathomorphology and proteomics of epilepsy, apoptosis, structural and metabolic changes of skeletal muscles in intensive care patients, morphological evaluation of the effectiveness of fluorescence navigation with chlorin e6 in surgery for gliomas.

In 1997, I defended my PhD thesis "Pathomorphological characteristics of changes in the articulations of the arteries of the base of the brain (to the problem of the origin of aneurysms)", which describes the previously unknown phenomenon of segmental (metameric) structure of the arterial circle of the brain and morphogenesis of brain aneurysms - stretching of the articulations of the arterial circle of the human brain, studied the structural changes of the arteries in vasospasm after rupture of aneurysms.

In 2012, I defended my doctoral dissertation on the topic "Pathological anatomy of a surgical wound of the brain with modern methods of surgical treatment", which presents the structure of the perifocal zone of brain tumors as an area of the surgical wound, the morphogenesis of the wound process, new data on the peritumorous zone were obtained.

Alongside with the research I performed duties of a clinical pathologist.

Professional Appointments:

1992-1995 - postgraduate studies at the Russian Polenov Scientific Research Neurosurgical Institute, pathologist by profession.

In 1995, after my postgraduate study I got the position of a scientific research on a competitive basis. For 30 years of my professional activity, I have gone from an ordinary researcher to the head of a laboratory.

Since 2008, Head of the Research Laboratory of Pathomorphology of the Nervous system of the Polenov Russian Neurosurgical Research Institute.

I am a Professor at the Department of Pathology of the Institute of Medical Education of the Almazov National Medical Research Center.

Honours: I am awarded three medals named after P. L. Kapitsa "To the author of a scientific discovery", the medal "For contribution to the development of medical genomics named after Yu. B. Yurov".

Publications from the Last 3 Years:

Gerasimov A.P., Khachatryan W.A., Ivanova N.E., Kondratev S.A., Zabrodskaya Y.M. Genetic examination for emergency situations: Time, distance, and logistics. *Lecture Notes in Civil Engineering.* 2023, 257: 61–65.

Zabrodskaya Y.M., Gaykov O.N., Alexandrov M.V. et al. Epileptic focus in drug-resistant epilepsy: Structure, organization, and pathophysiology. In *Epilepsy - Seizures Without Triggers [Working Title].* (2022) IntechOpen. https://doi.org/10.5772/intechopen.108395, WoS

Sokolova T.V., Zabrodskaya Y.M., Litovchenko, et al. Relationship between neuroglial apoptosis and neuroinflammation in the epileptic focus of the brain and in the blood of patients with drug-resistant epilepsy. *International Journal of Molecular Sciences.* 2022, 23: 12561. https://doi.org/10.3390/ijms232012561

Savvina I.A., Petrova A.O., Zabrodskaya Y.M. General anesthesia and autonomic nervous system: Control and management in neurosurgery. In *Autonomic Nervous System.* Ed. Intech Open; 2021, p. 24. https://doi.org/10.5772/intechopen.101829.

Savvina I.A., Zabrodskaya Y.M., Sebelev K.I., et al. Septic encephalopathy: Pathophysiology, pathomorphology, clinical syndromes, therapeutic tactics. *Neurosurgery and Neurology of Childhood.* 2017, 4 (54): 20–33. https://doi.org/10.17116/hirurgia202207158.

Kondratyev S.A., Skiteva E.N., Zabrodskaya Y.M. et al. Structural and metabolic changes in skeletal muscles of patients with chronic disorders of consciousness—To the issue of critical illness polyneuromyopathies (a PET/CT pathomorphological study). *Journal of Evolutionary Biochemistry and Physiology.* 2021, 57: 913–924. https://doi.org/10.1134/S0022093021040153

Vorobeva O.M., Sitovskaya D.A., Kukanov K.K., Zabrodskaya Yu.M. The phenomenon of pseudotumorous cross immunohistochemical reactivity of glia in progressive multifocal leukoencephalopathy. *Arkhiv Patologiithis.* 2022, 84(2): 36–43.

Rynda A.Yu., Zabrodskaya Yu.M., Olyushin V.E. et al. Morphological evaluation of the effectiveness of fluorescence navigation with chlorin e6 in surgery for malignant gliomas. *Arkhiv Patologii*. 2021, 83(5): 13–20.

Bodareva N.V., Zabrodskaya Y.M., Savvina I.A. Pathomorphological signs of encephalopathy in sepsis in neurosurgical patients. In *The Collection: Science and Innovation - Modern Concepts*. Moscow; 2021, p. 71–78.

Rynda A.Yu., Olyushin V.E., Rostovtsev D.M., Tastanbekov M.M., Papayan G.V. Intraoperative fluorescence control with chlorin e6 in resection of glial brain tumors. *Zhurnal Voprosy NejrokhirurgiiI meni N.N. Burdenkothis*. 2021, 85(4): 20–26.

Sitovskaya D.A., Zabrodskaya Y., Sokolova T.V., Nezdorovina V.G., Dobrogorskaya L.N. Structural heterogeneity of epileptic foci in local drug-resistant epilepsy. *ArkhivPatologiithis*. 2020, 82(6): 5–15.

Sazhina T.A., Sitovskaya D.A., Zabrodskaya Y.M., Bazhanova E.D. Functional imbalance of glutamate- and GABAergic neuronal systems in the pathogenesis of focal drug-resistant epilepsy in humans. *Bulletin of Experimental Biology and Medicinethis*. 2020, 168(4): 529–532.

Rynda A.Yu., Rostovtsev D.M., Olyushin V.E., Zabrodskaya Yu.M. Therapeutic pathomorphosis in malignant glioma tissues after photodynamic therapy with chlorin e6 (Reports of two clinical cases). *Biomedical Photonicsthis*. 2020, 9(2): 45–54.

Rynda A., Olyushin V.E., Rostovtsev D.M., Zabrodskaya Y. Complex treatment of a patient with neurofibromatosis type 2. *Zhurnal Nevrologii i Psihiatriiimeni S.S. Korsakova*. 2020, 120(8): 98–104.

Sidorin, V.S., Zabrodskaya, Y.M., Dobrogorskaya, L.N. Tanatogenetic role of type 2 diabetes in neurosurgical patients. *ArkhivPatologiithis*. 2020, 82(1): 38–46.

Emelyanov, A., Shtam, T., Kamyshinsky, R., Pchelina, S., Konevega, A. Cryo-electron microscopy of extracellular vesicles from cerebrospinal fluid. *PLoS ONE*. 2020, 15(1): e0227949.

Name: Elena Nikolaevna Zharova

Affiliation: Polenov Neurosurgical Institute - a branch of "Almazov National Medical Research Centre" of the Ministry of Health of the Russian Federation

Education:Leningrad Pediatric Medical Institute, qualification of a paediatrician. Specialist training in regenerative medicine, physiotherapy and sports medicine. Postgraduate course in neurology.

Business Address: 12 Mayakovskogo Street, Saint Petersburg, 191014, Russian Federation

Research and Professional Experience:
A highly qualified neurologist and neurophysiologist with more than 25 years of experience. Specialist in the field of neurophysiological methods for diagnosing diseases of the nervous system and neuro-oncology.

I am also involved in scientific research in this field.

My scientific interests are neurophysiological diagnostics of patients with neurological diseases and after neurosurgical operations. Intraoperative neurophysiological monitoring of conduction in functionally significant areas to avoid complications. Examination of patients treated in the Institute's neurosurgical clinic and rehabilitation.

In 2007, I defended my PhD thesis "Post-traumatic visual disturbances in the acute and remote periods of brain injury"," in which he described a previously unknown method of treating post-traumatic visual disturbances using LED radiation under the control of visual evoked potentials.

In 2019, I defended my PhD thesis "Optimisation of patient rehabilitation in the acute phase of brain injury with the help of physical factors", which presents a new concept of early rehabilitation involving certain physical factors that are well tolerated by patients and improve the prognosis of the disease.

Parallel to my scientific work, I performed the duties of the head of the department for rehabilitation and neurophysiologist of the institute.

Professional appointments:

2000-2002 - Residency at : Polenov Neurosurgical Institute, specialising in rehabilitation medicine, remedial gymnastics and sports medicine. Since 2001 I have been the head of the Rehabilitation Department at : Polenov Neurosurgical Institute. After completing my postgraduate studies in neurology and defending my doctorate, I obtained a position as a scientist on a competitive basis in 2007. In my 30 years of professional activity, I have made the journey from a simple researcher to the head of the department.

Publications in the last 3 years:

Rynda AY, Zabrodskaya YM, Olyushin VE, Rostovtsev DM, Sokolova TV, Papayan GV. Morfologicheskaya otsenka effektivnosti fluorestsentnoi navigatsii s khlorinom e6 v khirurgii zlokachestvennykh gliom [Morphological evaluation of the effectiveness of fluorescence navigation with chlorin e6 in surgery for malignant gliomas]. *Arkh Patol.* 2021;83(5):13–20. doi:10.17116/patol20218305113

Rynda AYu, Olyushin VE, Rostovtsev DM, Zabrodskaya YuM, Tastanbekov MM, Papayan GV. Intraoperative fluorescence control with chlorin E6 in resection of glial brain tumors. *Zhurnal Voprosy Neirokhirurgii Imeni N.N. Burdenko.* 2021;85(4):20–28. (In Russ., In Engl.) https://doi.org/10.17116/neiro20218504120

Sitovskaya DA, Zabrodskaya YM, Sokolova TV, Kuralbaev AK, Nezdorovina VG, Dobrogorskaya LN. Strukturnaya geterogennost' epilepticheskikh ochagov pri lokal'noi farmakorezistentnoi epilepsii [Structural heterogeneity of epileptic foci in local drug-resistant epilepsy]. *Arkh Patol.* 2020;82(6):5–15. doi:10.17116/patol2020820615

Sazhina TA, Sitovskaya DA, Zabrodskaya YM, Bazhanova ED. Functional Imbalance of Glutamate- and GABAergic Neuronal Systems in the Pathogenesis of Focal Drug-Resistant Epilepsy in Humans. *Bull Exp Biol Med.* 2020;168(4):529–532. doi:10.1007/s10517-020-04747-3

Rynda AYu, Rostovtsev DM, Olyushin VE, Zabrodskaya YuM.Therapeutic pathomorphosis in malignant glioma tissues after photodynamic therapy with chlorin E6 (reports of two clinical cases). *Biomedical Photonics.* 9(2):45–54.

Rynda AY, Olyushin VE, Rostovtsev DM, Zabrodskaya YM. Kompleksnoe lechenie patsienta s neirofibromatozom 2-go tipa [Complex treatment of a patient with neurofibromatosis type 2]. *Zh Nevrol Psikhiatr Im S S Korsakova.* 2020;120(8):98–104. doi:10.17116/jnevro202012008198

Sidorin VS, Zabrodskaya YM, Dobrogorskaya LN. Tanatogeneticheskaia rol' sakharnogo diabeta 2-go tipa u neĭrokhirurgicheskikh bol'nykh [Tanatogenetic role of type 2 diabetes in neurosurgical patients]. *Arkh Patol.* 2020;82(1):38–46. doi:10.17116/patol20208201138

Emelyanov A, Shtam T, Kamyshinsky R, et al. Cryo-electron microscopy of extracellular vesicles from cerebrospinal fluid. *PLoS One.* 2020;15(1):e0227949. Published 2020 Jan 30. doi:10.1371/journal.pone.0227949

Emelyanov A, Shtam T, Kamyshinsky R, et al. Cryo-electron microscopy of extracellular vesicles from cerebrospinal fluid. *PLoS One.* 2020;15(1):e0227949. Published 2020 Jan 30. doi:10.1371/journal.pone.0227949

INDEX

T

U

V

W